Cancer Treatment and Research

Series Editor

Steven T. Rosen, Chicago, IL, USA

For further volumes:
http://www.springer.com/series/5808

Jane Y. Wu
Editor

RNA and Cancer

Springer

Editor
Jane Y. Wu
Department of Neurology
Center for Genetic Medicine
Robert H. Lurie Cancer Center
Chicago, IL
USA

ISSN 0927-3042
ISBN 978-3-642-31658-6 ISBN 978-3-642-31659-3 (eBook)
DOI 10.1007/978-3-642-31659-3
Springer Heidelberg New York Dordrecht London

Library of Congress Control Number: 2012946188

Printed on acid-free paper

Springer is part of Springer Science+Business Media (www.springer.com)

Foreword

The experimental approaches and methodologies of genomics have revolutionized cancer research. The ability to scan the entire genome for relevant changes in DNA sequence, copy number, and location has generated staggering amounts of information about the derangements occurring in the genomes of cancer cells of individual patients. However, with a few welcome and notable exceptions, this information has not yet yielded major insights into the vulnerabilities of cancer cells, nor has it provided clues leading to widely effective therapies. This is partly due to the fact that, until recently, much of the information gathered has focused primarily on the ultimate effect of mutations on the proteins encoded by genes responsible for key metabolic and regulatory pathways in cells. Other major areas of the genome and its homeostasis were relatively understudied.

Fortunately, this situation has changed. During the past few years, there has been an explosion of information about "epigenomic" alterations in cancer cells, including abnormalities in DNA methylation, histone acetylation, telomere size and organization, subtleties of copy number variation, etc. As nicely summarized in this volume, edited by a distinguished RNA biologist, Professor Jane Wu, the most recent area of excitement and new information in this effort focuses on a comprehensive interrogation of the varied RNA products of DNA transcription, their metabolism, and their functional impact. For lack of a better or more original term, I will use the shorthand "RNA'omics" to refer to this broad area of research

It is well established that most eukaryotic genes that ultimately encode proteins in human are transcribed as modular pre-mRNA initial transcripts. Alternative pre-mRNA processing (alternative splicing), selects which combinations of modules (exons) are ultimately selected for inclusion in the mature mRNA. In humans, alternative splicing increases the diversity of unique protein products arising from the 20,000 human genes to greater than 100,000. Moreover, many individual alternative splicing pathways are regulated differently in different tissues and at different stages of development and differentiation. Thus, a single gene can give rise varying arrays of related but distinctive isoforms in tissue-specific, differentiation stage-specific, and physiologic state-specific patterns, as well as changing at during embryonic, fetal, and adult stages of development. The spliceoforms can change in ways that modify the protein's functions, localization, and catabolism, or even produce forms with unique or antagonistic functions.

Pre-mRNA's are also altered by polyadenylation stability at their 3′ end, and the addition of a 5′ CAP structure that facilitates initiation of translation. They also contain untranslated sequences (UTR's) at each end of the mature mRNA molecule. These govern stability and efficiency of translation, and their properties can be modified by interaction with RNA-binding proteins. All of these features interact with complex systems that modulate the efficiency of transport to the cytoplasm, efficiency of translation, and degradation. The net result is that sequence features built into mRNA and its precursors impact the quantity of protein produced from its template as well as the amino acid sequence. High throughput sequencing for mutations and gene expression arrays, which can measure only sequence alterations and the amount of the mRNA's produced thus miss much that governs the ultimate impact of an expressed gene on the cell.

Finally, there are at least 1,000 small RNA molecules (micro RNA's or miRNA's, inhibitory RNA's or RNA's, etc.) and the ribosomal and transfer RNA's that are actively transcribed but do not code for proteins. Abnormalities in almost all of these components and processes have been described in various cancers or cancer cell line but little is yet known about whether and how they affect the neoplastic state. Nonetheless, it is clear that the collections of various small nuclear RNA's play a major role in regulating chromatin structure, transcription, RNA stability, splicing, and translation, and that these steps are modified in many cancer cells. miRNA's have been shown to participate in the modulation of gene expression, mRNA stability, and translatability. Some small nuclear RNA's are also critical for the formation of the spliceosomes that support constitutive and alternative mRNA splicing pathways. Mutations in key protein factors that regulate alternative mRNA splicing have been recently found to be highly prevalent in many hematologic malignancies. It is thus increasingly clear that any attempt to form a comprehensive vision of the molecular abnormalities important in cancer cells will require the inclusion of thorough analyses of the RNA'ome.

The chapters in this volume provide highly informative and readable summaries of recent progress in many of these areas. Dr. Wu is an internationally renowned expert in the regulation of alternative mRNA splicing and its abnormalities in human disease. This interest is reflected in the fact that chapters about mRNA splicing are the most abundant in this volume. However, she has not neglected other considerations such as miRNA's, mRNA stability, the perinucleolar body, and ribosomal RNA's. The volume is thus unique in the current snapshot it provides of work that is being pursued in the role of RNA metabolism in cancer, and the evolving insights into that role. Each chapter provides a good overview and much specific information that is current and to the point of the book. It is a volume to be commended to students of molecular cancer pathobiology.

I congratulate Dr. Wu and her colleagues on the production of a high quality and timely monograph about an important topic in cancer research.

Boston, MA, March 2012

Edward J. Benz Jr.
Dana-Farber Cancer Institute

Preface

In the last decade, it has become increasingly clear that RNA (ribonucleic acid) is not simply a messenger molecule (mRNA) directing protein synthesis. RNA has multiple versatile functional roles in cells, especially in mammalian gene regulation to influence almost every aspect of cellular life.

This volume reviews recent progresses in the selected areas of RNA processing, especially data related to cancer development and therapy. It is not our intention to cover comprehensively all areas of RNA processing. Instead, we have focused on several areas in which more information with cancer relevance has been obtained.

Cancer is a group of highly complex, multifactorial genetic diseases. In cancer, genetic defects may affect each step of gene expression: from transcription, splicing to translational regulation, mRNA stability control, and post-translational modifications. With the rapid development in technologies in gene expression profiling and sequencing, we now have much more comprehensive knowledge about the entire collection of different transcripts encoded by the human genome. The vast majority of human protein-coding genes use a mechanism known as alternative pre-mRNA splicing to generate more than one transcript from single genes. This alternative splicing process, in which different combinations of different regions of the primary gene transcript (pre-mRNA) are selected to form different mRNA species, is one of most robust mechanisms to achieve genetic diversity. Alternative splicing pattern changes have been detected in many types of cancer in genes critical for various aspects of tumor development and cancer metastasis. Such alternative splicing perturbations are being systematically investigated not only for the underlying mechanisms but also as potential biomarkers for diagnosis and therapeutic development.

In addition to protein coding genes, a large number of non-protein coding transcripts (ncRNAs) are produced by the human genome. This recent discovery has grown into a very active area of research. Evidence is accumulating that ncRNAs including microRNAs play important roles in regulating signal transduction pathways involved in cancer development and progression. In addition, small RNAs and oligonucleotes are becoming promising tools for cancer therapy development.

This book begins with the coupling between transcription and splicing. Three subsequent chapters describe in detail cancer-associated aberrant RNAs, new methodology for their detection, and the functional impact on expression of important genes including oncogenes and tumor suppressor genes. The following chapter focuses on microRNAs in cancer. The possible involvement of particular subcellular compartment, such as perinucleolar compartment (PNC), in cancer is reviewed. Implications of mRNA stability regulation in cancer are also discussed. In addition to genes controlling cell proliferation, cell death genes are tightly regulated by alternative splicing. Splicing defects in regulation of cell death genes have been discovered in many types of cancer. Potentials of developing therapeutics using oligonucleotides to modulate cancer-associated RNA defects are then reviewed. Finally, clinical perspectives of studying RNA defects in cancer are discussed together with their relevance to cancer diagnosis, therapies, and treatment resistance.

The target readers of this book are primarily those interested in gene regulation and cancer biology, especially those who are not directly working on RNA biology, including clinicians and medical students.

We are very fortunate to have internationally renowned experts to contribute to this book. We hope that this book will stimulate further innovative research collaborations between RNA biologists and cancer researchers, improving cancer diagnosis and treatment in the future.

Chicago, USA, March 2012

Jane Y. Wu
Department of Neurology
Charles Louis Mix Professor of Neurology
Lurie Comprehensive Cancer Center
and Center for Genetic Medicine
Northwestern University
Feinberg School of Medicine

Contents

Coupling Between Transcription and Alternative Splicing

Ignacio E. Schor, Luciana I. Gómez Acuña and Alberto R. Kornblihtt

Abstract

The scenario of alternative splicing regulation is far more complex than the classical picture of a pre-mRNA being processed post-transcriptionally in more than one way. Introns are efficiently removed while transcripts are still being synthesized, supporting the idea of a co-transcriptional regulation of alternative splicing. Evidence of a functional coupling between splicing and transcription has recently emerged as it was observed that properties of one process may affect the outcome of the other. Co-transcriptionality is thought to improve splicing efficiency and kinetics by directing the nascent pre-mRNA into proper spliceosome assembly and favoring splicing factor recruitment. Two models have been proposed to explain the coupling of transcription and alternative splicing: in the recruitment model, promoters and pol II status affect the recruitment to the transcribing gene of splicing factors or bifunctional factors acting on both transcription and splicing; in the kinetic model, differences in the elongation rate of pol II would determine the timing in which splicing sites are presented, and thus the outcome of alternative splicing decisions. In the later model, chromatin structure has emerged as a key regulator. Although definitive evidence for transcriptionally coupled alternative splicing alterations in tumor development or cancer pathogenesis is still missing, many alternative splicing events altered in cancer might be subject to transcription-splicing coupling regulation.

I. E. Schor · L. I. Gómez Acuña · A. R. Kornblihtt (✉)
Laboratorio de Fisiologia y Biologia Molecular, Departmento de Fisiologia, Biologia Molecular y Celular, IFIBYNE-CONICET, Facultad de Ciencias Exactas y Naturales, Universidad de Buenos Aires, Ciudad Universitaria, PAB. II, 20 Piso, Buenos Aires 1428, Argentina
e-mail: ark@fbmc.fcen.uba.ar

J. Y. Wu (ed.), *RNA and Cancer*, Cancer Treatment and Research,
DOI: 10.1007/978-3-642-31659-3_1, © Springer-Verlag Berlin Heidelberg 2013

Keywords
Alternative splicing · Co-transcriptional splicing · Transcription-splicing coupling · RNA polymerase II-CTD · Kinetic model · Chromatin

Contents

1 Introduction

Transcription and splicing are two processes that occur simultaneously in the eukaryotic nucleus and that can functionally influence each other, due to coupling mechanisms.

Several reports in which alterations of either of the two processes are associated with cancer progression can be found. In the case of alternative splicing, examples of cancer associated-mutations that change splicing patterns [1] include tumor supp-resor genes like Klf6, where a mutation that originates a binding site for the regulatory protein SRSF5 (formerly SRp40) originates isoforms that presumably act as dominant-negative mutants. Another example is the Brca1 gene, where mutations are thought to eliminate a splicing enhancer on exon 18. In other cases, mutations might not affect the alternatively spliced gene product itself, but can alter the levels and activity of trans-acting splicing regulators instead. This is probably the case of the Ron alternative isoform ΔRon, an inductor of invasive phenotype in gastric carcinomas, whose splicing is regulated by the binding of the SR protein SRSF1.

As it will be shown in this chapter, the transcriptional status can modulate the recruitment of splicing regulators to splice sites. Also, kinetic considerations of transcription must be taken into account, especially in cases of long genes (for example, Brca1 gene is 81kbp-long).

Although we do not have definitive evidence of transcriptionally coupled alternative splicing alterations responsible for tumor development or cancer pathogenesis, recent evidence suggests that the influence of transcription on alternative splicing might determine cell fate decision between apoptosis and cell cycle progression. DNA damage results in changes in RNA polymerase II elongation rate, which ultimately affects the alternative splicing patterns of the *Bcl-*

X and *Caspase9* genes toward the proapoptotic isoforms [2]. In this context, alterations in the DNA damage response that lead to changes in transcription and, as a consequence, in alternative splicing, might provoke cell cycle progression, and oncogenic transformation.

Another intriguing issue is the existence of genes with multiple alternative promoters in addition to alternative splicing events. In these cases, such as the gene coding for p53 tumor-suppresor protein, interaction between altered promoter choice and altered alternative splicing pattern in cancer is a suggestive possibility deduced from the coupling between transcription and splicing.

In the following pages, we will summarize the evidence for coupling accumulated mainly during the last decade.

2 Alternative Splicing and Its Regulation

We will review here some concepts that will apply to understand the coupling between transcription and alternative splicing that is covered in detail in Chap. 3 of this book.

Understanding alternative splicing regulation requires first a description of the way the splicing machinery identifies exons and introns. Constitutive splice sites are defined by consensus sequences (3′ splice donor, 5′ splice acceptor, polypyrimidine tract, and branching point) that recruit constitutive splicing factors, primarily the small nuclear ribonucleoprotein particles (snRNPs) and several auxiliary factors that mark the boundaries between introns and exons. In order to get accurate splicing, these intron–exon boundaries have to be paired. This pairing can occur across an intron (marking the intron that has to be removed) or across an exon (specifying the exon that must be joined to the adjacent exon). In the first case, we are in the presence of splicing via intron definition, typical of yeast where introns are short; in the second one, splicing takes place via exon definition as can be seen in higher eukaryotes that have small exons separated by much longer introns [3].

Both circumstances (recognition of intron–exon boundaries and pairing of the splicing complexes) are prerequisites for the spliceosome to carry out the splicing reaction. Any interference with this recognition (for example, due to mutation of the consensus sequences or increase in the length of an exon in exon definition) can affect splicing efficiency leading to complete inhibition of the splicing event, or, in milder cases, to alternative splicing. In these cases, strong splices sites would compete against weaker ones leading to a less frequent use of the inefficient splice site.

Using high-throughput sequencing approaches, it is now estimated that more than 90 % of the human genes with multiple exons have alternatively spliced mRNA isoforms [4, 5] and that nearly 86 % of all human genes undergo alternative splicing to generate appreciable levels of two or more mRNA isoforms [4]. Why are not these mutations that decrease splicing efficiency of a given splice site eliminated by negative selection? One possible answer is that new splicing events are created as alternative ones and go through a “test” period before they are

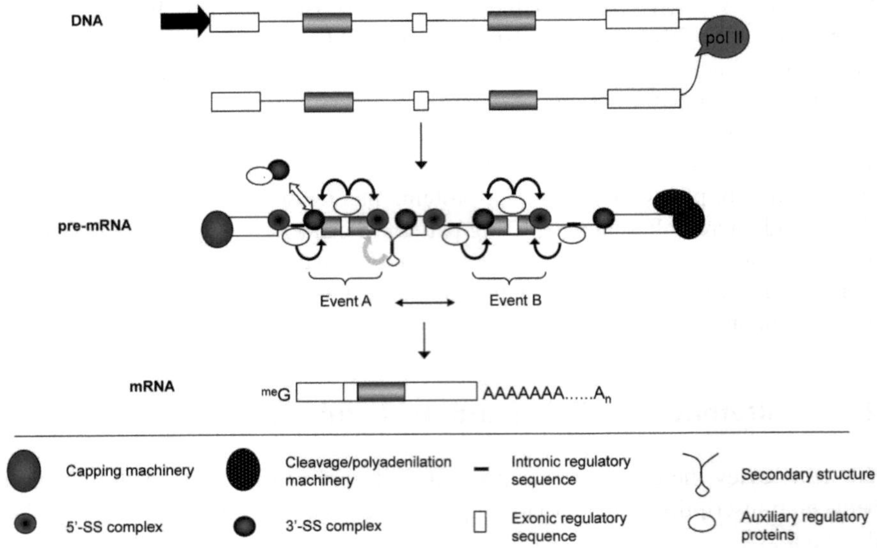

Fig. 1 Combinatorial regulation of alternative splicing, considering post-transcriptional RNA processing. An example of a pre-mRNA with two alternative exon cassettes is presented. Auxiliary proteins can help to recruit basal splicing factors (*light blue arrow*). Auxiliary proteins binding to exonic or intronic sequences modulate the use of the suboptimal splice sites of alternative exons (*black arrows*). Secondary structures of pre-mRNA can inhibit binding of factors to some of these sequences (*gray arrow*). The interaction can either promote of inhibit inclusion of the exons. In addition, splicing outcome of one event (e.g. Event A) can affect splicing of the other (Event B) and viceversa. The final mRNA results from the interaction of all these factors

eliminated by negative selection or stabilized as constitutive [6]. Another explanation would be that the result of these apparently harmful mutations (alternative splicing) is sometimes very useful. The most obvious favorable consequence is that if the exon was part of the coding region of the gene, and the proteins produced by the different mRNAs generated by alternative splicing were stable, that cell would be able to increase its proteomic diversity by means of a very simple and economic way. But perhaps the most important advantage of this process is the ability to control and regulate the relative amounts of the different protein products through alternative splicing regulation. Accordingly to the latter hypothesis, it was estimated that nearly 60 % of the human alternative splicing events have tissue specific regulation [4]. This observation also supports the hypothesis that phenotypic complexity in mammals can be explained, at least partially, by alternative splicing, and that such a mechanism clearly contributes to cell lineage and tissue identity.

If we think in the classical picture of a precursor messenger RNA (pre-mRNA) that has just been transcribed and is waiting to be processed (capped, spliced, and polyadenylated), there should be several ways in which splicing efficiency or recognition of poor splicing targets can be modulated: [7–9].

1. Auxiliary proteins (that would recognize *cis*-acting elements in the RNA molecule) can help or inhibit recruitment of basal splicing factors.
2. Auxiliary proteins interacting with the 3′ and 5′ splicing complexes of the spliceosome can help or inhibit pairing between contiguous exon–intron boundaries.
3. A secondary structure of the pre-mRNA can block the access of the splicing machinery to certain important sequence element, so it would be necessary to recruit additional factors that change the secondary structure.

The picture is even more complex if we consider the existence of pre-mRNAs with more than one event of alternative splicing (it is estimated that this occurs in 25 % of the human genes). The fibronectin (FN) gene is a paradigmatic example [10] as it contains three regions of alternative splicing that display cell type- and development-specific regulation. The combination of splicing events can eventually give rise up to 20 mRNA isoforms in humans, 12 in rodents, and 8 in chicken [11]. In that situation, it is expected that the outcome of one alternative splicing choice can affect the other/s, and that is indeed what is seen within this gene [12]. This effect (known as coordination) is likely to have influence on the processing of several transcripts, as bioinformatics searches detect a strong bias in the splicing isoforms of ESTs (sequences derived from mRNAs) annotated in genomic databases. Other examples of long distance regulation of splice site selection have been reported in equine ß-casein intron 1, [13] and in the human thrombopoietin gene [14].

These levels of modulation can exert their effects alone or in combination with each other, to give some degree of regulation complexity (Fig. 1).

3 Splicing Co-Transcriptionality and Coupling

The classical view of the pre-mRNA as a full length molecule that will be processed (capped, spliced, and polyadenylated) only after transcription is completed has been long known to be incorrect. It is becoming clearer that the nucleus is a highly organized organelle and that nuclear processes occur in coordinated complexes of different proteins and ribonucleoproteins acting in the same region. The concept of co-transcriptional processing has been widely accepted in the case of capping. However, it is now clear that it applies also to splicing and polyadenylation [15–21].

Electron microscopy visualization of *Drosophila* embryo nascent transcripts clearly demonstrated that splicing occurs co-transcriptionally with a reasonable frequency and that splice site selection precedes polyadenylation [22]. Co-transcriptional splicing was also demonstrated for the dystrophin gene [23]. Since transcription of this 2,400 kb-gene, the largest in the human genome, would take approximately 16 h to be completed, co-transcriptional splicing of its pre-mRNA appears as a very intuitive concept. In fact, it is very difficult to conceive that the splicing of the dozens of dystrophin introns would "wait" until the synthesis of a huge 2,400 kb pre-mRNA substrate molecule is finished.

More recently, nascent RNA associated with actively transcribed chromatin was analyzed in comparison with RNA found in nucleoplasm, no longer associated with the transcribing machinery [24]. As predicted for co-transcriptional splicing, introns are efficiently removed within the chromatin-associated RNA fraction suggesting that they are excised while still associated with a transcribing RNA polymerase II (pol II). Moreover, the presence of introns in the pre-mRNA increases toward the 5′end of the two genes analyzed, *c-Src,* and *FN,* suggesting that they are removed as they are transcribed. Exceptions can be found, however, as the 3′terminal *FN* intron is excised, co-transcriptionally, with higher efficiency that the upstream ones.

It should be noted, then, that co-transcriptionality of splicing is not strict, in the sense that introns are not necessarily removed in the exact order they are transcribed. If that was the case, the competition among splicing sites that leads to alternative splicing would be impossible. What really happens is that introns in a transcript can be eliminated in different orders, and some can be processed co-transcriptionally while others are processed post-transcriptionally. This is exemplified by studies with the Balbiani ring 1 (BR1) gene where intron 3, located 3 kb from the 5′ end of the 40-kb-pre-mRNA, is excised mostly co-transcriptionally, but intron 4, located 0.6 kb from the poly A site, is excised co-transcriptionally in only 10 % of the molecules [25]. As in the case of constitutive splicing, alternative splicing was also found to be co-transcriptional, in the sense that it occurs mainly when the transcript is still being synthesized, but the order of the flanking intron removal is not strict [24]. When analyzing alternative splicing events that differ in their regulation mechanisms, flanking introns were removed in different orders [24, 26], indicating the existence of diverse splicing pathways. In the case of the *FN* alternative exon E33, the downstream intron is removed prior to the upstream one and the rate of intron removal is altered by *cis* acting mutations of splicing factors binding sites or SR proteins abundance changes that affect the alternative exon inclusion levels [26]. Overall, this evidence suggests that intron order removal of an alternative splicing event is a reflection of the underlying regulation mechanism.

All the evidence mentioned above suggest that the reaction of splicing occurs while transcripts are still being synthesized, i.e., co-transcriptionally. However, this does not imply, *per se*, that transcription and splicing are two processes that are functionally coupled in terms that one alters the properties or the outcome of the other [27, 28]. On the other hand, the fact that these processes occur at the same time and in the same place seems to be a prerequisite for their machineries to functionally interact in a coordinated manner.

Recently, two reports showed some evidence that strongly suggest coupling between constitutive splicing and transcription in yeast. In one of them [29], inducible reporter minigenes with or without an intron were stably integrated into *S. cereviciae* genome. Upon induction, and at the time point when spliced mRNA was first detected, a transient pol II accumulation, indicating transcriptional pausing, was observed around the 3′ splice site (3′SS) of the intron bearing minigene. When mutating the 3′SS or the 5′SS, pol II signal became lower at the promoter, suggesting reduced transcriptional activity, and its accumulation around the 3′SS was no longer detected. Moreover, in the case of the 3′SS mutation, pol II accumulation was observed around the 5′SS. Overall, this work indicates that the dynamics of pol II elongation along a gene depend on the presence of a splicing event. In agreement, several splicing factors were found to affect transcription. SC35, for example, stimulates pol II elongation by interacting with P-TEFb, a complex that phosphorilates Ser2 of the CTD, engaging pol II to active elongation [30]. In the second study [31], a genome wide approach was used to provide evidence of a functional association between splicing and transcription. Total RNAs purified from the chromatin associated fraction (i.e. nascent pre-mRNAs) were analyzed with high density tilling microarrays, looking for intronic under, or overrepresentation. The majority of intron bearing genes (taking into account that in yeast most intron containing genes have only one intron) showed co-transcriptional intron removal. In silico simulations, assuming no coupling, predicts a positive correlation between co-transcriptionallity and terminal exon length. However, this did not correlate with the experimental observations as genes with higher efficiency in co-transcriptional splicing than predicted bear shorter terminal exons. Accordingly, this group of genes showed a significant increase in pol II density within the gene body, downstream the intron, in opposition to genes that display lower efficiency than predicted in co-transcriptional splicing [31].

This evidence suggests a selective pressure toward co-transcriptionality in splicing, perhaps to allow the functional coupling between both mechanisms. This raises the question of the possible benefits on nuclear metabolism and gene expression fine tuning. Currently, transcription and processing of mRNAs is thought to be carried out by coordinated complexes of proteins and ribonucleoproteins that link the two steps in the genesis of mature mRNAs, so the efficiency of the general process is greatly improved [15]. As a general principle that can be deduced intuitively, the transcriptional elongation complex might provide a scaffold over which the splicing machinery is recruited or assembled, so that the sequence of events is established in order and there is less chance for mistakes [28]. The general result could be both improved efficiency and enhanced splicing kinetics.

4 Molecular Mechanisms of Coupling

The coordination between transcription and processing seems to be a specific feature of RNA polymerase II. Indeed, when protein-encoding genes are placed under the control of either pol I, pol III, or T7 RNA polymerase promoters, transcription takes place, but pre-mRNA processing is deeply affected, and in particular the resulting transcripts are poorly spliced [32–35]. In vitro assays show that nascent pre-mRNA synthesized by pol II is stabilized and efficiently spliced [36] apparently, because it is immediately and quantitatively directed into the spliceosome assembly pathway. In contrast, nascent pre-mRNA synthesized by T7 phage RNA polymerase is quantitatively assembled into nonspecific hnRNP complexes which are inhibitory for spliceosome assembly, indicating that pol II mediates the functional coupling of transcription to splicing by directing the nascent pre-mRNA into proper spliceosome assembly [37]. However, other in vitro assays reported no changes in splicing efficiency or kinetics between pol II synthesized RNA and presynthesized pre-mRNA [27]. This apparent contradiction may be due to the fact that RNA stability is not properly measured and taken into account as a possible cause of the splicing efficiency improvement [27]. This brings us back to the notion that a concurrent splicing reaction along with transcription, which appears to be the case in these assays, does not necessarily imply coupling. We must consider, nevertheless, the limitations of in vitro systems, consisting mainly on nuclear extracts that do not reproduce nuclear organization and architecture and in which DNA is necessarily short and not packed into chromatin [27]. More recently, the Reed lab demonstrated that a large group of proteins interacts with RNA pol II in vivo. This includes almost all known SR proteins and U1snRNP, but not other splicing factors or hnRNPs. Futhermore, using nuclear extracts that perform both transcription and splicing in vitro, they showed that SR proteins are necessary for pol II-mediated coupling, as efficient splicing of extracts depleted of SR proteins is restored if these are added before but not after transcription [38].

A key player in the coupling appears to be the carboxy-terminal domain (CTD) of the catalytic subunit of RNA pol II. In fact, association of splicing factors to sites of transcription is dependent on pol II CTD [39] and deletion of CTD causes defects in capping, cleavage/polyadenylation, and splicing of the β-globin transcript [40].Besides, isolated CTD fragments [41] as well as the entire purified phosphorylated pol II [42] are able to activate splicing in vitro. Nevertheless, isolated CTD fragments cannot duplicate the whole pol II effect unless the precursor RNA is recognized via exon definition. These findings support a direct role for the CTD in exon recognition and lead to the speculation that the CTD would bring consecutive exons closer, which would then facilitate spliceosome assembly. Consistently, Dye and Proudfoot [43] showed that exons flanking an intron that has been engineered to be co-transcriptionally cleaved by inserting a ribozyme in the middle are accurately and efficiently spliced together. These data suggest that a continuous transcript is not required for pre-mRNA splicing in vivo and provide evidence for a molecular tether connecting emergent splice sites in the pre-mRNA to transcribing pol II.

The structure of the CTD is quite unique: it is composed of 52 tandem repeats in mammals (26 in yeasts) of the consensus heptad YSPTSPS. CTD serines at positions 2 and 5 within each heptad are subject to regulatory phosphorylations. Phosphorylation of Ser5 by TFIIH is linked to transcriptional initiation, whereas phosphorylation of Ser2 by P-TEFb is associated to transcriptional elongation [44, 45]. However, it is becoming clearer now that this might be an oversimplification as the mammalian CTD bear 46 Ser2 and 51 Ser1 residues and it can be subjected to other post translational modifications [46]. In this scenario, post-translational modifications are likely to act in a combinatory way to exert different effects to the properties of the pol II in terms of elongation and protein recruitment.

It has been shown that changes in the structure and phosphorylation pattern of CTD modulate co-transcriptional but not post-transcriptional processing [47, 48]. It is worth mentioning that the roles of CTD in splicing may vary depending on the gene. Transcription by a pol II mutant lacking the CTD causes a dramatic enhancement in the inclusion levels of the FN E33 alternative cassette exon without affecting the efficiency of general splicing [49, 50]. The use of pol II CTD variants with different numbers of repeats revealed that the length of the CTD correlates inversely with E33 inclusion levels, with 19 heptads being the minimum number of repeats necessary to sustain normal E33 splicing. This is in agreement with reports showing that 22 tandem repeats are sufficient to support wild-type levels of splicing of pre-mRNAs containing constitutively spliced introns or introns that depend on an exonic splicing enhancer for efficient splicing [51].

Another feature that should be considered as a link between transcription and alternative splicing is chromatin, since some splicing factors are known to be recruited to the transcription site by interacting with specific histone post-translational modifications. Histone H3 lysine 4 tri-methylation (H3K4me3), for example, was shown to associate to major spliceosomal snRNPs, with U2 snRNP being the strongest interaction, through binding to the CHD1 adaptor protein. Downregulation of either CHD1 or H3K4me3 exerted a reduction of the IRF1 pre-mRNA splicing efficiency [52]. A similar adaptor system seems to be relevant in genes whose alternative splicing regulation is dependent on the polypyrimidine tract binding protein (PTB) splicing factor. In such genes, tri-methylated H3 lysine 36 (H3K36me3) recruits PTB via binding the adaptor protein MRG15 [53]. H3K36me3 is a mark associated with transcription as the H3K36 methyltransferase Set1 is known to bind pol II CTD [54, 55].

All this evidence points to a temporal and functional coupling between pol II mediated transcription and mRNA processing, with a central role for the CTD. However, while this is a pre-requisite for an influence of transcription quality on splicing choices, it does not imply this influence *per se*.

5 Evidence of Functional Coupling Between Transcription and Alternative Splicing

Although the results mentioned above strongly suggest that the quality of transcription would influence alternative splicing choices, they do not provide a direct evidence of this "functionally-coupled regulation". The first direct evidence came from experiments of promoter swapping using a minigene containing the extra domain I alternative exon (E33, also known as EDI or EDA) of the FN gene as a splicing reporter [56, 57]. E33 is 270 bp-long and contains an exonic splicing enhancer (ESE) with the core sequence GAAGAAGA, which is targeted by the SR proteins SRSF1 and SRSF7. When transcription of the minigene is driven by the α-globin promoter; for example, E33 inclusion levels in the mature mRNA are about 10 times lower than when transcription is driven by the FN or cytomegalovirus (CMV) promoters. In other genes, similar effects can be observed. Alternative splicing reporter minigenes corresponding to the CD44 and the calcitonin gene-related product (CGRP) genes were placed under the control of steroid sensitive promoters or promoters that do not respond to steroid hormones. Steroid hormones affected splice site selection only of pre-mRNAs produced by the first type of promoters [58]. However, the effects are not the trivial consequence of different mRNA levels produced by each promoter (promoter strength) but depend on some qualitative properties conferred by promoters to the transcription/RNA processing machinery. Promoter dependent alternative splicing patterns have been also found in the cystic fibrosis transmembrane regulator [59] and in the fibroblast growth factor receptor 2 genes [60].

Promoter swapping is not likely to be found in nature (although alternative promoter usage might resemble it), but this artificial situation may reflect differences in the transcriptional machinery that physiologically are modulated via transcription factor and co-regulator recruitment. In agreement with this view, targeting of different transcription factors to a minigene promoter, using a Gal4-fusion system, differentially affects splicing choices [61]. Constitutive splicing can be modulated also by transcriptional activators, in a pol II CTD-dependent manner [62]. Transcriptional co-regulators have been also implicated in the control of alternative splicing. Several co-regulators of steroid hormone nuclear receptors showed differential effects on alternative splicing in a promoter-dependent manner [63]. Transcriptional co-regulators are proteins recruited to gene promoters through protein–protein interactions with transcription factors that bind directly to DNA. They can act as transcriptional co-activators or co-repressors or both, depending on the promoter context on which they are recruited. For example CoAA (co-activator activator), recruited by TRBP, which is, in turn, recruited to promoters through direct interactions with activated nuclear receptor, can regulate alternative splicing in a promoter-dependent manner. It similarly enhances transcriptional activities fired by the steroid sensitive or insensitive promoters, but only affects alternative splicing of transcripts synthesized from the progesterone-activated MMTV promoter [64].

6 Consequence of Co-Transcriptionality in Splicing

Regulation of splicing, as summarized in Fig. 1, becomes even more complex as we add the dimension of time.

Splicing complexes must be recruited to all introns and exons in a time window that begins when the target sequence is transcribed and extends to the moment of transcription termination (or even after, if we take into account post-transcriptional processing) [20]. Thanks to the powerful chromatin immunoprecipitation technique, co-transcriptional assembly of splicing factors can be examined in vivo. In both yeast and mammalian cells it has been observed that snRNPs and other processing factors accumulate at positions along intron-containing genes, coincidently with the appearance of their target splicing sequences in nascent pre-mRNA [65–68]. As said before, analysis of RNA associated to actively transcribed chromatin showed that both spliced and unspliced forms are detected, which tells us that splicing has already undergone in some of the RNA molecules [24, 68]. Furthermore, the proportion of spliced mRNA associated with chromatin is increased when transcription is paused

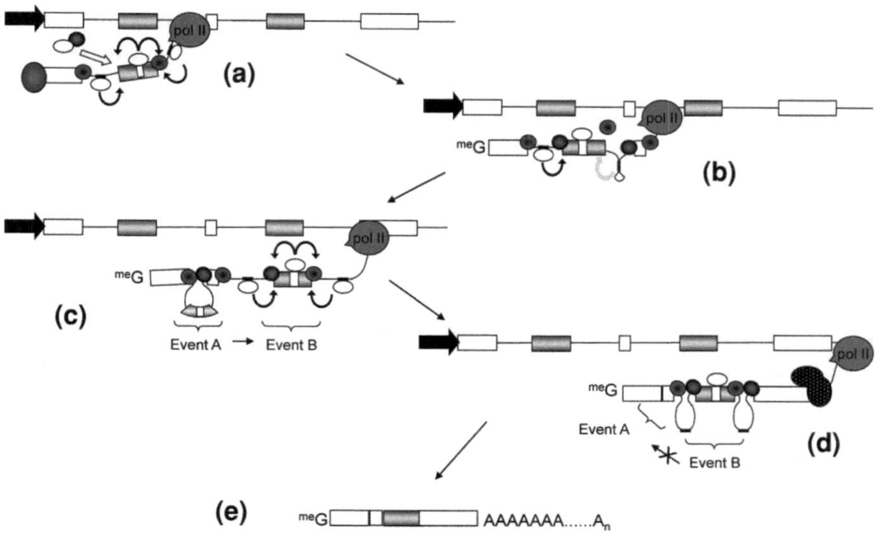

Fig. 2 Example of regulation of alternative splicing in time, considering co-transcriptional RNA processing. (**a**). First alternative exon has recently been transcribed and its fate is being determined by a combination of *cis*-acting sequences and *trans*-acting factors, as described for Fig. 1. The downstream intronic sequence can be targeted by a regulatory factor that is able to regulate 5′ SS use. (**b**). As the downstream intron continues being transcribed, a secondary structure forms that inhibits binding of factors to the intronic regulator, preventing its participation in splicing regulation if the alternative exon fate has not been determined yet. Also, the downstream constitutive exon is now transcribed, enabling competition for the upstream splicing donor. (**c**). The first alternative splicing event (Event A) is already commited for exon exclusion while the second alternative splicing event (Event B) is in an earlier step. In this situation, the outcome of the first event is likely to influence the second. (**d**). When the Event B is commited to exon inclusion, is not possible for it to influence the outcome of Event A, since the later is already spliced. This situation explains the polarity observed in coordination phenomena. (**e**). The final mRNA is the result of the combination of the different regulation steps and the kinetics of transcription

by application of the drug camptothecin (an inhibitor of DNA topoisomerase I) [68]. Therefore, splicing sequences exist that are transcribed in time following a predetermined order, splicing complexes are recruited to these sequences in a different order and splicing catalysis occurs in another order, depending on the quality of splicing complexes and the interaction between them. Processing complexes are also interacting with the transcription machinery (mainly RNA pol II CTD), which might affect co-transcriptional splicing.

The relevance of this situation to alternative splicing is obvious: the timing of these different steps would either favor or disfavor the competition between splicing sites, altering the outcome of alternative splicing. At the same time, exonic and intronic splicing enhancer or silencers are being transcribed and secondary structures in the precursor RNA (that could inhibit or enhance splicing) are changing, further influencing the result of alternative splicing choices. To add an extra level of complexity, the coordination of different alternative splicing events within a same transcript (the influence of one event in the outcome of the other) would be influenced by the degree of co-transcriptionality.

Bearing these new considerations in mind, we surely need to upgrade our model of alternative splicing regulation by including co-transcriptionality as a key factor (Fig. 2). In the following sections, we will present evidence for the different models of functional coupling between transcription and alternative splicing regulation.

7 Models for Co-Transcriptional Regulation of Alternative Splicing

Two different models have been proposed to deal with the promoter influence on alternative splicing [18]. On the one hand, the promoter might affect the recruitment to the transcribing gene of splicing factors or bifunctional factors acting on both transcription and splicing. On the other hand, the promoter might affect the rate of pol II elongation, affecting, in turn, the timing of co-transcriptional splicing. It must be taken into account that these models do not exclude each other, as they can both act physiologically at different times, in different exons or even together on the same alternative splicing event. However, for the sake of simplicity, we discuss in depth the evidence for the two models separately.

7.1 The Recruitment Model

There are several examples of transcription factors with effects in alternative splicing, such as the transcriptional activator of the human papilloma virus [69], and the thermogenic coactivator PGC-1. Interestingly, PGC-1 affects alternative splicing, but only when it is recruited to complexes that interact with gene promoters [70]. Another example is the transcription factor Spi-1, required for myeloid and B lymphoid differentiation. Spi-1 is able to regulate alternative splicing of a pre-mRNA for a gene whose transcription it regulates. Guillouf et al. [71]. demonstrated that, similarly to PGC-1, Spi-1 must bind and transactivate its cognate promoter to favor the use of a proximal 5′ alternative site. Other mammalian cell candidates to act as bifunctional factors include the product of the WT-1 gene, which is essential for normal kidney development, [72] SAF-B, which mediates chromatin attachment to the nuclear matrix [73], CA150, a human nuclear factor with characteristic WW and FF domains implicated in transcriptional elongation [74, 75] and a group of proteins known as SCAFs (SR-like CTD associated factors) which interact with the CTD and, similarly to SR proteins, contain an RS domain and an RNA binding domain [76].

There are other DNA-binding proteins, with function in transcriptional regulation, which can exert some effects on splicing regulation. One example is the methyl-CpG-binding protein 2 (MeCP2), originally reported to participate in

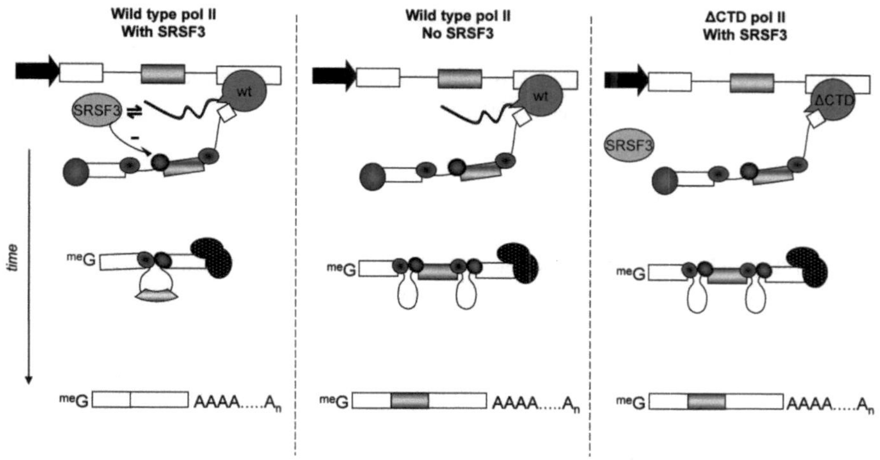

Fig. 3 An example of how the transcription complex can affect alternative splicing by recruitment of splicing factors. The carboxy terminal domain (CTD) of RNA polymerase II mediates the inhibitory effect of the SR protein SRp20 on the inclusion of the alternatively spliced fibronectin E33 exon. Transcription by a WT pol II (*left*) allows recruitment of SRSF3 to the transcription machinery which stimulates E33 skipping. Either absence of SRSF3 or transcription by a mutated pol II lacking the CTD (ΔCTD, right) causes higher E33 inclusion because in both cases SRSF3 is not recruited

transcriptional repression of methylated genes in part via recruitment of histone deacetylases. Young et al. showed that MeCP2 is able to promote the inclusion of a CD44 minigene reporter. Interestingly, this effect does not depend on binding to the DNA, but on interaction with the YB-1 splicing regulator [77].

Based on the experiments that determined the important role of RNA pol II CTD for efficient mRNA processing, some lines of research pointed to the possibility that splicing factors were "loaded" on the CTD and delivered to the splicing sites by the pol II holoenzyme. New insights into this possible mechanism came from in vitro experiments in which the CTD was fused at the C terminus of the splicing factor SRSF1 (formerly called SF2/ASF). Compared to SRSF1 alone, SRSF1-CTD increased the reaction rate during the early stages of splicing. Both the RNA-targeting domain of SRSF1 and phosphorylation of the CTD moiety were necessary for the stimulation of splicing by the chimerical protein [78].

Using a combination of siRNA knockdown, inducible reporter systems and transfection of different RNA polymerases, de la Mata et al. determined that the requirement of CTD coupling differs among splicing factors. Whereas activation of E33 inclusion by the SR protein SRSF1 is not affected by the absence of the CTD, inhibition of E33 inclusion by another SR protein, SRSF3 (formerly SRp20), is completely abolished when transcription is carried out by a ΔCTD pol II, indicating that SRSF3 needs the CTD to be recruited to the transcription/splicing machinery (Fig. 3) [48]. Interestingly, the CTD influences alternative splicing in a way that is independent of capping and 3′ end processing. Although no direct physical interaction between SRSF3 and the CTD or the whole pol II large subunit could be detected, it should probably exist, perhaps weak or indirect, because SRSF3 has been found in a transcription complex known as "mediator", together with the large subunit of RNA pol II [79].

7.2 The Kinetic Model

As we stated, when we first considered the consequences of co-transcriptionality in alternative splicing, differences in the elongation rate of pol II would determine the timing in which splicing sites are presented, and thus the outcome of alternative splicing decisions. Accordingly, it is expected that regulators of pol II elongation would also act as alternative splicing regulators. A kinetic role for transcription on alternative splicing was originally suggested by Eperon et al. [80], who found that the rate of RNA synthesis affects its secondary structure, which in turn affects splicing. A similar mechanism involving a kinetic link was suggested from experiments in which pol II pause sites affect alternative splicing by delaying the transcription of an essential splicing inhibitory element (DRE) required for regulation of tropomyosin exon 3 [81].

7.2.1 Control of RNA pol II Elongation

Further evidences for a role of pol II elongation rates in regulating alternative splicing came from a series of experiments using fibronectin E33 exon as a model. For example, it was showed that transcription factors that stimulate mostly transcriptional initiation, such as Sp1 and CTF/NF1, have little effect on alternative splicing, whereas factors (such as VP16) and transcriptional regulatory elements (such as the SV40 enhancer) that activate pol II elongation provoke skipping of the E33 [61, 82, 83]. Also, the use of a pharmacological inhibitor of the kinase that promotes pol II elongation phosphorylating ser 2 on CTD (p-TEFb) increased E33 inclusion by threefold [61, 84].

Given that, E33 (and most alternative exon cassettes) is alternatively spliced due to a suboptimal 3′ splice site that competes with the stronger 3′ splice site of the downstream exon, a highly processively elongating pol II, or the absence of internal pauses, would favor the simultaneous presentation of both introns to the splicing machinery, a situation in which the stronger 3′ splice site of the downstream intron outcompetes the weaker 3′ splice site of the upstream intron, resulting in exon skipping. On the contrary, in the case of a slow polymerase or the presence of pauses anywhere between these two sites, only elimination of the upstream intron can take place. Once the pause is passed or the polymerase proceeds, there is no option for the splicing machinery but to eliminate the downstream intron, which leads to exon inclusion. This dependence on competing splice sites for splicing response to elongation was supported by mutation analysis showing that the better the E33 alternative exon is recognized by the splicing machinery, the less its degree of inclusion is affected by factors that modulate transcriptional elongation [84].

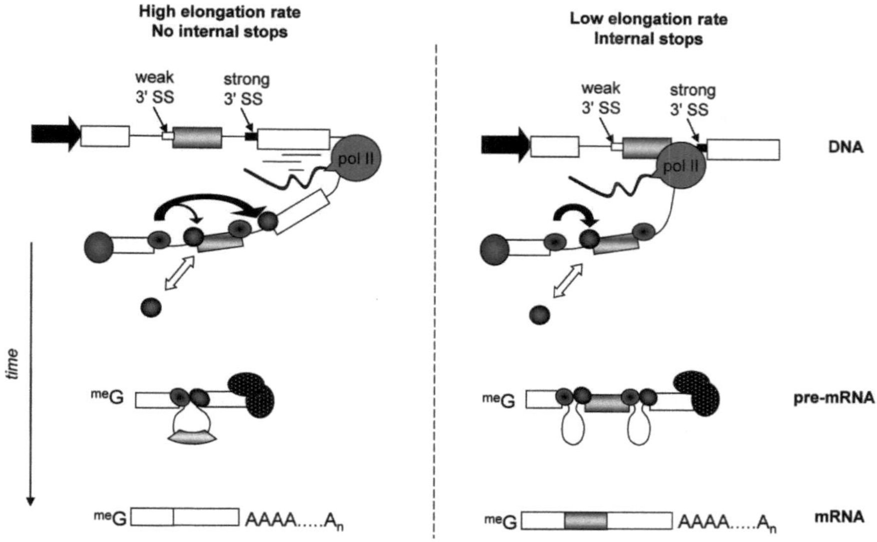

Fig. 4 Kinetic coupling model for the regulation of alternative splicing by pol II elongation. The 3′ splice site (SS) by the alternative cassette exon (*white*) is weaker than the 3′ SS of the downstream intron (*black*). Low transcriptional elongation rates (*right*) favor exon inclusion because it gives time for the weaker 3′ SS to be used, whereas high elongation rates (*left*) favor skipping as it results in almost simultaneous presentation of both 3′ SS

Therefore, in theory, low pol II elongation rates or internal pauses for elongation would favor the inclusion of alternative exons governed by an exon skipping mechanism (such as E33), whereas a highly elongating pol II, or the absence of internal pauses, would favor exclusion of these kinds of exons (Fig. 4). This hypothesis was tested directly using a mutant form of RNA pol II (called C4) with lower elongation rates [85]. The result supported the hypothesis: when a E33 reporter minigene is transcribed by the C4 pol II, the inclusion is 4-fold higher than the same reporter transcribed by a wild-type pol II. Most importantly and of physiological relevance, *Drosophila* flies carrying the C4 mutation show changes in the alternative splicing profile of the large ultrabithorax (Ubx) endogenous gene. The observed changes are consistent with a kinetic mechanism which allows more time for early splicing events. Interestingly, *Drosophila* with the C4 allele in heterozygosis but being wild-type for both Ubx alleles show a mutant phenotype called "Ubx effect" that resembles the one seen in flies haploinsufficient for the Ubx protein. Similar effects of pol II elongation rates on splicing were found in yeast. Alternative splicing is a very rare event in yeast. By mutating the branch point upstream of the constitutive internal exon of the DYN2 gene, an artificial cassette exon that becomes alternatively spliced was created. Skipping of this exon is prevented when expressed in a yeast mutant carrying a slow pol II or in the presence elongation inhibitors [86]. This supports the hypothesis that relative rates of spliceosome formation and pol II processivity are important to the balance between exon skipping and exon inclusion.

More recent evidence called for a revision of the original kinetic model. Using the E33 reporter minigen, it was observed that, when the alternative exon is included, the downstream intron is removed prior to the upstream one. Alterations on splicing factors recruitment that changed E33 inclusion levels, affects the relative rate of intron removal according to the respective splicing factors mechanism of action, as discussed above. However, changes in pol II elongation, caused either by DRB (an inhibitor of the elongation factor pTEFb) treatment or by transcribing the minigene with the C4 mutant, did not alter the rate of intron removal [26]. Therefore, reducing pol II elongation might not necessarily affect the kinetics of intron removal itself, but the early recruitment of splicing factors and commitment to splice.

The kinetics of transcription can also affect the coordination between different splicing events in the same pre-mRNA molecule. According to the model, when the elongation rate is high, both events are processed almost simultaneously so they can influence each other equaly. However, if pol II elongation is slower, polarity is expected as the proximal event can modulate the distal one, but no viceversa. This is because when the second event is transcribed, the first one will already be commited to splice or even spliced. In fact, when coordination and polarity were tested transfecting human cells with minigenes carrying two alternative E33 regions in tandem, separated by 3,400 bp spanning three constitutive exons and the corresponding introns, coordination was observed with transcription driven by different promoters, but polarity was abolished when using a promoter known to transcribe at higher elongation rates. More strikingly, polarity was restored with this promoter if the cells were treated with an inhibitor of pTEF-b that disfavor pol II elongation [12].

Recently, changes in the alternative splicing outcome due to alterations of pol II elongation properties were reported in a more physiologically relevant cellular context. In Muñoz et al. study [2], UV treatment caused an increase in the inclusion levels of E33 into the endogenous FN mRNA, independently of DNA damage in *cis*. Such increase is explained by pol II CTD hyper phosphorylation of Ser2 and Ser5 residues and subsequent transcription elongation inhibition, in agreement with the kinetic model. The same inclusion level increase was observed, without UV treatment, using a mutant pol II that mimics the hyperphosphorylated state (Ser2 and Ser5 are replaced by a negatively charged glutamate). By a similar mechanism, UV treatment also leads to an increase of the Bcl-x and C9 proapoptotic isoforms. Interestingly, this UV effect is independent of p53, a factor shown to be a key player in the apoptotic response. Overexpression of the Bcl-x antiapoptotic long isoform abolished the UV response toward apoptosis, suggesting that modulation on Bcl-x alternative splicing through this mechanism is a key part of the p53-independent apoptotic response.

7.2.2 Chromatin Structure

Modification of the transcription machinery is not the only way to alter elongation rates. The characteristics of the transcription template can be very important as well. In particular, chromatin structure is known to affect elongation. Being dynamically regulated in vivo (by chromatin remodeling factors or post-transcriptional modifications of histones—such as acetylation and methylation), the modification of chromatin can be an important step of regulation of transcription and transcription-coupled alternative splicing. Accordingly, Trichostatin A, a potent inhibitor of histone deacetylation, favors E33 skipping [61]. This is consistent with the idea that acetylation of the core histones would facilitate the passage of the transcribing polymerase leading to a situation of higher elongation rates. On the other hand, replication of the transfected minigene reporters, after which these template plasmids adopt a more compact chromatin structure which resists the pass of the polymerase, causes a 10 to 30-fold increase in E33 exon inclusion levels in the transcript [82]. It is worth noting that intragenic DNA methylation provokes a close chromatin structure and subsequently reduces the efficiency of pol II elongation, [87] suggesting an additional role of DNA methylation in alternative splicing regulation as it might not only be involved in transcriptional silencing when located at promoter regions.

Batsché et al. [88]. revealed a new role in alternative splicing for the chromatin remodeling factor SWI/SNF whose mechanism of action involves the regulation of pol II elongation. SWI/SNF is known to interact with pol II, splicing factors and spliceosome associated proteins. Overexpression of Brahma (Brm), the key subunit of SWI/SNF, favors inclusion of a block of consecutive alternative exons (v1 to v10) in the CD44 gene, which is a target for SWI/SNF transcriptional activation. Brm interacts with Sam68, a nuclear RNA-binding protein that, in turn, binds splicing regulatory elements present in the CD44 variable exons and to stimulate their inclusion upon activation of the ERK MAP kinases. ChIP experiments showed that Brm is not only present at the gene promoter but appears distributed along the whole transcription unit with levels that decrease gradually toward the 3′ end. Although also concentrated at the promoter region, pol II molecules display a different distribution inside the gene with a clear accumulation within the variable region, peaking on exon v4. This peak disappears when endogenous Brm is knocked down by RNAi, but is higher when cells are treated with phorbol esthers, that activate ERKs. Furthermore, in this region the phosphorylation status of the CTD shows an enrichment of the non-elongating phospho-ser5 form of RNA pol II (typical of promoters). These findings strongly suggest that activation of Sam68 by ERK triggers the formation of macromolecular complexes together with pol II and Brm at the central block of variable exons where the nascent transcript is exposing binding sites for Sam68, resulting in the stalling of pol II molecules and the subsequent inclusion of the variable exons into mature mRNA, in agreement with the kinetic coupling model. This work suggests the existence of internal road-blocks regulated in vivo by external signals, that can affect alternative splicing according to the kinetic model (Fig. 5) [89].

It is clear now, that modulation of histone post-translational modification patterns can affect the outcome of alternative splicing, bringing into our attention a new field of research with the premise that chromatin structure is likely to be a key player in the effects of transcription over alternative splicing regulation. In a neuronal depolarization model, for instance, it was found that depolarization triggers the skipping of

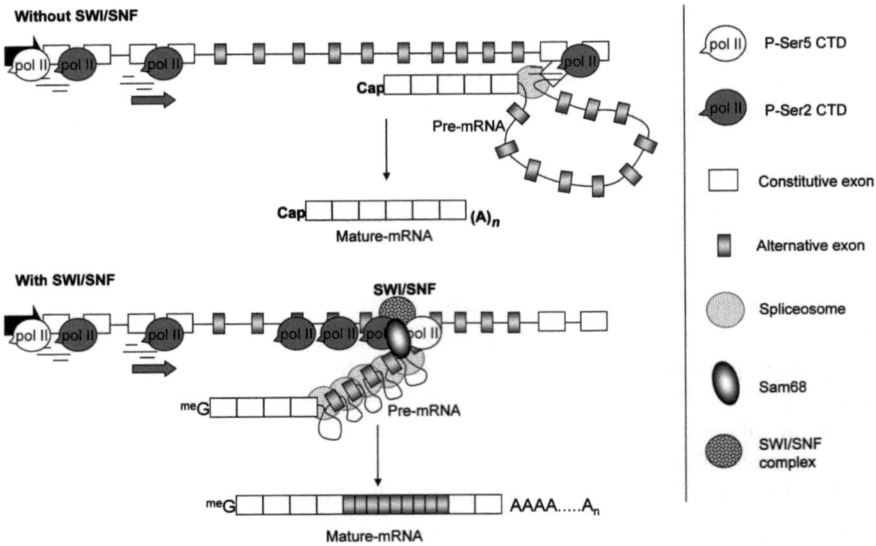

Fig. 5 SWI/SNF stimulates inclusion of alternative exons in the CD44 gene by creating a "road block" to pol II elongation at the variable region. The pause is the consequence of multiple protein interactions involving SWI/SNF, pol II, the splicing regulator Sam68 and spliceosomal components. The phosphorylation pattern of pol II CTD associated to Brm is changed from phospho-Ser2 to phospho-Ser5. This might cause the stalling of pol II molecules coming behind, even if they are phosphorylated at the elongation-competent Ser2

exon 18 from the neuronal cell adhesion molecule (NCAM) mRNA and that this correlates with increased acetylation of lysine 9 of Histone H3 (H3K9ac) between exons 17 and 19, with no parallel increase at the promoter region [90]. Another histone mark associated with transcription elongation, [54, 55] H3 lysine 36 tri-methylation (H3K36me3) was also found to increase in distal regions of the *ncam* gene upon depolarization. This is consistent with an increase in RNA pol II pocessivity observed at the area affected by the acetylation changes which explains the decreased recognition of the alternative exon [90].

In a different work [91], targeting transfected small interfering RNAs (siRNAs) to intronic regions downstream of the fibronectin alternative exon E33, increased its inclusion into the mRNA due to local facultative heterochromatin formation, in a mechanism resembling transcriptional gene silencing [92–94]. Moreover, this effect was abolished by treating cells with drugs that favors chromatin relaxation: TSA and the DNA methyltransferase inhibitor 5-azadeoxycytidine, implying a causal relationship between the local repressive chromatin structure and the splicing outcome. In light of these observations, then, it would not be surprising to find out that endogenous noncoding RNAs have a relevant role in alternative splicing regulation through epigenetic modulation.

Recently, genome-wide analysis of nucleosome positioning and histone marks distribution, has revealed striking patterns that can be understand, at least partially, from the perspective of pre-mRNA processing. In several metazoan organisms, nucleosomes were found to be preferentially positioned on exons, strongly suggesting a role of nucleosome occupancy in exon definition [95, 96]. Accordingly, pseudoexons (nonincluded intronic sequences flanked by strong splice sites) were depleted of nucleosomes, whereas exons flanked by weaker splice sites showed more nucleosome enrichment than those with strong splice sites [96] and included alternative exons were more highly enriched in nucleosomes than excluded ones [95], suggesting a role in alternative splicing regulation as well. Consistently with the kinetic model of coupling, pol II levels were shown to be increased along exons, suggesting that positioned nucleosomes might slow its elongation rate, favoring exon definition [95]. Regarding histone marks, genome-wide analysis revealed a nonrandom distribution as several modifications are enriched in exons but not in introns [95, 96]. The H3K36me3 mark, for instance, was enriched along exons of active genes, [95–97] although this pattern partially reflects underlying nucleosome occupancy [96]. Interestingly, H3K36me3 signal was reduced on alternative exons in comparison with constitutive ones [97]. Altogether, this compelling evidence suggests a role of nucleosome positioning, chromatin structure, and histone modifications in alternative splicing regulation. This influence can be achieved through pol II elongation rate modulation or, alternatively, by recruitment of splicing factors through direct or indirect recognition of the different chromatin marks [52, 53].

8 Concluding Remarks

The combinatorial model once proposed to explain alternative splicing regulation was initially thought to deal with post-transcriptional processing. During this chapter, we wanted to introduce new insights into the complexity of this model when considering transcription-coupled alternative splicing. Although the resulting model is far from being simple, there is little doubt in that it represents a much more realistic picture of the process.

The first issue that must be taken into account is that different splicing events will differ in their degree of co-transcriptionality, and that a specific splicing event can be processed at different relative times depending on the transcriptional status. This degree of co-transcriptionality would affect splicing choices *per se* (according to the elongation model) and would also modulate the effect of *trans*-acting factors (especially those that interact with the transcription machinery) and secondary structures on alternative splicing.

This complex picture can be seen as an epi-phenomenon of the necessity to couple transcription and splicing (an advantageous situation itself as it would facilitate a more efficient processing of the pre-mRNA). However, it is also an opportunity for a multi-step subtle regulation of the alternative splicing process, a physiologically relevant issue when considering different splicing patterns in different tissues or in response to external signals. For example, it is known that the epigenetic status of particular sequences is altered during tissue differentiation, resulting in specific template and transcription patterns for each cell type. It is expected that these transcriptional differences would impact on alternative splicing choices. In addition, cell signaling can induce changes in transcriptional status of specific genes and localized remodeling of chromatin and epigenetic marks, further affecting alternative splicing.

We also should reconsider previous reports of altered genes or gene expression in some cancer types in light of the generalization of transcription/splicing coupling. One example could be the fusion protein originated in human myeloid leukemia between TLS and ERG proteins. Whereas both normal and fused TLS can interact with RNA pol II, only TLS recruits splicing regulators such as TASR1, also known as SRSF10 (formerly SRp38). This makes TLS/ERG fusion protein act as an inhibitor of TASR-mediated splicing [98].

At this point, it should be noticed that there are plenty of levels where the coupling between transcription and alternative splicing is probably altered in cancer cells, resulting in abnormal expression patterns. The ongoing effort of scientists to put all the regulatory processes together will test and clarify this possibility and define its role in the disease.

Acknowledgments We thank the members of our lab and Anabella Srebrow for criticisms and helpful discussions. This work was supported by grants from the Fundación Antorchas, the Agencia Nacional de Promoción de Ciencia y Tecnología of Argentina, the European Union Network of Excellence on Alternative Splicing (EURASNET), and the University of Buenos Aires. I.E.S. and L.G.A. are recipients of fellowships from the Consejo Nacional de Investigaciones Científicas y Técnicas of Argentina (CONICET). A.R.K. is a Howard Hughes Medical Institute international research scholar and a career investigator of the CONICET.

References

1. Srebrow A, Kornblihtt AR (2006) The connection between splicing and cancer. J Cell Sci 119(13):2635–2641
2. Muñoz MJ, Perez Santángelo MS, Paronetto MP, de la Mata M, Pelisch F, Boireau S, Glover-Cutter K, Ben-Dov C, Blaustein M, Lozano JJ, Bird G, Bentley D, Bertrand E, Kornblihtt AR (2009) DNA damage regulates alternative splicing through inhibition of RNA Polymerase II elongation. Cell 137:708–720
3. Berget SM (1995) Exon recognition in vertebrate splicing. J Biol Chem 270(6):2411–2414
4. Wang ET, Sandberg R, Luo S, Khrebtukova I, Zhang L, Mayr C, Kingsmore SF, Schroth GP, Burge CB (2008) Alternative isoform regulation in human tissue transcriptomes. Nature 456(27): 470–476
5. Pan Q, Shai o, Lee LJ, Frey BJ, Blencowe BJ (2008) Deep surveying of alternative splicing complexity in the human transcriptome by high throughput sequencing. Nat Genet 40(12):1413–1415
6. Ermakova EO, Nurtdinov RN, Gelfand MS (2006) Fast rate of evolution in alternative spliced coding regions of mammalian genes. BMC Genomics 7:84–93
7. Smith CW, Valcárcel J (2000) Alternative pre-mRNA splicing: the logic of combinatorial control. Trends Biochem Sci 25(8):381–388
8. Cáceres JF, Kornblihtt AR (2002) Alternative splicing: multiple control mechanisms and involvement in human disease. Trends Genet 18:186–193
9. Black DL (2003) Mechanisms of alternative pre-messenger RNA splicing. Annu Rev Biochem 72:291–336
10. Sharp PA (1994) Split genes and RNA splicing. Cell 77(6):805–815

11. Kornblihtt AR, Pesce CG, Alonso CR et al (1996) The fibronectin gene as a model for splicing and transcription studies. FASEB J 10(2):248–257
12. Fededa JP, Petrillo E, Gelfand MS et al (2005) A polar mechanism coordinates different regions of alternative splicing within a single gene. Mol Cell 19(3):393–404
13. Lenasi T, Peterlin BM, Dovc P (2006) Distal regulation of alternative splicing by splicing enhancer in equine beta-casein intron 1. RNA 12(3):498–507
14. Romano M, Marcucci R, Baralle FE (2001) Splicing of constitutive upstream introns is essential for the recognition of intra-exonic suboptimal splice sites in the thrombopoietin gene. Nucleic Acids Res 29(4):886–894
15. Bentley D (2002) The mRNA assembly line: transcription and processing machines in the same factory. Curr Opin Cell Biol 14(3):336–342
16. Bentley DL (2005) Rules of engagement: co-transcriptional recruitment of pre-mRNA processing factors. Curr Opin Cell Biol 17(3):251–256
17. Maniatis T, Reed R (2002) An extensive network of coupling among gene expression machines. Nature 416(6880):499–506
18. Kornblihtt AR (2005) Promoter usage and alternative splicing. Curr Opin Cell Biol 17(3):262–268
19. Zorio DA, Bentley DL (2004) The link between mRNA processing and transcription: communication works both ways. Exp Cell Res 296(1):91–97
20. Neugebauer KM (2002) On the importance of being co-transcriptional. J Cell Sci 115(Pt 20):3865–3871
21. Proudfoot NJ, Furger A, Dye MJ (2002) Integrating mRNA processing with transcription. Cell 108(4):501–512
22. Beyer AL, Osheim YN (1988) Splice site selection, rate of splicing, and alternative splicing on nascent transcripts. Genes Dev 2(6):754–765
23. Tennyson CN, Klamut HJ, Worton RG (1995) The human dystrophin gene requires 16 hours to be transcribed and is cotranscriptionally spliced. Nat Genet 9(2):184–190
24. Pandya-Jones A, Black DL (2009) Co-transcriptional splicing of constitutive and alternative exons. RNA 15:1896–1908
25. Bauren G, Wieslander L (1994) Splicing of Balbiani ring 1 gene pre-mRNA occurs simultaneously with transcription. Cell 76(1):183–192
26. de la Mata M, Lafaille C, Kornblihtt AR (2010) First come, first served revisited: Factors affecting the same alternative splicing events have different effects on the relative rates of intron removal. RNA 16:904–912
27. Lazarev D, Manley JL (2007) Concurrent splicing and transcription are not sufficient to enhance splicing efficiency. RNA 13:1546–1557
28. Perales R, Bentley D (2009) "Cotranscriptionality": the transcription elongation complex as a Nexus for nuclear transactions. Mol Cell 36:178–191
29. Alexander RD, Innocente SA, Barrass JD, Beggs JD (2010) Splicing-dependent RNA Polymerase pausing in yeast. Mol Cell 40:582–593
30. Lin S, Coutinho-Mansfield G, Wang D, Pandit S, Fu XD (2008) The splicing factor SC35 has an active role in transcriptional elongation. Nat Struct Mol Biol 15(8):819–826
31. Carrillo Oesterreich F, Preibisch S, Neugebauer KM (2010) Global analysis of nascent RNA reveals transcriptional pausing in terminal exons. Mol Cell 40:571–581
32. Smale ST, Tjian R (1985) Transcription of herpes simplex virus tk sequences under the control of wild-type and mutant human RNA polymerase I promoters. Mol Cell Biol 5(2):352–362
33. Sisodia SS, Sollner-Webb B, Cleveland DW (1987) Specificity of RNA maturation pathways: RNAs transcribed by RNA polymerase III are not substrates for splicing or polyadenylation. Mol Cell Biol 7(10):3602–3612
34. McCracken S, Rosonina E, Fong N et al (1998) Role of RNA polymerase II carboxy-terminal domain in coordinating transcription with RNA processing. Cold Spring Harb Symp Quant Biol 63:301–309

35. Dower K, Rosbash M (2002) T7 RNA polymerase-directed transcripts are processed in yeast and link 3′ end formation to mRNA nuclear export. RNA 8(5):686–697
36. Hicks MJ, Yang CR, Kotlajich MV, Hertel KJ (2006) Linking splicing to Pol II transcription stabilizes pre-mRNAs and influences splicing patterns. PLoS Biol 4(6):e147
37. Das R, Dufu K, Romney B, Feldt M, Elenko M, Reed R (2006) Functional coupling of RNAP II transcription to spliceosome assembly. Genes Dev 20(9):1100–1109
38. Das R, Yu J, Zhang Z, Gygi MP, Krainer AR, Gygi SP, Reed R (2007) SR proteins function in coupling RNAP II trancription to pre-mRNA splicing. Mol Cell 26:867–881
39. Misteli T, Spector DL (1999) RNA polymerase II targets pre-mRNA splicing factors to transcription sites in vivo. Mol Cell 3(6):697–705
40. McCracken S, Fong N, Yankulov K et al (1997) The C-terminal domain of RNA polymerase II couples mRNA processing to transcription. Nature 385(6614):357–361
41. Zeng C, Berget SM (2000) Participation of the C-terminal domain of RNA polymerase II in exon definition during pre-mRNA splicing. Mol Cell Biol 20(21):8290–8301
42. Hirose Y, Tacke R, Manley JL (1999) Phosphorylated RNA polymerase II stimulates pre-mRNA splicing. Genes Dev 13(10):1234–1239
43. Dye MJ, Gromak N, Proudfoot NJ (2006) Exon tethering in transcription by RNA polymerase II. Mol Cell 21(6):849–859
44. Sims RJ 3rd, Belotserkovskaya R, Reinberg D (2004) Elongation by RNA polymerase II: the short and long of it. Genes Dev 18(20):2437–2468
45. Saunders A, Core LJ, Lis JT (2006) Breaking barriers to transcription elongation. Nat Rev Mol Cell Biol 7(8):557–567
46. Muñoz MJ, de la Mata M, Kornblihtt AR (2010) The carboxy terminal domain of RNA polymerase II and alternative splicing. Trends Biochem Sci 35:497–504
47. Xu YX, Hirose Y, Zhou XZ, Lu KP, Manley JL (2003) Pin1 modulates the structure and function of human RNA polymerase II. Genes Dev 17(22):2765–2776
48. Bird G, Zorio DA, Bentley DL (2004) RNA Polymerase II Carboxy-Terminal domain phosphorylation is required for Cotranscriptional Pre-mRNA Splicing and 3′-End formation. Mol Cell Biol 24(20):8963–8969
49. de la Mata M, Kornblihtt AR (2006) Pol II CTD mediates SRp20 regulation of alternative splicing. Nat Struct Mol Biol 13(11):973–980
50. Laurencikiene J, Kallman AM, Fong N, Bentley DL, Ohman M (2006) RNA editing and alternative splicing: the importance of co-transcriptional coordination. EMBO Rep 7(3): 303–307
51. Rosonina E, Blencowe BJ (2004) Analysis of the requirement for RNA polymerase II CTD heptapeptide repeats in pre-mRNA splicing and 3′-end cleavage. RNA 10(4):581–589
52. Sims RJ III, Millhouse S, Chen CF, Lewis BA, Erdjument-Bromage H, Tempst P, Manley JL, Reinberg D (2007) Recognition of Trimethylated Histone H3 Lysine 4 facilitates the recruitment of transcription postinitiation factors and Pre-mRNA splicing. Mol Cell 28:665–676
53. Luco RF, Pan Q, Tominaga K, Blencowe BJ, Pereira-Smith OM, Misteli T (2010) Regulation of alternative splicing by histone modifications. Science 327:996–1000
54. Edmunds JW, Mahadevan LC, Clayton AL (2008) Dynamic histone H3 methylation during gene induction: HYPB/Setd2 mediates all H3K36 trimethylation. EMBO J 27:406–420
55. Krogan NJ, Kim M, Tong A, Golshani A, Cagney G, Canadien V, Richards DP, Beattie BK, Emili A, Boone C, Shilatifard A, Buratowski S, Greenblatt J (2003) Methylation of Histone H3 by Set2 in *Saccharomyces cerevisiae* Is Linked to Transcriptional Elongation by RNA Polymerase II. Mol Cell Biol 23(12):4207–4218
56. Cramer P, Pesce CG, Baralle FE, Kornblihtt AR (1997) Functional association between promoter structure and transcript alternative splicing. Proc Natl Acad Sci U S A 94(21):11456–11460

57. Cramer P, Caceres JF, Cazalla D et al (1999) Coupling of transcription with alternative splicing: RNA pol II promoters modulate SF2/ASF and 9G8 effects on an exonic splicing enhancer. Mol Cell 4(2):251–258
58. Auboeuf D, Honig A, Berget SM, O'Malley BW (2002) Coordinate regulation of transcription and splicing by steroid receptor coregulators. Science 298(5592):416–419
59. Pagani F, Stuani C, Zuccato E, Kornblihtt AR, Baralle FE (2003) Promoter architecture modulates CFTR exon 9 skipping. J Biol Chem 278(3):1511–1517
60. Robson-Dixon ND, Garcia-Blanco MA (2004) MAZ elements alter transcription elongation and silencing of the fibroblast growth factor receptor 2 exon IIIb. J Biol Chem 279(28):29075–29084
61. Nogues G, Kadener S, Cramer P, Bentley D, Kornblihtt AR (2002) Transcriptional activators differ in their abilities to control alternative splicing. J Biol Chem 277(45):43110–43114
62. Rosonina E, Bakowski MA, McCracken S, Blencowe BJ (2003) Transcriptional activators control splicing and 3′-end cleavage levels. J Biol Chem 278(44):43034–43040
63. Auboeuf D, Dowhan DH, Kang YK et al (2004) Differential recruitment of nuclear receptor coactivators may determine alternative RNA splice site choice in target genes. Proc Natl Acad Sci U S A 101(8):2270–2274
64. Auboeuf D, Dowhan DH, Li X et al (2004) CoAA, a nuclear receptor coactivator protein at the interface of transcriptional coactivation and RNA splicing. Mol Cell Biol 24(1):442–453
65. Kotovic KM, Lockshon D, Boric L, Neugebauer KM (2003) Cotranscriptional recruitment of the U1 snRNP to intron-containing genes in yeast. Mol Cell Biol 23(16):5768–5779
66. Lacadie SA, Rosbash M (2005) Cotranscriptional spliceosome assembly dynamics and the role of U1 snRNA:5′ss base pairing in yeast. Mol Cell 19(1):65–75
67. Gornemann J, Kotovic KM, Hujer K, Neugebauer KM (2005) Cotranscriptional spliceosome assembly occurs in a stepwise fashion and requires the cap binding complex. Mol Cell 19(1):53–63
68. Listerman I, Sapra AK, Neugebauer KM (2006) Cotranscriptional coupling of splicing factor recruitment and precursor messenger RNA splicing in mammalian cells. Nat Struct Mol Biol 13(9):815–822
69. Lai MC, Teh BH, Tarn WY (1999) A human papillomavirus E2 transcriptional activator. The interactions with cellular splicing factors and potential function in pre-mRNA processing. J Biol Chem 274(17):11832–11841
70. Monsalve M, Wu Z, Adelmant G, Puigserver P, Fan M, Spiegelman BM (2000) Direct coupling of transcription and mRNA processing through the thermogenic coactivator PGC-1. Mol Cell 6(2):307–316
71. Guillouf C, Gallais I, Moreau-Gachelin F (2006) Spi-1/PU.1 oncoprotein affects splicing decisions in a promoter binding-dependent manner. J Biol Chem 281(28):19145–19155
72. Davies RC, Calvio C, Bratt E, Larsson SH, Lamond AI, Hastie ND (1998) WT1 interacts with the splicing factor U2AF65 in an isoform-dependent manner and can be incorporated into spliceosomes. Genes Dev 12(20):3217–3225
73. Nayler O, Stratling W, Bourquin JP et al (1998) SAF-B protein couples transcription and pre-mRNA splicing to SAR/MAR elements. Nucleic Acids Res 26(15):3542–3549
74. Goldstrohm AC, Albrecht TR, Sune C, Bedford MT, Garcia-Blanco MA (2001) The transcription elongation factor CA150 interacts with RNA polymerase II and the pre-mRNA splicing factor SF1. Mol Cell Biol 21(22):7617–7628
75. Lin KT, Lu RM, Tarn WY (2004) The WW domain-containing proteins interact with the early spliceosome and participate in pre-mRNA splicing in vivo. Mol Cell Biol 24(20): 9176–9185
76. Yuryev A, Patturajan M, Litingtung Y et al (1996) The C-terminal domain of the largest subunit of RNA polymerase II interacts with a novel set of serine/arginine-rich proteins. Proc Natl Acad Sci U S A 93(14):6975–6980

77. Young JI, Hong EP, Castle JC et al (2005) Regulation of RNA splicing by the methylation-dependent transcriptional repressor methyl-CpG binding protein 2. Proc Natl Acad Sci U S A. 102(49):17551–17558
78. Millhouse S, Manley JL (2005) The C-terminal domain of RNA polymerase II functions as a phosphorylation-dependent splicing activator in a heterologous protein. Mol Cell Biol 25(2):533–544
79. Sato S, Tomomori-Sato C, Parmely TJ et al (2004) A set of consensus mammalian mediator subunits identified by multidimensional protein identification technology. Mol Cell 14(5):685–691
80. Eperon LP, Graham IR, Griffiths AD, Eperon IC (1988) Effects of RNA secondary structure on alternative splicing of pre-mRNA: is folding limited to a region behind the transcribing RNA polymerase? Cell 54(3):393–401
81. Roberts GC, Gooding C, Mak HY, Proudfoot NJ, Smith CW (1998) Co-transcriptional commitment to alternative splice site selection. Nucleic Acids Res 26(24):5568–5572
82. Kadener S, Cramer P, Nogues G et al (2001) Antagonistic effects of T-Ag and VP16 reveal a role for RNA pol II elongation on alternative splicing. EMBO J 20(20):5759–5768
83. Kadener S, Fededa JP, Rosbash M, Kornblihtt AR (2002) Regulation of alternative splicing by a transcriptional enhancer through RNA pol II elongation. Proc Natl Acad Sci U S A 99(12):8185–8190
84. Nogues G, Munoz MJ, Kornblihtt AR (2003) Influence of polymerase II processivity on alternative splicing depends on splice site strength. J Biol Chem 278(52):52166–52171
85. de la Mata M, Alonso CR, Kadener S et al (2003) A slow RNA polymerase II affects alternative splicing in vivo. Mol Cell 12(2):525–532
86. Howe KJ, Kane CM, Ares M Jr (2003) Perturbation of transcription elongation influences the fidelity of internal exon inclusion in Saccharomyces cerevisiae. RNA 9(8):993–1006
87. Lorincz MC, Dickerson DR, Schmitt M, Groudine M (2004) Intragenic DNA methylation alters chromatin structure and elongation efficiency in mammalian cells. Nat Struct Mol Biol 11(11):1068–1075
88. Batsche E, Yaniv M, Muchardt C (2006) The human SWI/SNF subunit Brm is a regulator of alternative splicing. Nat Struct Mol Biol 13(1):22–29
89. Kornblihtt AR (2006) Chromatin, transcript elongation and alternative splicing. Nat Struct Mol Biol 13(1):5–7
90. Schor IE, Rascovan N, Pelisch F, Alló M, Kornblihtt AR (2009) Neuronal cell depolarization induces intragenic chromatin modifications affecting NCAM alternative splicing. Proc Natl Acad Sci USA 106(11):4325–4330
91. Alló M, Buggiano V, Fededa JP, Petrillo E, Schor I, de la Mata M, Agirre E, Plass M, Eyras E, Elela SA, Klinck R, Chabot B, Kornblihtt AR (2009) Control of alternative splicing through siRNA-mediated transcriptional gene silencing. Nat Struct Mol Biol 16(7):717–724
92. Suzuki K, Juelich T, Lim H, Ishida T, Watanebe T, Cooper DA, Rao S, Kelleher AD (2008) Closed Chromatin architecture Is induced by an RNA Duplex targeting the HIV-1 promoter region. J Biol Chem 283:23353–23363
93. Kim DH, Villeneuve LM, Morris KV, Rossi JJ (2006) Argonaute-1 directs siRNA-mediated transcriptional gene silencing in human cells. Nat Struct Mol Biol 13:793–797
94. Morris KV, Chan SW, Jacobsen SE, Looney DJ (2004) Small interfering RNA-induced transcriptional gene silencing in human cells. Science 305:1289–1292
95. Schwartz S, Meshorer E, Ast G (2009) Chromatin organization marks exon-intron structure. Nat Struct Mol Biol 16(9):990–995
96. Tilgner H, Nikolaou C, Althammer S, Sammeth M, Beato M, Valcárcel J, Guigó R (2009) Nucleosome positioning as a determinant of exon recognition. Nat Struct Mol Biol 16(9):996–1001
97. Kolosinska-Zwierz P, Down T, Latorre I, Liu T, Liu XS, Ahringer J (2009) Differential chromatin marking of introns and expressed exons by H3K36me3. Nat Genet 41(3):376–381
98. Yang L, Embree LJ, Hickstein DD (2000) TLS-ERG leukemia fusion protein inhibits RNA splicing mediated by serine-arginine proteins. Mol Cell Biol 20(10):3345–3354

Detection of Alternatively Spliced or Processed RNAs in Cancer Using Oligonucleotide Microarray

Marieta Gencheva, Lixin Yang, Gong-Biao Lin and Ren-Jang Lin

Abstract

Deregulation of gene expression plays a pivotal role in tumorigenesis, so the ability to detect RNA alterations is of great value in cancer diagnosis and management. DNA microarrays have been used to measure changes in mRNA or microRNA level, but less often the change of RNA isoforms. Here we appraise the utilization of microarray in detecting alternatively processed RNAs, which have alternative splice forms, retained introns, or altered 3′ untranslated regions. We cover the methodology and focus on cancer studies. Recent development in parallel or deep sequencing used in transcriptome analysis is also discussed.

Keywords

Alternative splicing · Splice variants · Intron retention · Alternative 3′ processing · Splicing-sensitive microarray · Genomic tiling microarray · Parallel or deep sequencing

Contents

M. Gencheva · L. Yang · G.-B. Lin · R.-J. Lin (✉)
Department of Molecular Biology, Beckman Research Institute of the City of Hope, 1500 East Duarte Road, Duarte CA 91010-3000, USA
e-mail: rlin@coh.org

J. Y. Wu (ed.), *RNA and Cancer*, Cancer Treatment and Research,
DOI: 10.1007/978-3-642-31659-3_2,

1 Introduction

Cancer is a genetic disease and it is the expression of genetic information, dictated by intrinsic genetic content and by extrinsic influences, that ultimately determines the disease status. Thus, knowing the entire gene activities of cancer cells would have tremendous value to cancer diagnosis and treatment. Gene expression changes are a key feature of cancer development. The changes can be at the level of expression, but they can also be in the forms of RNA due to alternative RNA processing. In this chapter, we illustrate the detection of form changes in RNA due to alternative splicing or 3′ end processing. We include studies that use genomic tiling array to detect unspliced or partially spliced RNA. We also describe parallel or deep sequencing techniques that are recently used to analyze gene expression, and compare them with the microarray approaches.

2 Detection of Alternatively Spliced RNA

2.1 Exon-Junction Microarray

Exon junction microarray is composed of DNA oligos that span the exon–exon junction of a splicing event. Only correctly spliced RNA will stably hybridize to the junction oligo, and thus allowing detection of that splicing event. Exon junction microarray is the first type of array specifically designed to detect alternatively spliced RNA isoforms. The first reported design is used to detect splice events in *S. cerevisiae* and comprises three oligos per gene: one exon probe, one intron probe, and one splice junction probe [1].

To detect exon skipping events in human cells, Shoemaker and colleagues use an array that contains exon junction probes targeting all splice junctions in ~10,000 multi-exon genes [2]. This microarray is used to profile 52 human tissues; they discover evidence of exon skipping in 74 % of those human multi-exon genes, and they also detect a number of previously unidentified splice isoforms. Subsequent microarray designs include exon-body probes, together with exon-junction probes [3–5]. These improved microarrays permit better measurements of RNA isoform quantities. For example, to detect a cassette exon, a probe set typically consists of exon-body probes to detect the alternative exon and the two flanking exons, as well as probes that monitor each of the three splice junctions. Quantification in the exon-junction arrays depends on the optimal oligo design and probe length, as well as on the data analysis algorithms [4–6]. The design of the junction probe is particularly challenging, since flexibility in choosing the oligo sequences is restricted.

Exon junction microarray is used to determine alternative splicing changes in cell lines derived from Hodgkin lymphoma tumors at different disease stages [7]. Selected genes involved in apoptosis, cell signaling, proliferation, and regulation of splicing are included in the array. Constitutive exons, alternative exons, and splice junctions are monitored by oligonucleotide pairs, one has perfect match and the other contains a single mismatch. Unsupervised clustering of the array data illustrates a clear separation of Hodgkin cell lines and a normal B cell line, with about 20–30 % of the splicing events showing a change in splice isoforms.

In collaboration with the Ares group, we employ exon-junction microarrays to detect alternative splicing changes in two breast cancer cell lines, MCF7 and MDA-MB-231 [8]. We elect to study 64 genes whose alternative splicing is well documented or linked to cancer. For a cassette exon, each alternative splicing event is monitored by oligonucleotide probes, three targeting the splice junctions and three exon-body probes targeting the alternative exon and the two adjacent constitutive exons. For each cassette exon, a skipping index and an inclusion index are calculated, based on the ratio of the signal from junction probes and the signal from constitutive exon probes. A cutoff of 1.5-fold change in the skipping or inclusion indexes is used to detect alternative splicing events. We first compare the two breast cancer cell lines to human mammary epithelial cells (HMEC) and detect a change in splicing pattern in the cancer cell lines for a number of genes, including *hnRNPA/B*, *RBM9*, *FAS*, and *MYL6*. We also identify differentially spliced isoforms between MCF7 and MDA-MB-231 cell lines for *HRMT1L1*, *APLP2*, *CD44*, *VEGF*, *ESR1*, and *EEF1D*. Our microarray study also shows that alternative splicing in tumor xenograft is more closely related to splicing in three dimensional Matrigel cultures than to splicing in two dimensional flat dish cultures.

The use and design improvement of exon junction microarray for detecting alternative splicing have since been described recently including lung cancer studies [9], analysis of the human transcriptome [10], and ABC transporter splicing in drug development [11].

2.2 Ligation-PCR Followed by Microarray Detection

A different method to detect alternatively spliced transcripts is to take advantage of accurate and specific ligation of oligonucleotides hybridizing at the splice junction [12]. The RASL assay (RNA-mediated annealing, selection, and ligation) does not involve prior RNA purification or cDNA synthesis, but is based on detecting a RNA splice junction by annealing to it in solution two oligos complementary to the two respective exonic sequences which create the junction. The correctly annealed oligos are then ligated and become templates for PCR, which are amplified using universal primers, labeled by either biotin or a dye. The products of the RASL reaction are then hybridized to a fiber optic bead array. This approach has great specificity of detecting a defined set of transcripts by virtually eliminating the problems of cross-hybridization. The method is also more sensitive compared to exon or splice junction arrays that rely on direct hybridization, especially when monitoring small differences between different samples. RASL can detect a well-expressed RNA transcript isolated from less than ten cells, as well as to specifically amplify a transcript from a highly complex RNA mixture.

The RASL method is further improved by first converting mRNA to cDNA in a method called DASL (cDNA-mediated annealing, selection, extension and ligation) [13]. The oligo-annealing and ligation steps are also modified to include a locus-specific oligonucleotide extension. Rather than ligating two oligos at the splice junction as in the case of RASL, this approach permits a gap of 1–20 nt between them, thus providing flexibility for choosing optimal sequences for the oligos and resulted in increasing specificity. The assay is automated and used to detect considerably degraded mRNAs from formalin-fixed and paraffin-embedded tumor samples [14]. The assay is used to profile both transcript abundance and alternatively spliced isoforms in prostate cancer tissues and cell lines [15]. The study identifies a panel of 104 RNA isoforms, the majority of which displays differential expression between normal and tumor prostate tissue and thus can be used as biomarkers. In addition, many alternatively spliced genes linked to prostate tumors are revealed, and differential splicing in *MAPT*, *CACNA1D*, and *AMACR* is validated by RT-PCR. The DASL assay is commercialized by Illumina, which assembles a DASL panel of 502 genes linked to cancer for monitoring gene expression and alternative splicing [16]. The company also supports custom probe panel creation and can profile up to 1,536 targets.

2.3 Exon Microarray

2.3.1 Design and Analysis of Exon Microarray

Since alternatively spliced RNAs have different combinations of exons, one could use quantity changes of individual exons as indicators of alternative splicing. Exon microarrays to detect individual exons in humans and other organisms have been produced. For example, the Affymetrix human exon array contains 5.3 million features (oligo probes) grouped into 1.4 million probe sets. One probe set is typically designed to detect one exon, although some exons have more than one probe set. The array can detect approximately 1.1 million exons or exon clusters, which can be grouped into more than 300,000 different RNAs or transcript clusters. Apart from targeting exons of well known genes, the array also includes probes that map to exons and transcripts supported only by EST or gene prediction algorithms; about half of the probes on the array are based on ESTs or GENESCAN only and offering an opportunity to discover unannotated exons or novel transcripts. The probes are grouped together according to supporting evidence and the user can choose to look at the signal from only well-annotated exons (core exons, supported by RefSeq and full length GenBank mRNAs), the extended set (ESTs, syntenic rat and mouse mRNAs), or the full set of probes (gene predictions). Exons of less than 25 bases are not represented on the array due to hybridization requirements, so some short exons as well as some alternative 5 or 3′ splice sites are not interrogated by this array.

The exon array can also be used to derive gene level expression data, which is important when analyzing alternative splicing. Since there are no mismatch probes for background estimation, the exon array has to use a different algorithm to estimate nonspecific hybridization by using genomic or antigenomic background probes with defined GC content. Several groups have actually used the human exon array to obtain reliable gene expression data comparable to those from conventional gene arrays [17–20]. Gene expression estimates from the exon array are further improved by selecting only probes with a reliable signal, while removing probes that perform poorly or cross-hybridize to more than one target in the genome [21, 22].

2.3.2 Alternative Splicing in Cancer Detected by Exon Microarray

The exon array has been used to assess alternative splicing in cancer. A study to compare colon tumors with normal tissues has been reported [17]. The authors filter the data both at exon level and at gene level to eliminate outliers and retain exons/transcripts with signal above background. Then they calculate a Splicing Index (SI), which represents the log ratio of exon signals between normal tissue and tumors after normalization to the gene signal. The SI index is used in the MIDAS algorithm (ExACT program, http://www.affymetrix.com/products/software/specific/exact.affx) to test the hypothesis that no alternative splicing occurs for a given exon. This approach identifies a list of potentially differentially spliced genes between normal and tumor colon tissues. Among the 43 genes identified, 9 (*ACTN1*, *VCL*, *CALD1*, *CTTN*, *TPM1*, *FN1*, *COL6A3*, *SLC3A2*, and *ITGB4*) are validated by RT-PCR. Five of these genes, *ACTN1*, *VCL*, *CALD1*, *CTTN*, and *TPM1*, code for proteins linked to cytoskeleton organization. *FN1* and *COL6A3* are important for the extracellular matrix and *SLC3A2* has a function in integrin signaling. For some of these genes, cancer-specific alternative splice variants have been previously identified. For example *TPM1*, *ACTN1*, and *ITGB4* show similar splicing pattern in colon tumors [23] and *ITGB4* and *TPM1* are identified as differentially spliced in several tumors by computational analysis [24].

A more recent study uses human exon arrays to identify differences in alternative splicing in colon, bladder, and prostate cancer and reports seven genes as differentially spliced: *ACTN1*, *CALD1*, *COLA3*, *LRRFIP2*, *PIK4CB*, *TPM1*, and *VCL* [25]. The validation rate in this study was 67 % (7 out of 15 candidates confirmed by RT-PCR) and the identified genes match the previous studies, including the prevalence of genes involved in the cytoskeletal organization.

Cancer-specific alternative splice forms are identified using exon arrays in tumors of the nervous system. One study [26] reports that *ATP2B4*, *CaMKII*, *NLGN4Y*, *UNC84A*, *BIN1*, *MPZL1*, and *NRCAM* are differentially spliced in glial brain tumors. Glioblastoma samples are used in another study that discovers 14 glioma-specific alternative splicing changes, seven of them novel: *A2BP1*, *BCAS1*, *CACNA1G*, *CLTA*, *KCNC2*, *SNCB*, and *TPD52L2* [27].

The use of exon microarray in detecting alternative splicing has grown in the past few years [28], including studies of breast cancer [29] and method refinements [30].

2.3.3 Improvement in Data Analysis for Alternative Splicing Discovery

The studies based on the Affymetrix exon array analysis tools achieve a relatively low validation rate for detection of differentially spliced exons. Substantial improvements of alternative splicing detection are achieved by two groups using different type of array analysis. One develops a regression-based algorithm for analyzing the array data (REAP), and achieves a validation rate of 60 % for randomly chosen differential splicing events [31]. The other method, MADS (microarray analysis of differential splicing), attempts to remove the major sources of false positives in detecting alternative splicing [32]. The authors incorporate in the analysis algorithm background correction of probes intensities, iterative probe selection for gene expression index calculation, and a procedure to remove sequence-specific cross-hybridization. The method leads to a detection of 25 % more true positive differentially expressed exons compared to Affymetrix's ExACT algorithm, with a validation rate of 90 %. The study also compares the sensitivity of the Affymetrix Exon 1.0 array to a custom spotted oligonucleotide array with splice junction probes [33], and concludes that the latter is more sensitive to small changes in alternative splicing.

3 Detection of Alternatively Processed RNA Using Genomic Tiling Microarray

3.1 The Design of Genomic Tiling Microarray

Genomic tiling arrays aim to interrogate transcripts from a whole genome, using regularly spaced oligonucleotide probes in an unbiased way except for repetitive sequences (reviewed in [34–36]). Three companies offer tiling arrays, with different resolution and hybridization protocols. The Affymetrix protocol uses biotin labeling and one-color assay, while Agilent and NimbleGen produce tiling arrays that use dual-color hybridization and longer oligo probes (60-mer for Agilent, and 50–75-mer for NimbleGen, both tiled at about 100-bp intervals). The Affymetrix tiling arrays are probably the most popular to date and offer the highest resolution. Its human tiling array consists of 25-mer probes with approximately a 10-bp gap between adjacent probes (Fig. 1a). The array has two variants. The GeneChip Human Tiling 1.0 R Array Set includes perfect match (PM) and mismatch (MM) probes in 14 arrays, each having over 6.5 million probes. The GeneChip Tiling 2.0R Array Set has seven arrays, for which the mismatch probes are omitted.

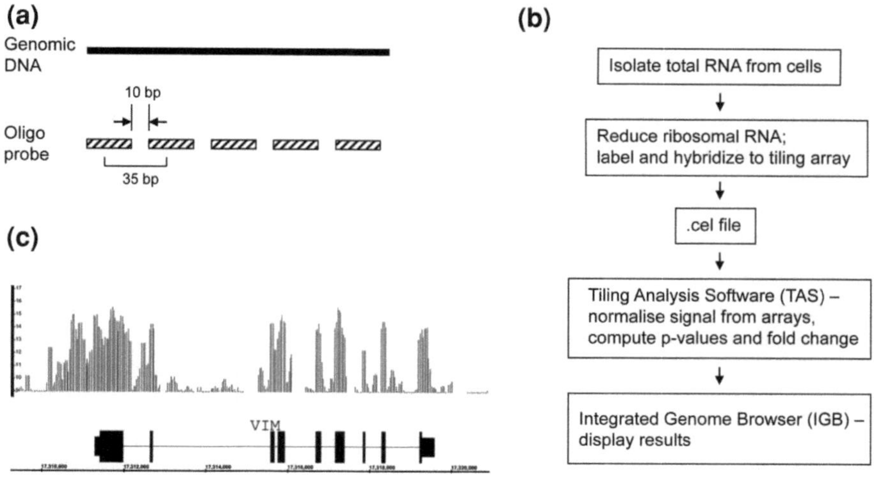

Fig. 1 Design and analysis of a genomic tiling array. (**a**) Probes of 25-mer on a genomic tiling array are spaced at 35 base pairs on the average, with a gap of about 10 bp between adjacent probes. (**b**) Flowchart for tiling array analysis. (**c**) Expression of *VIM* in HEK293 cells transfected with wild type DHX16 cDNA, detected by Affymetrix human tiling array. Exons are represented as boxes and introns as lines. The graph above the gene shows the normalized signal from individual oligo probes as vertical lines, on a log2 scale

Affymetrix has developed Tiling Analysis Software (TAS) for analyzing the arrays, which can perform quantile normalization of the array signal, sliding window analysis of the signal intensities, and subsequent region definition according to user-defined parameters for length and threshold (minimum run and maximum gap). Figure 1b illustrates the steps in a typical experiment involving Affymetrix tiling arrays, and Fig. 1C demonstrates the signal visualization for a single gene, vimentin (*VIM*), taken from an experiment performed in our group (see Sect. 3.3).

3.2 Tiling Microarray Used in the Transcriptome Mapping and the ENCODE Project

The tiling array is unique among the different microarray designs in the fact that it systematically interrogates transcription outside known or predicted genes. Initial experiments to assess transcription across human chromosomes 21 and 22 using tiling arrays are performed with 11 tumor tissues and fetal cell lines and reveal surprising complexity [37, 38]. About an order of magnitude more of the genomic sequence is detected as transcripts than what has been assumed on the basis of annotated and predicted exons. This finding is confirmed and extended by using a tiling array of 36-mer probes at a resolution of 46 base pairs on the average, covering the entire human genome [39]. The study detects numerous transcriptionally active regions (TARs) in addition to unannotated genes, antisense transcription, and previously undetected exons of known genes. A study using arrays with a high resolution of five base pairs further provides evidence of an extensive network of overlapping transcripts with almost half of all transcribed sequences not polyadenylated [40]. The massive unannotated transcription is not unique to human cells, since similar findings are documented in mouse [41], fly [42], and *Arabidopsis* [43].

Tiling arrays are also used in the ENCODE project [44] to assess transcription of ~1 % of the human genome. The ENCODE tiling array has ~750,000 25-mer PM and MM oligo probes, spaced at 21-bp intervals. The ENCODE study detects transcription fragments (TxFrags) from 14.7 % of the nucleotides represented on the arrays, with 63 % of the TxFrags residing in intronic or intergenic regions. By a combination of 5′RACE and tiling array hybridization, more than 60 % of the annotated protein-coding genes show evidence of new alternative exons in their introns, and 68 % exhibit a potential new transcription start site upstream of their first annotated exon [45]. The distal 5′ exons often overlap with adjacent genes, thus creating chimeric transcripts. Many of the novel exons are expressed in a tissue-specific manner, which underlines the importance of whole-genome transcriptome studies in disease models.

3.3 Detection of Unspliced or Partially Spliced RNA by Tiling Microarray

While alternative cassette exons and many 5 or 3′ alternative splice sites can be detected by exon or exon-junction arrays, unspliced or partially spliced transcripts are best followed by probes that cover the intron regions. The genomic tiling arrays thus provide an opportunity to systematically assess intron retention events arising from perturbation of the splicing machinery. Such types of splicing changes may be important for cancer, since miss-splicing is linked to cancer [46, 47]. While alternative splicing involving exon skipping is underrepresented in tumor cells than in normal cells, intron retention events are at a higher level [48].

Detection of introns by tiling arrays is reported by comparing wild-type *S. cerevisiae* and a mutant strain deficient in processing of excised introns [49]. The study confirms previously predicted introns and discovers new intron-containing genes. A recent study also uses tiling arrays to investigate the effect of nonsense-mediated decay and nuclear exosome on the intron content in *S. cerevisiae* [50]. The study shows that about a third of the yeast introns increase upon inactivation of the nonsense-mediated decay pathway, an effect which is not observed when analyzing yeast intron content by other types of microarrays. The sensitivity of the tiling array detection in this experiment is comparable to Northern blot data.

Our group has used the Affymetrix human tiling array to detect transcripts affected by a human DExH-box spliceosomal protein, DHX16 [51]. RNA samples from cells expressing wild type DHX16 and from cells expressing a dominant negative mutant were removed of ribosomal RNA, labeled, and hybridized to probes on the array. The data were analyzed using TAS to integrate neighboring oligo signals and to identify RNA fragments or intervals. In this analysis, we included only

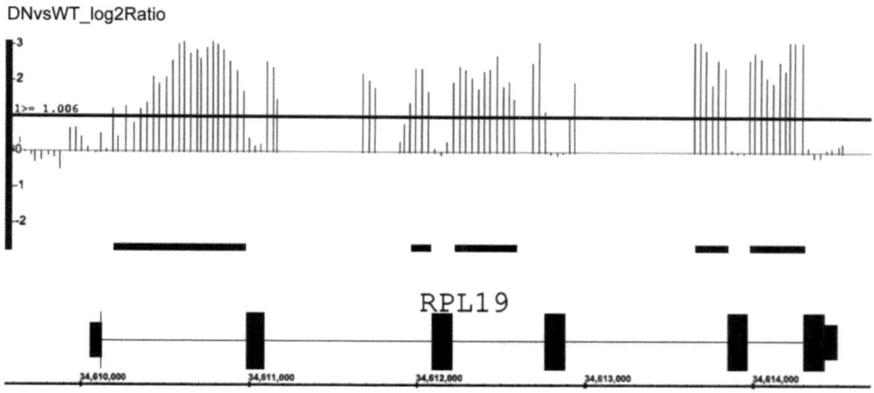

Fig. 2 Comparing RNA from mutant and wild type DHX16-expressing cells using genomic tiling microarray. HEK293 cells were transfected with a dominant negative DHX16 mutant cDNA (DN) or with a wild type DHX16 cDNA (WT). RNA was extracted and analyzed on tiling microarray. Shown here is the genomic region containing *RPL19* gene, which is transcribed from left to right. Log2 of the signal ratio between DN and WT are shown as vertical lines above the gene. Signals that are lower in DN have lines pointing downward. Intervals with a 2-fold increase are depicted with thick bars

intervals with a minimum length of 100 nucleotides, since an average human intron is longer than 4,000 nt and few introns are shorter than 100 nt [52]. We detected a number of genes showing clear evidence of intron retention in the transcripts. *RPL19* is an example of a gene whose transcripts retain introns in the mutant-expressing cells (Fig. 2). The array data indicate that many of those genes have elevated signal from the majority of their introns, a pattern which is possible to detect with the unbiased tiling array. Thus, genomic tiling microarray is effective in identifying gene transcripts that retain introns when splicing is impaired.

3.4 Detection of Alternatively Processed RNAs in Breast Cancer Using Tiling Array

We also used the aforementioned Affymetrix genomic tiling microarray to compare RNA samples from breast tumors and from normal tissues [53]. Breast tumors were biopsies from patients and normal breast tissues were taken from plastic surgery of normal individuals for cosmetic purpose. In this analysis, we included intervals with a minimum length of 50 bases, since the median of human exons is only 124 bases [54]. Intervals representing increase in breast tumors by more than 2-fold with a p value less than 0.01 were further analyzed.

Most of the up-regulated intervals were coincided with annotated mRNA exons. For example, *KPNA2* has 11 exons; five of the exons were identified as up-regulated intervals (Fig. 3a). The remaining six exons of *KPNA2* had probes showing significant increase in signals. KPNA2, karyopherin alpha2, is a potential prognostic marker in breast tumors and predicts poor survival in breast cancer patients [55, 56].

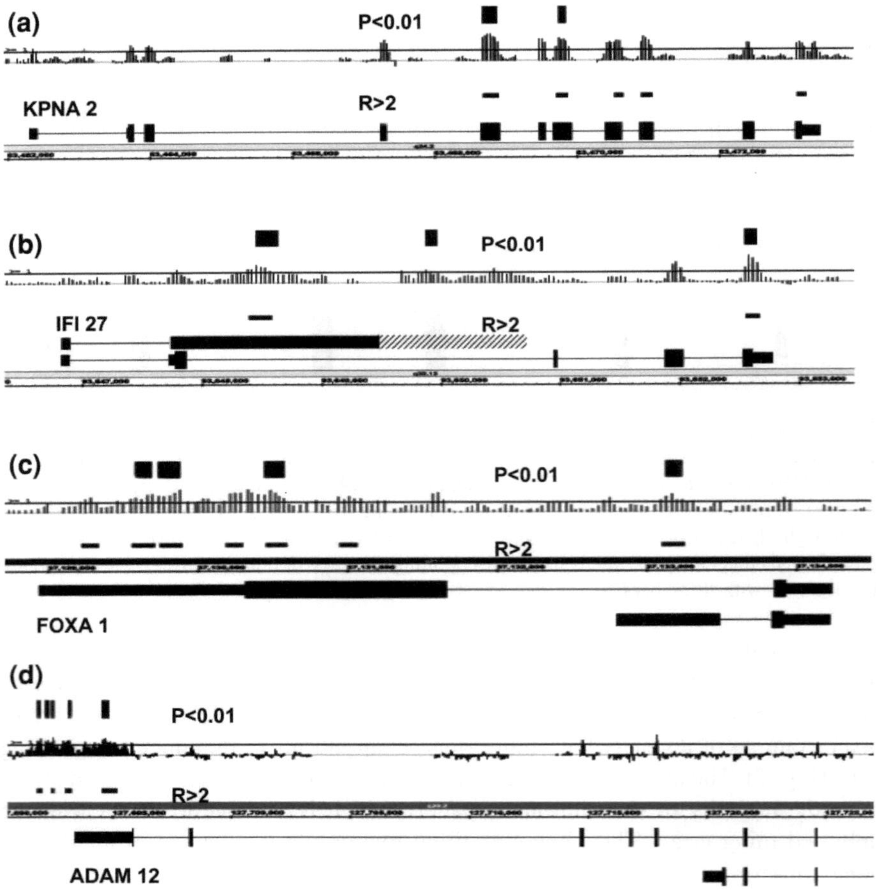

Fig. 3 Comparing the tiling microarray signals between breast tumors and the normal tissues. Four genes are depicted: (**a**) *KPNA2*, (**b**) *IFI27*, (**c**) *FOXA1*, and (**d**) *ADAM12*. The exons and introns are depicted as in Fig. 1; KPNA2 and IFI27 are transcribed from *left* to *right*, while the other two genes are *right* to *left*. The vertical lines above the gene represent log2 of the signal ratio between tumors and normal tissues, with a horizontal line representing 2-fold up-regulation. Intervals with a ratio greater than 2 ($R > 2$) are shown as bars below the ratio lines and intervals with a p value less than 0.01 ($p < 0.01$) are shown above the ratio lines

A few upregulated intervals fell into introns of known genes. For example, an intronic interval was found in intron 2 of the *IFI27* gene. Further analysis indicates that this intragenic interval is part of a novel transcript with a long exon 2 that ends within the intron 2 of the standard, longer transcript (Fig. 3b). Another interval was found in the intron of *FOXA1* gene, which is shown to be an alternative exon (Fig. 3c). IFI27, interferon alpha-inducible protein 27, is up-regulated in a number of epithelial cancers, although its association with breast cancer is less clear [57, 58]. FOXA1, forkhead-box A1, is expressed in breast cancer, although its value in prognostic prediction is still being investigated [59, 60].

Several intergenic intervals were found to locate near the 3′ end of a protein-coding gene. These RNA segments could represent a 3′ extension of the nearby gene or a complete separate transcript. For example, RefSeq database shows transcripts of the *ADAM12* gene having two different 3′ ends (Fig. 3d). The tiling array data indicated that the short form was not well expressed in breast tumor. Moreover, the intervals found 3′ to the *ADAM12* gene, upon further analysis, represent a transcript that is longer than the long form. ADAM12, a disintegrin and metalloprotease 12, is associated with several cancers including breast [61, 62], however, this "extra" long transcript has never been described.

Recently, genomic tiling microarray was used to detect aberrant processing of RNA transcripts at cryptic polyadenylation sites in introns when U1 snRNP was knockdown [63].

4 Transcriptome Analysis by Direct Sequencing

Whole genome direct sequencing of transcripts has emerged as a powerful alternative to microarray analysis [64–69]. It is based on a new generation of massive parallel sequencing technologies. Currently three deep sequencing platforms have gained popularity. The first platform was introduced by 454 Life Sciences (available trough Roche) and relies on pyrosequencing by synthesis. The 454 platform can read 200–400 bases from each molecule and can achieve 1 million reads per run. Illumina offers a bead-based sequencing by synthesis employing reversible fluorescent terminators. The technology was developed by Solexa and can achieve ~3 billion bases per run, with read length of 35–70 bases. A relatively new system is SOLiD (Applied Biosystems), based on massive, parallel sequential ligation technology. SOLiD can map 4–6 billion bases per run, with a read length of 50 bases. Although the length of the reads in all three cases is short compared to the Sanger sequencing, the new technologies provide very high accuracy and ultra-high throughput, making the sequencing of whole transcriptome fast and increasingly affordable.

Analysis of transcripts by sequencing has important advantages compared to microarrays. First, sequencing can discover new isoforms without prior knowledge of the exact sequence. Second, sequencing bypasses hybridization and thus eliminates problems associated with background and cross-hybridization, a major cause of signal variability in microarray analysis [70, 71]. Third, transcript detection achieved by deep sequencing and RNA-Seq protocol is shown to be quantitative with a linear range over five orders of magnitude [65, 66]. Furthermore, it is reported that about 40 million reads of ~25 bases are sufficient to accurately detect splice isoforms for transcripts with high- or moderate expression [65]. Detecting alternatively spliced RNAs, for nearly all of the multi-exon RefSeq human genes with an accuracy of detection comparable to quantitative PCR have also been reported [66].

Massive parallel sequencing has been used to detect cancer-specific transcripts in two comprehensive studies of pancreatic cancer and glioblastoma [72, 73]. In both studies, deep sequencing on an Illumina/Solexa platform is combined with SAGE to quantitate gene expression. This approach identifies 541 genes differentially expressed in prostate cancers compared to normal cells. On average, these genes have 88-fold higher expression in primary pancreatic tumors. In the case of glioblastoma, 143 genes are determined to be expressed at 10-times the level in normal brain. Many of these genes encoded proteins which are secreted or expressed on the cell surface, thus making them potential diagnostic markers or therapy targets.

5 Summary and Conclusion

In this chapter, we evaluate microarrays that are used to detect alternatively spliced or processed RNA. Ligation of junction-hybridizing oligos followed by PCR and array detection is most sensitive, although the number of splicing events it can simultaneously measure is somewhat limited. Exon junction microarray can measure splice variants with a potential to be genome-wide; however, its accuracy can be affected by the hybridization behaviors of the restricted exon junction probes. All-exon microarray has already reached genome-wide scale and is commercially available; however, there is still a need to develop an algorithm for analyzing most if not all alternatively splicing events reliably.

No microarray is specifically designed to discern RNA with intron retention or alternative 3′ processing in human cells. We describe here our studies using genomic tiling microarray from Affymetrix for these purposes. Although novel alternatively spliced RNA is detected in our studies, the recognition relies on visual examination of the intervals on Integrated Genome Browser and additional molecular assays. The suitability of using genomic tiling microarray for alternative splicing studies remains to be further evaluated. Parallel or deep sequencing has shown great promise in identifying novel transcripts and obtaining quantitative information. However, the storage and computation power needed to handle the massive data generated from sequencing still post a major challenge to its general applications.

The role of alternative or aberrant splicing in cancer is quite evident [74], but more investigations are warranted [75]. The 3′ untranslated region is critical for the translation, stability, localization of the RNA, and microRNA regulation [76, 77], and the length regulation of 3′ UTR in cancer has just gained momentum [78]. Thus, detecting and studying alteration in splicing/processing shall remain a focus in cancer biology.

References

1. Clark TA, Sugnet CW, Ares M Jr (2002) Genome-wide analysis of mRNA processing in yeast using splicing-specific microarrays. Science 296:907–910
2. Johnson JM, Castle J, Garrett-Engele P et al (2003) Genome-wide survey of human alternative pre-mRNA splicing with exon junction microarrays. Science 302:2141–2144
3. Pan Q, Shai O, Misquitta C et al (2004) Revealing global regulatory features of mammalian alternative splicing using a quantitative microarray platform. Mol Cell 16:929–941

4. Fehlbaum P, Guihal C, Bracco L et al (2005) A microarray configuration to quantify expression levels and relative abundance of splice variants. Nucleic Acids Res 33:e47
5. Srinivasan K, Shiue L, Hayes JD et al (2005) Detection and measurement of alternative splicing using splicing-sensitive microarrays. Methods 37:345–359
6. Castle J, Garrett-Engele P, Armour CD et al (2003) Optimization of oligonucleotide arrays and RNA amplification protocols for analysis of transcript structure and alternative splicing. Genome Biol 4:R66
7. Relogio A, Ben-Dov C, Baum M et al (2005) Alternative splicing microarrays reveal functional expression of neuron-specific regulators in Hodgkin lymphoma cells. J Biol Chem 280:4779–4784
8. Li C, Kato M, Shiue L et al (2006) Cell type and culture condition-dependent alternative splicing in human breast cancer cells revealed by splicing-sensitive microarrays. Cancer Res 66:1990–1999
9. Pio R, Blanco D, Pajares MJ et al (2010) Development of a novel splice array platform and its application in the identification of alternative splice variants in lung cancer. BMC genomics 11:352
10. Zhou W, Calciano MA, Jordan H et al (2009) High resolution analysis of the human transcriptome: detection of extensive alternative splicing independent of transcriptional activity. BMC Genet 10:63
11. Srinivasan S, Bingham JL, Johnson D (2009) The ABCs of human alternative splicing: a review of ATP-binding cassette transporter splicing. Curr Opin Drug Discov Devel 12:149–158
12. Yeakley JM, Fan JB, Doucet D et al (2002) Profiling alternative splicing on fiber-optic arrays. Nat Biotechnol 20:353–358
13. Fan JB, Yeakley JM, Bibikova M et al (2004) A versatile assay for high-throughput gene expression profiling on universal array matrices. Genome Res 14:878–885
14. Zhang C, Li HR, Fan JB et al (2006) Profiling alternatively spliced mRNA isoforms for prostate cancer classification. BMC Bioinformatics 7:202
15. Li HR, Wang-Rodriguez J, Nair TM et al (2006) Two-dimensional transcriptome profiling: identification of messenger RNA isoform signatures in prostate cancer from archived paraffin-embedded cancer specimens. Cancer Res 66:4079–4088
16. Fan JB, Gunderson KL, Bibikova M et al (2006) Illumina universal bead arrays. Methods Enzymol 410:57–73
17. Gardina PJ, Clark TA, Shimada B et al (2006) Alternative splicing and differential gene expression in colon cancer detected by a whole genome exon array. BMC Genomics 7:325
18. Robinson MD, Speed TP (2007) A comparison of Affymetrix gene expression arrays. BMC Bioinformatics 8:449
19. Abdueva D, Wing MR, Schaub B, Triche TJ (2007) Experimental comparison and evaluation of the Affymetrix exon and U133Plus2 Gene Chip arrays. PLoS ONE 2:e913
20. Okoniewski MJ, Hey Y, Pepper SD, Miller CJ (2007) High correspondence between Affymetrix exon and standard expression arrays. Biotechniques 42:181–185
21. Xing Y, Kapur K, Wong WH (2006) Probe selection and expression index computation of Affymetrix Exon Arrays. PLoS ONE 1:e88
22. Kapur K, Xing Y, Ouyang Z, Wong WH (2007) Exon arrays provide accurate assessments of gene expression. Genome Biol 8:R82
23. Okumura M, Kondo S, Ogata M et al (2005) Candidates for tumor-specific alternative splicing. Biochem Biophys Res Commun 334:23–29
24. Xu Q, Lee C (2003) Discovery of novel splice forms and functional analysis of cancer-specific alternative splicing in human expressed sequences. Nucleic Acids Res 31:5635–5643
25. Thorsen K, Sorensen KD, Brems-Eskildsen AS et al (2008) Alternative splicing in colon, bladder, and prostate cancer identified by exon array analysis. Mol Cell Proteomics 7:1214–1224

26. French PJ, Peeters J, Horsman S et al (2007) Identification of differentially regulated splice variants and novel exons in glial brain tumors using exon expression arrays. Cancer Res 67:5635–5642
27. Cheung HC, Baggerly KA, Tsavachidis S et al (2008) Global analysis of aberrant pre-mRNA splicing in glioblastoma using exon expression arrays. BMC Genomics 9:216
28. Hallegger M, Llorian M, Smith CW (2010) Alternative splicing: global insights. The FEBS J 277:856–866
29. Lapuk A, Marr H, Jakkula L et al (2010) Exon-level microarray analyses identify alternative splicing programs in breast cancer. Mol Cancer Res 8:961–974
30. Subbaram S, Kuentzel M, Frank D et al (2010) Determination of alternate splicing events using the Affymetrix Exon 1.0 ST arrays. Method Mol Biol 632:63–72
31. Yeo GW, Xu X, Liang TY et al (2007) Alternative splicing events identified in human embryonic stem cells and neural progenitors. PLoS Comput Biol 3:1951–1967
32. Xing Y, Stoilov P, Kapur K et al (2008) MADS: a new and improved method for analysis of differential alternative splicing by exon-tiling microarrays. RNA 14:1470–1479
33. Boutz PL, Stoilov P, Li Q et al (2007) A post-transcriptional regulatory switch in polypyrimidine tract-binding proteins reprograms alternative splicing in developing neurons. Genes Dev 21:1636–1652
34. Mockler TC, Chan S, Sundaresan A et al (2005) Applications of DNA tiling arrays for whole-genome analysis. Genomics 85:1–15
35. Johnson JM, Edwards S, Shoemaker D, Schadt EE (2005) Dark matter in the genome: evidence of widespread transcription detected by microarray tiling experiments. Trends Genet 21:93–102
36. Yazaki J, Gregory BD, Ecker JR (2007) Mapping the genome landscape using tiling array technology. Curr Opin Plant Biol 10:534–542
37. Kapranov P, Cawley SE, Drenkow J et al (2002) Large-scale transcriptional activity in chromosomes 21 and 22. Science 296:916–919
38. Kampa D, Cheng J, Kapranov P et al (2004) Novel RNAs identified from an in-depth analysis of the transcriptome of human chromosomes 21 and 22. Genome Res 14:331–342
39. Bertone P, Stolc V, Royce TE et al (2004) Global identification of human transcribed sequences with genome tiling arrays. Science 306:2242–2246
40. Cheng J, Kapranov P, Drenkow J et al (2005) Transcriptional maps of 10 human chromosomes at 5-nucleotide resolution. Science 308:1149–1154
41. Okazaki Y, Furuno M, Kasukawa T et al (2002) Analysis of the mouse transcriptome based on functional annotation of 60,770 full-length cDNAs. Nature 420:563–573
42. Stolc V, Gauhar Z, Mason C et al (2004) A gene expression map for the euchromatic genome of *Drosophila melanogaster*. Science 306:655–660
43. Yamada K, Lim J, Dale JM et al (2003) Empirical analysis of transcriptional activity in the *Arabidopsis* genome. Science 302:842–846
44. Birney E, Stamatoyannopoulos JA, Dutta A et al (2007) Identification and analysis of functional elements in 1 % of the human genome by the ENCODE pilot project. Nature 447:799–816
45. Denoeud F, Kapranov P, Ucla C et al (2007) Prominent use of distal 5' transcription start sites and discovery of a large number of additional exons in ENCODE regions. Genome Res 17:746–759
46. Le Hir H, Charlet-Berguerand N, de Franciscis V, Thermes C (2002) 5'-End RET splicing: absence of variants in normal tissues and intron retention in pheochromocytomas. Oncology 63:84–91
47. Lee MP, Feinberg AP (1997) Aberrant splicing but not mutations of TSG101 in human breast cancer. Cancer Res 57:3131–3134
48. Kim E, Goren A, Ast G (2008) Insights into the connection between cancer and alternative splicing. Trends Genet 24:7–10

49. Juneau K, Palm C, Miranda M, Davis RW (2007) High-density yeast-tiling array reveals previously undiscovered introns and extensive regulation of meiotic splicing. Proc Natl Acad Sci USA 104:1522–1527
50. Sayani S, Janis M, Lee CY, Toesca I, Chanfreau GF (2008) Widespread impact of nonsense-mediated mRNA decay on the yeast intronome. Mol Cell 31:360–370
51. Gencheva M, Lin TY, Wu X et al (2010) Nuclear retention of unspliced pre-mRNAs by mutant DHX16/hPRP2, a spliceosomal DEAH-box protein. J Biol Chem 285:35624–35632
52. Sakharkar MK, Perumal BS, Sakharkar KR, Kangueane P (2005) An analysis on gene architecture in human and mouse genomes. In Silico Biol 5:347–365
53. Yang L, Lin G, Wu X, Yen Y, Lin R-J Novel RNAs overexpressed in breast tumors as revealed by genomic tiling microarray. (In Preparation)
54. Gudlaugsdottir S, Boswell DR, Wood GR, Ma J (2007) Exon size distribution and the origin of introns. Genetica 131:299–306
55. Dahl E, Kristiansen G, Gottlob K et al (2006) Molecular profiling of laser-microdissected matched tumor and normal breast tissue identifies karyopherin alpha2 as a potential novel prognostic marker in breast cancer. Clin Cancer Res 12:3950–3960
56. Gluz O, Wild P, Meiler R et al (2008) Nuclear karyopherin alpha2 expression predicts poor survival in patients with advanced breast cancer irrespective of treatment intensity. Int J Cancer 123:1433–1438
57. Suomela S, Cao L, Bowcock A, Saarialho-Kere U (2004) Interferon alpha-inducible protein 27 (IFI27) is upregulated in psoriatic skin and certain epithelial cancers. J Invest Dermatol 122:717–721
58. Wenzel J, Tomiuk S, Zahn S et al (2008) Transcriptional profiling identifies an interferon-associated host immune response in invasive squamous cell carcinoma of the skin. Int J Cancer 123:2605–2615
59. Badve S, Turbin D, Thorat MA, Morimiya A, Nielsen TO, Perou CM, Dunn S, Huntsman DG, Nakshatri H (2007) FOXA1 expression in breast cancer-correlation with luminal subtype A and survival. Clin Cancer Res 13:4415–4421
60. Habashy HO, Powe DG, Rakha EA, Ball G, Paish C, Gee J, Nicholson RI, Ellis IO (2008) Forkhead-box A1 (FOXA1) expression in breast cancer and its prognostic significance. Eur J Cancer 44:1541–1551
61. Mochizuki S, Okada Y (2007) ADAMs in cancer cell proliferation and progression. Cancer Sci 98:621–628
62. Rocks N, Paulissen G, El Hour M et al (2008) Emerging roles of ADAM and ADAMTS metalloproteinases in cancer. Biochimie 90:369–379
63. Kaida D, Berg MG, Younis I, Kasim M, Singh LN, Wan L, Dreyfuss G (2010) U1 snRNP protects pre-mRNAs from premature cleavage and polyadenylation. Nature 468:664–668
64. Sultan M, Schulz MH, Richard H et al (2008) A global view of gene activity and alternative splicing by deep sequencing of the human transcriptome. Science 321:956–960
65. Mortazavi A, Williams BA, McCue K, Schaeffer L, Wold B (2008) Mapping and quantifying mammalian transcriptomes by RNA-Seq. Nat Methods 5:621–628
66. Wang ET, Sandberg R, Luo S, Khrebtukova I, Zhang L, Mayr C, Kingsmore SF, Schroth GP, Burge CB (2008) Alternative isoform regulation in human tissue transcriptomes. Nature 456:470–476
67. Lister R, O'Malley RC, Tonti-Filippini J, Gregory BD, Berry CC, Millar AH, Ecker JR (2008) Highly integrated single-base resolution maps of the epigenome in *Arabidopsis*. Cell 133:523–536
68. Wilhelm BT, Marguerat S, Watt S, Schubert F, Wood V, Goodhead I, Penkett CJ, Rogers J, Bahler J (2008) Dynamic repertoire of a eukaryotic transcriptome surveyed at single-nucleotide resolution. Nature 453:1239–1243
69. Cloonan N, Forrest AR, Kolle G et al (2008) Stem cell transcriptome profiling via massive-scale mRNA sequencing. Nat Methods 5:613–619

70. Okoniewski MJ, Miller CJ (2006) Hybridization interactions between probe sets in short oligo microarrays lead to spurious correlations. BMC Bioinformatics 7:276
71. Hoen PAt, Ariyurek Y, Thygesen HH, et al (2008) Deep sequencing-based expression analysis shows major advances in robustness, resolution and inter-lab portability over five microarray platforms. Nucleic Acids Res 36(21):e141
72. Parsons DW, Jones S, Zhang X et al (2008) An integrated genomic analysis of human glioblastoma multiforme. Science 321:1807–1812
73. Jones S, Zhang X, Parsons DW, Lin JC et al (2008) Core signaling pathways in human pancreatic cancers revealed by global genomic analyses. Science 321:1801–1806
74. Venables JP (2006) Unbalanced alternative splicing and its significance in cancer. Bioessays 28:378–386
75. Pajares MJ, Ezponda T, Catena R, Calvo A, Pio R, Montuenga LM (2007) Alternative splicing: an emerging topic in molecular and clinical oncology. Lancet Oncol 8:349–357
76. Moore MJ (2005) From birth to death: the complex lives of eukaryotic mRNAs. Science 309:1514–1518
77. Jan CH, Friedman RC, Ruby JG, Bartel DP (2011) Formation regulation and evolution of Caenorhabditis elegans 3'UTRs. Nature 469:97–101
78. Sandberg R, Neilson JR, Sarma A, Sharp PA, Burge CB (2008) Proliferating cells express mRNAs with shortened 3' untranslated regions and fewer microRNA target sites. Science 320:1643–1647

Cancer-Associated Perturbations in Alternative Pre-messenger RNA Splicing

Lulzim Shkreta, Brendan Bell, Timothée Revil, Julian P. Venables, Panagiotis Prinos, Sherif Abou Elela and Benoit Chabot

Abstract

For most of our 25,000 genes, the removal of introns by pre-messenger RNA (pre-mRNA) splicing represents an essential step toward the production of functional messenger RNAs (mRNAs). Alternative splicing of a single pre-mRNA results in the production of different mRNAs. Although complex organisms use alternative splicing to expand protein function and phenotypic diversity, patterns of alternative splicing are often altered in cancer cells. Alternative splicing contributes to tumorigenesis by producing splice isoforms that can stimulate cell proliferation and cell migration or induce resistance to apoptosis and anticancer agents. Cancer-specific changes in splicing profiles can occur through mutations that are affecting splice sites and splicing

L. Shkreta · B. Bell · T. Revil
Département de microbiologie et d'infectiologie,
Faculté de Médecine et des sciences de la santé,
Université de Sherbrooke, Québec, Canada

J. P. Venables
Institut de Génétique Moléculaire de Montpellier,
Laboratoire de Génomique Fonctionnelle de l'Université de Sherbrooke,
Montpellier, France

P. Prinos · S. A. Elela
Laboratoire de Génomique Fonctionnelle de l'Université de Sherbrooke,
Université de Sherbrooke, Québec, Canada

B. Chabot (✉)
Département de microbiologie et d'infectiologie,
Faculté de Médecine et des sciences de la santé,
Laboratoire de Génomique Fonctionnelle, Université de Sherbrooke,
3201, rue Jean-Mignault Sherbrooke, Québec, J1E 4K8, Canada
e-mail: benoit.chabot@usherbrooke.ca

J. Y. Wu (ed.), *RNA and Cancer*, Cancer Treatment and Research,
DOI: 10.1007/978-3-642-31659-3_3,

control elements, and also by alterations in the expression of proteins that control splicing decisions. Recent progress in global approaches that interrogate splicing diversity should help to obtain specific splicing signatures for cancer types. The development of innovative approaches for annotating and reprogramming splicing events will more fully establish the essential contribution of alternative splicing to the biology of cancer and will hopefully provide novel targets and anticancer strategies. Metazoan genes are usually made up of several exons interrupted by introns. The introns are removed from the pre-mRNA by RNA splicing. In conjunction with other maturation steps, such as capping and polyadenylation, the spliced mRNA is then transported to the cytoplasm to be translated into a functional protein. The basic mechanism of splicing requires accurate recognition of each extremity of each intron by the spliceosome. Introns are identified by the binding of U1 snRNP to the 5′ splice site and the U2AF65/U2AF35 complex to the 3′ splice site. Following these interactions, other proteins and snRNPs are recruited to generate the complete spliceosomal complex needed to excise the intron. While many introns are constitutively removed by the spliceosome, other splice junctions are not used systematically, generating the phenomenon of alternative splicing. Alternative splicing is therefore the process by which a single species of pre-mRNA can be matured to produce different mRNA molecules (Fig. 1). Depending on the number and types of alternative splicing events, a pre-mRNA can generate from two to several thousands different mRNAs leading to the production of a corresponding number of proteins. It is now believed that the expression of at least 70 % of human genes is subjected to alternative splicing, implying an enormous contribution to proteomic diversity, and by extension, to the development and the evolution of complex animals. Defects in splicing have been associated with human diseases (Caceres and Kornblihtt, Trends Genet 18(4):186–93, 2002, Cartegni et al., Nat Rev Genet 3(4):285–98, 2002, Pagani and Baralle, Nat Rev Genet 5(5):389–96, 2004), including cancer (Brinkman, Clin Biochem 37(7):584–94, 2004, Venables, Bioessays 28(4):378–86, 2006, Srebrow and Kornblihtt, J Cell Sci 119(Pt 13):2635–2641, 2006, Revil et al., Bull Cancer 93(9):909–919, 2006, Venables, Transworld Res Network, 2006, Pajares et al., Lancet Oncol 8(4):349–57, 2007, Skotheim and Nees, Int J Biochem Cell Biol 39:1432–1449, 2007). Numerous studies have now confirmed the existence of specific differences in the alternative splicing profiles between normal and cancer tissues. Although there are a few cases where specific mutations are the primary cause for these changes, global alterations in alternative splicing in cancer cells may be primarily derived from changes in the expression of RNA-binding proteins that control splice site selection. Overall, these cancer-specific differences in alternative splicing offer an immense potential to improve the diagnosis and the prognosis of cancer. This review will focus on the functional impact of cancer-associated alternative splicing variants, the molecular determinants that alter the splicing decisions in cancer cells, and future therapeutic strategies.

Keywords

Oncogene · Mutations · Apoptosis · RNA binding proteins · Anticancer strategies · Splice variants

Contents

1 Introduction

For most of our 25,000 genes, the removal of introns by pre-messenger RNA (pre-mRNA) splicing represents an essential step toward the production of functional messenger RNAs (mRNA). Alternative splicing of a single pre-mRNA results in the production of different mRNAs. Although complex organisms use alternative splicing to expand protein function and phenotypic diversity, patterns of alternative splicing are often altered in cancer cells. Alternative splicing contributes to tumorigenesis by producing splice isoforms that can stimulate cell proliferation and cell migration or induce resistance to apoptosis and anticancer agents. Cancer-specific changes in splicing profiles can occur through mutations that are affecting splice sites and splicing control elements, and also by alterations in the expression of proteins that control splicing decisions. Recent progress in global approaches that interrogate splicing diversity should help to obtain specific splicing signatures for cancer types. The development of innovative approaches for annotating and reprogramming splicing events will more fully establish the essential contribution of alternative splicing to the biology of cancer and will hopefully provide novel targets and anticancer strategies.

Metazoan genes are usually made up of several exons interrupted by introns. The introns are removed from the pre-mRNA by RNA splicing. In conjunction with other maturation steps, such as capping and polyadenylation, the spliced mRNA is then transported to the cytoplasm to be translated into a functional protein. The basic mechanism of splicing requires accurate recognition of each extremity of each intron by the spliceosome. Introns are identified by the binding of U1 snRNP to the 5′ splice site and the U2AF65/U2AF35 complex to the 3′ splice site. Following these interactions, other proteins and snRNPs are recruited to generate the complete spliceosomal complex needed to excise the intron.

While many introns are constitutively removed by the spliceosome, other splice junctions are not used systematically, generating the phenomenon of alternative splicing. Alternative splicing is therefore the process by which a single species of pre-mRNA can be matured to produce different mRNA molecules (Fig. 1). Depending on the number and types of alternative splicing events, a pre-mRNA can generate from two to several thousands different mRNAs leading to the production of a corresponding number of proteins. It is now believed that the expression of at least 70 % of human genes is subjected to alternative splicing, implying an enormous contribution to proteomic diversity, and by extension, to the development and the evolution of complex animals.

Defects in splicing have been associated with human diseases [1–3], including cancer [4–10]. Numerous studies have now confirmed the existence of specific differences in the alternative splicing profiles between normal and cancer tissues. Although there are a few cases where specific mutations are the primary cause for these changes, global alterations in alternative splicing in cancer cells may be primarily derived from changes in the expression of RNA-binding proteins that control splice site selection. Overall, these cancer-specific differences in alternative splicing offer an immense potential to improve the diagnosis and the prognosis of cancer.

This review will focus on the functional impact of cancer-associated alternative splicing variants, the molecular determinants that alter the splicing decisions in cancer cells, and future therapeutic strategies.

2 Function of Cancer-Associated Splice Variants

Alternative splicing is part of the normal expression program of the majority of human genes. The initial reports describing the importance of alternative splicing in the control of sex determination in *Drosophila* [11] were followed by several examples linking splicing to the regulation of gene expression in human cells. For example, it was shown that alternative splicing controls the production of membrane-associated or secreted forms of immunoglobulins [12], and the synthesis of hormones with distinct physiological functions [13]. The most striking examples of the effect of splicing on gene expression are found in the nervous system where alternative splicing is used to expand the functional repertoire of receptor molecules. One notable example is the alternative splicing of the Slo gene that leads to the production of different proteins playing a role in the perception of different sound frequencies during audition [14].

The contribution of alternative splicing to gene expression is not always to expand protein diversity. Indeed, alternative splicing can also regulate the level of gene expression by producing mRNA isoforms containing premature stop codons that activate nonsense-mediated RNA decay (NMD). However, a global analysis

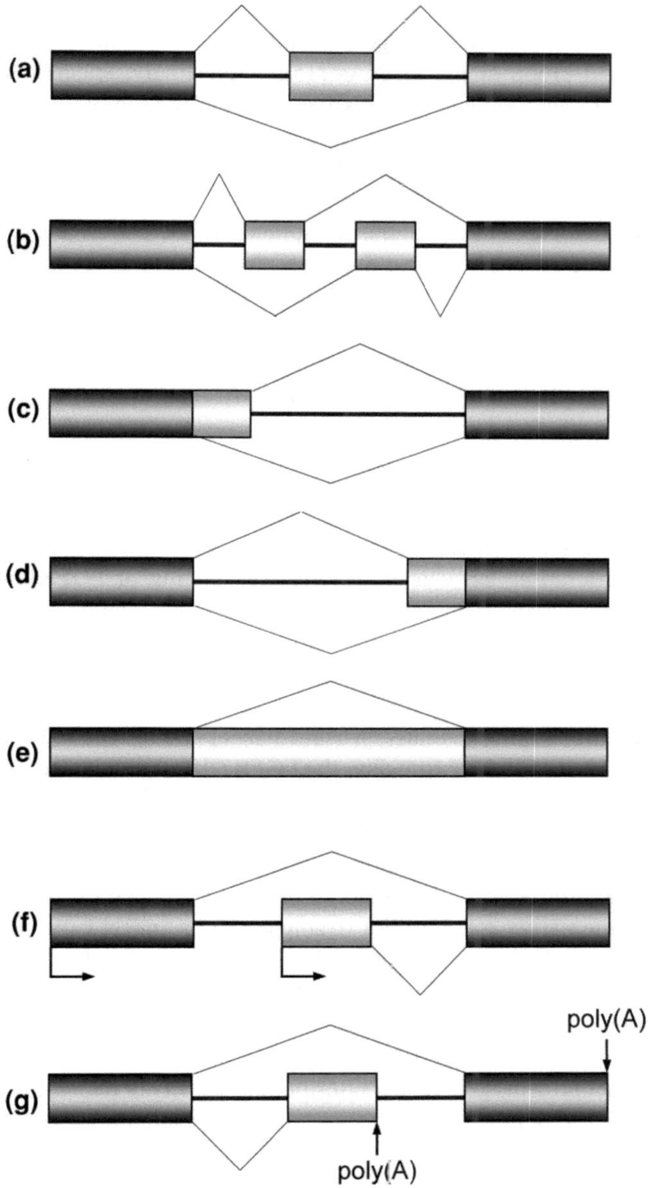

Fig. 1 Patterns of alternative splicing. *Gray* boxes represent exons or exonic fragments that are alternatively spliced. **a** cassette exon, **b** mutually exclusive exons, **c** alternative 5′ splice sites, **d** alternative 3′ splice sites, **e** intron retention, **f** alternative promoters can affect the identity of the first exon, and **g** alternative polyadenylation sites can impact the structure of the terminal exon

of the effect of knocking-down a specific NMD component on the abundance of 3126 alternative splicing events suggests that this pathway is not general but rather affects a selected group of pre-mRNAs [15]. Interestingly, splicing factors such as PTB and SC35 autoregulate their own expression by promoting the production of the NMD-sensitive isoforms [16–18]. Recent studies indicate that this mode of regulation is a hallmark of many splicing regulatory factors that belong to the SR and hnRNP family of proteins [17, 19].

Despite the involvement of alternative splicing in the expression and diversity of selective sets of genes, the global impact of the functional diversity imparted by alternative splicing still remains incomplete and controversial [20]. However, some of the best available evidence documenting the breadth and significance of alternative splicing has been provided by the study of cancer cells. Selected examples ordered by cellular functions are presented below.

2.1 Cellular Proliferation

Expression of the fibroblast growth factor receptor (FGFR) family is closely linked to cellular proliferation and cancer. Alternative splicing of FGFR1 and FGFR2 pre-mRNAs produce splice variants that have different affinities for their respective ligands. The FGFR2-IIIc splice isoforms is overexpressed in advanced stages of prostate cancers and transforms human mammary epithelial cells when expressed ectopically [21, 22]. FGFR2-IIIc accumulates in mesenchymal cells while FGFR2-IIIb is preferentially produced in epithelial cells. In a rat model system, prostate cancer cells expressing the FGFR2-IIIc-specific exon in a reporter construct revealed unexpected mesenchymal-epithelial transitions in primary tumors and lung micrometastastases, revealing their phenotypic plasticity [23].

Proto-oncogenes and tumor-suppressor genes are essential players in the regulation of cellular proliferation. The majority of these genes express isoforms that are generated by alternative splicing. For example, the pre-mRNA encoding the p53 protein is alternatively spliced to produce isoforms whose abundance vary in breast tumors [24]. Other members of the p53 family such as p73 and p63 are alternatively spliced leading to the inclusion or the exclusion of the transcription transactivation domain. Inclusion of the transactivation domain transforms these tumor-suppressor proteins into oncoproteins [25]. The transcriptional activity of p53 is itself controlled via the alternative splicing of MDM2. Variations in the splicing of MDM2 in cancer tissues influence its accumulation in the nucleus and therefore affect its capacity to repress the transcription of p53 [26, 27]. Other examples of cancer-associated changes in alternative splicing are listed in Table 1.

2.2 Cellular Invasion

Integrins are a family of cell adhesion transmembrane proteins. Their expression modulates the invasive properties of cancer cells. Numerous integrin splice

Table 1 Examples of genes expressing splicing variants that are relevant to various aspects of cell transformation and cancer

Gene	Splice variants	Cancer type	Functional impact	References
Cellular proliferation				
FGFR1 (Fibroblast growth factor receptor 1)	FGFR1-α FGFR1-β FGFR1-IIIb FGFR1-IIIc	Brain, breast, colon and pancreas, PANC-1 cells	FGFR1-β correlates with pancreatic adenocarcinoma cell growth and resistance to chemotherapy. FGFR1-β has a 10-fold higher affinity for the FGF ligand, which may provide a growth advantage to tumors. FGFR1-β is the dominant splice variant found in glial cell and pancreatic tumors. FGFR1-α inhibits adenocarcinoma cell growth in vivo and restores cytotoxic response to chemotherapy. FGFR1-IIIc expressed in pancreatic cancer cells can enhance pancreatic ductal cell transformation.	[202, 220–222]
FGFR2	FGFR2-IIIb FGFR2-IIIc	Prostate, lung metastasis, breast, urothelial, and cervical carcinomas	In prostate cancers, the expression of FGFR2-IIIc is upregulated while that of FGFR2-IIIb is downregulated. Restoration of FGFR2-IIIb to malignant cells expressing FGFR1 represses tumor growth rate and re-establishes responsiveness to stromal cells.	[21–23]
FGFR3	FGFR3-Δ8-10 FGFR3IIIc FGFR3IIIS	Bladder, colorectal cancer, various	FGFR3-Δ8-10 acts as a dominant negative regulator of FGFR3 signaling in bladder cancer. FGFR3IIIS functions as a dominant negative inhibitor of FGFR3-induced growth arrest. FGFR3IIIS may regulate FGF and FGFR trafficking and function, thus contributing to the development of a malignant phenotype.	[223, 224]
FGFR4	FGFR4-s	Gastric, colon, and pancreatic cancer cell lines	The splice variant FGFR4-s encodes a soluble form of the receptor with a ligand binding affinity that is different from the transmembrane FGFR4 receptor.	[225]

(continued)

Table 1 (continued)

Gene	Splice variants	Cancer type	Functional impact	References
p53	p53β and p53γ Δ40p53 Δ40p53β and γ Δ133p53 Δ133p53β and γ	Breast cancer, various	N-terminally truncated splice variants (Δ40p53) suppress both transcriptional and growth inhibiting activities of p53. While full-length p53 efficiently induces apoptosis, p53β triggers a more attenuated apoptotic response and Δ133p53β inhibits apoptosis and acts as a dominant negative.	[24]
p63	ΔNp63α	Breast, squamous cell carcinoma of the esophagus	ΔNp63α promotes survival of breast cancer cells by binding to TAp73 and inhibiting its pro-apoptotic activity.	[226]
p73	p73α p73β ΔNp73 TAp73	Prostate, squamous cell carcinoma and adenocarcinoma of the esophagus, various	p73α is abundant in prostate cancer. It represses drug-induced apoptosis in two non-small cell lung cancer cell lines but not in other cancer cell lines. p73α and p73β isoforms have antagonistic functions on drug-induced apoptosis. ΔNp73 impairs the transcriptional activity of TAp73 and p53.	[25, 227, 228]
MDM2	>than 40 different isoforms	Various	Splice variants that lack the p53 binding domain but retain the RING domains are detected in various cancer cell lines and primary tumors. Many negatively regulate the MDM2 full-length protein and activate and upregulate p53. MDM2-b cannot bind p53 but can sequester the full-length MDM2 protein in the cytoplasm. Its overexpression inhibits apoptosis and enhances cell growth in cancer cell lines.	[26, 27, 229, 230]
MDM4 (HDMX)	HDMX-E HDMX-A HDMX-G HMDX211 XALT1 XALT2	Soft-tissue sarcomas	Expression of the HDMX-E splice variant correlates with decreased patient survival and is a stronger negative regulator of p53 than the full-length HDMX protein.	[231, 232]

(continued)

Table 1 (continued)

Gene	Splice variants	Cancer type	Functional impact	References
PTEN	PTEN-3a, 3b, 3c, PTEN-5a, 5b, 5c, DelE5, DelE6	Cowden syndrome, sporadic breast cancers	SV-5a decreases P-Akt level and cyclin D1 promoter activity, SV-5b and -5c increase Cyclin D1 promoter activity. SV-5b functionally counteracts the activity of PTEN.	[233]
HTERT	Several isoforms	Various	Telomerase is activated in 85–90 % of human tumors, which represents the single most frequent alteration associated with malignancy. Many shorter versions are inactive. hTERT-alpha is one of the four isoforms that are considered negative regulators of telomerase activity.	[234]
Cyclin D1	Cyclin D1a Cyclin D1b	Prostate	Expression of Cyclin D1a inhibits cell-cycle progression in androgen receptor-dependent prostate cancer cells while Cyclin D1b stimulates proliferation. The altered androgen receptor regulatory capacity of Cyclin D1b is associated with an increased risk of prostate cancer.	[235, 236]
CYP1A1 (Cytochrome P450 1A1)	CYP1A1v	Epithelial ovarian	In contrast to the ER localization for the wild-type enzyme, CYP1A1v is restricted to the nucleus and mitochondria. CYP1A1v induces anchorage-independent growth.	[237]
KAP (cyclin-dependent kinase associated protein phosphatase)	Four variants	Glioblastomas	A dominant negative KAP variant increases cell proliferation.	[238]
hMena (ENAH)	hMena(+11a)	Breast and breast cancer cell lines	Overexpression and phosphorylation of hMena (+11a) increases the activation of p42/44 mitogen-activated protein kinase (MAPK) and cell proliferation.	[239]

(continued)

Table 1 (continued)

Gene	Splice variants	Cancer type	Functional impact	References
APC	cAPC BS-APC 0.3-APC	Colorectal cancers, SW480 colon cancer cell line	All three splice variants alter cellular morphology and affect cell growth by elongating the G1 phase of the cell cycle. Overexpression of the full-length ACP in SW480 colon cancer cells impairs proliferation while the removal of the truncated APC reduces cell growth. The truncated splice variants enhance the migratory capacity of colon cancer cells. In contrast to 0.3-APC, the c-APC and brain-specific (BS) APC isoforms suppress the tumorigenic phenotype of cells in culture.	[240, 241]
β 1 integrin	β 1C	Endometrial cancers	β 1C acts as a growth modulator in cancer cells.	[28]
Cellular adhesion, invasion and angiogenesis				
CD44	>20 isoforms of CD44v	Gastric carcinomas urothelial cancer, metastatic lesions of gynecological cancers, various	CD44v4-v7 isoforms alter hyaluronate binding. CD44v8-v10 are associated with tumor progression. CD44v6 is involved in the progression of carcinoma, nodal metastasis, myometrial invasion and vascular invasion.	[29, 31, 242]
CD99	CD99wt CD99sh	Osteosarcoma, prostate and breast cancer cells	CD99wt inhibits anchorage-independent growth, migration, and metastasis, whereas the CD99sh markedly elevates motility, binding to fibronectin, MMP-9 expression, and invasiveness of MDA-MB-231 and MCF-7 cells.	[243, 244]
Fibronectin	EDA EDB IIICS-0, -95 and -120	Melanoma, prostate, lung, liver	Preferential inclusion of exon EDB was found in lung cancer and of both the EDB and EDA exons in liver cancer.	[245 246]
C-CAM1 (Cell–cell adhesion molecule)	L-C-CAM1 S–C-CAM1	Colorectal, breast, prostate carcinomas, non-small cell lung cancers (NSCLC) and cell lines	Tumor cells expressing L-C-CAM1 grow more slowly and are less tumorigenic, suggesting that L-form C-CAM1 is a tumor suppressor. NSCLC tissue and cell lines express predominantly S–C-CAM1.	[247, 248]

(continued)

Table 1 (continued)

Gene	Splice variants	Cancer type	Functional impact	References
CCK_2 R (Cholecystokinin-2/ gastrin receptor)	CCK_2R ΔCCK_2R $CCK_{2L}R$ $CCK_{2i4sv}R$	Esophageal, gastric, pancreatic and colorectal cancers	CCK_2R and $CCK_{2i4sv}R$ may regulate tumor growth and dissemination. Expression of the $CCK_{2i4sv}R$ isoform induces activation of the Src kinase with which it appears to form a signaling complex. $CCK_{2i4sv}R$ expression and activation of Src induce tumor cell growth and angiogenesis.	[37]
KLF6	KLF6-SV1 KLF6-SV2 KLF6-SV3	Epithelial ovarian cancer, prostate cancer, glioblastoma	KLF6-SV1 variant promotes cell proliferation and invasion. Its downregulation suppresses tumor formation. KLF6-SV1 and KLF6-SV2 are mislocalized to the cytoplasm and antagonize wtKLF6 function leading to decreased p21 expression and increased cell growth. Both splice variants are upregulated in tumor versus normal prostatic tissue. Decreased KLF6 and increased KLF6-SV1 expression are common primary glioblastomas. These changes have antagonistic effects on the growth of glioblastoma cell lines.	[88, 249, 250]
Rac1	Rac1b	Colorectal and breast cancer cells	The GTPase Rac1b is mostly expressed in its active and GTP-bound state, compromising activation of important signaling pathways that are classically stimulated by Rac1. Rac1b overexpression may facilitate tumor progression by enhancing Dishevelled-3-mediated Wnt signaling pathway and inducing Wnt target genes specifically involved in decreasing the adhesive properties of colorectal cells. Rac1b induces an increase in cellular reactive oxygen species leading to genomic instability and promotion of tumorigenesis.	[251, 252]
OPN (Osteoponin)	OPN-c	Hepatocellular carcinoma	Splice variant OPN-c promotes cellular invasion and correlates with metastatic potential.	[253]

(continued)

Table 1 (continued)

Gene	Splice variants	Cancer type	Functional impact	References
RON (Macrophage-stimulating protein receptor)	RonD RonD165 RonD160 RonD155	Gastric carcinoma breast and colorectal cancers	RonD mRNA lacks exon 11, which renders the protein constitutively active. RonD induces invasion and mobility properties to cancer cells and participates in malignant transformation of epithelial tumors by activating the epithelial-to-mesenchymal transition.	[33, 125]
HER2 (neu/c-erbB-2) receptor tyrosine kinase	At least five splice variants	Various epithelial tumors	Two variants encode soluble proteins that function as inhibitors of HER2 to inhibit the proliferation of cancer cells. The variant HER2-ECD that contains the extracellular domain is progressively downregulated in more advanced gastric tumors, suggesting that the soluble variants inhibit tumor progression.	[254]
VEGF	VEGF121 VEGF165 VEGF189 VEGF165b	Prostate, kidney, breast, colorectal carcinoma, different solid tumors	In contrast to the other pro-angiogenic variants, VEGF165b is anti-angiogenic. VEGF165b is downregulated in several carcinomas. An increase in the VEGF121/VEGF165-189 ratio enhances angiogenesis in prostate tumors.	[35, 255]
HYAL	HYAL1-v1	Bladder	HYAL expression in bladder cancers promotes tumor growth, invasion, and angiogenesis. HYAL1-v1 expression may negatively regulate bladder tumor growth, infiltration, and angiogenesis.	[256]
PTK2 Focal adhesion kinase (FAK)	FAK-related non-kinase (FRNK)	MTLn3 mammary adenocarcinoma cells	Expression of FRNK inhibits cell spreading and migration, and reduces phosphorylation of FAK.	[257]
IIp45 (Invasion inhibitory protein 45)	IIp45S	Infiltrating gliomas	A tumor-specific alternative splicing event generates an aberrant and unstable IIp45S splice variant that acts as a dominant negative.	[258]

(continued)

Table 1 (continued)

Gene	Splice variants	Cancer type	Functional impact	References
uPAR (cellular receptor for urokinase-type plasminogen receptor)	uPARdel4/5	Breast	Splice variant uPAR-del4/5 is predominantly expressed in various cancer cell lines and tumors and its expression is associated with shorter survival of cancer patients.	[259]
Resistance to apoptosis				
Fas (CD95)	Fas FasExo6 Del (sFas) FasExo3-4 Del FasExo3-4,6 Del FasExo4 Del FasExo4-6 Del	Lymphoma cell lines hepatocellular carcinoma, bladder, breast, ovarian, renal cell carcinoma, and melanoma	Shorter splice variants of Fas lack the membrane-anchoring transmembrane domain, therefore antagonizing the pro-apoptotic function of full-length FAS. sFas induces resistance to FAS-mediated apoptosis in human lymphoma cell lines. sFas levels increase in the serum of cancer patients and correlates with tumor stage and burden. Increased levels of sFas are observed in several cancers.	[260–263]
APAF1	APAF-1-ALT	LNCaP human prostate cancer cell line	The splice variant shows antagonistic functions during apoptosis and may contribute to resistance to DNA damage-induced treatment.	[264, 265]
BIRC5 (Survivin)	Survivin-ΔEX3, Survivin-2B Survivin-3B	Breast carcinoma, metastatic gastric cancer	Survivin-2B is pro-apoptotic and antagonises Survivin and Survivin-ΔEX3 (both with anti-apoptotic function) that are overexpressed in several tumors. Survivin-ΔEX3 forms a complex with Bcl-2 that inhibits the activity of caspase-3. Survivin-2B is downregulated in breast and gastric cancers.	[266, 267, 268]
Bcl-2	Bcl-2α Bcl-2β	Prostate and colon	Bcl-2α contributes to the resistance of cancer cells to chemotherapeutic drugs. Bcl-2β has minimal or no anti-apoptotic function.	[269, 270]

(continued)

Table 1 (continued)

Gene	Splice variants	Cancer type	Functional impact	References
Bcl-x	Bcl-xL Bcl-xS Bcl-xΔTM Bcl-xβ Bcl-xγ	Prostate, ovarian, leukemias	Bcl-xL is the major anti-apoptotic splice variant expressed in various tumors rendering cancer cells more resistant to chemotherapeutic drugs. Bcl-xS acts as the pro-apoptotic isoform, antagonizing the anti-apoptotic properties of Bcl-xL and sensitizing cancer cells to chemotherapeutic drugs. Bcl-xΔTM, Bcl-xβ, and Bcl-xγ exhibit various levels of anti-apoptotic activity.	[49, 271, 272]
Bax	Bax-α Bax-β Bax-γ Bax-δ Bax-ε Bax-σ Bax-ω	Breast Hodgkin lymphoma	Bax-α, the most frequent splice variant, and Bax-σ act as pro-apoptotic proteins, while Bax-ω has anti-apoptotic activity. Higher levels of Bax-α and lower levels of Bcl-2 in breast cancer tissue correlate with lower tumor grade. Bax-β may promote cancer cell growth. Bax-γ is considered a negative regulator of other Bax isoforms. Bax-ε induces apoptosis when expressed ectopically.	[273–275]
c-FLIP	c-$FLIP_L$ c-$FLIP_S$ c-$FLIP_R$	Colorectal cancer	c-$FLIP_L$ acts as a pro-apoptotic isoform while c-$FLIP_R$ is anti-apoptotic. c-$FLIP_L$ but not c-$FLIP_S$ can inhibit cell death induced by anticancer drugs.	[276, 277]
IG20 (Insulinoma-Glucagonoma)	IG20pa MADD IG20-SV2 DENN-SV	HeLa and PA-1 cancer cell lines	IG20-SVs play critical role in cell proliferation and apoptosis. IG20pa renders cells more susceptible to apoptosis and decreases cell proliferation while DENN-SV can increase the resistance to apoptosis and cell proliferation. MADD demonstrates antagonistic functions during apoptosis. MADD is sufficient and necessary for cancer cell survival.	[67, 278]
Mcl-1 (Myeloid cell leukemia)	MCL1-L MCL1-S	Leukemia	MCL1-L is the anti-apoptotic while MCL1-S is pro-apoptotic.	[279]

(continued)

Table 1 (continued)

Gene	Splice variants	Cancer type	Functional impact	References
Bim	BimL BimEL BimS Bimγ	Prostate, precursor B cell acute lymphoblastic leukemia cell line	All Bim isoforms promote apoptosis. BimS is the most potent pro-apoptotic isoform. BimL induces apoptosis by binding to and antagonizing anti-apoptotic Bcl-2 family members, such as Bcl-xL and BCL2L2. Bimγ inhibits clonal growth in prostate cancer cells. Induction of Bim by glucocorticoids is required for the complete apoptotic response in a precursor B cell acute lymphoblastic leukemia cell line.	[280–282]
CASP2	CASP-2L CASP-2S CASP-2L-Pro CASP-2S-Pro	Human B lymphoma, Namalwa and U937 human leukemic cells	CASP-2L is the most abundant pro-apoptotic splice variant while CASP-2S can function as anti-apoptotic isoform. CASP2-L expression sensitizes non-small cell lung cancer to cisplatin-induced apoptosis. CASP-2L-Pro functions as an endogenous apoptosis inhibitory protein that antagonizes caspase activation and cell death.	[283, 284]
CASP3	CASP-3S	Breast carcinomas and cancer cell lines	CASP-3S inhibits apoptosis and is associated with chemoresistance.	[285]
CASP8	CASP-8a CASP-8b CASP-8L	Neuroblastoma cell lines	CASP-8L and CASP-8a are dominant negative splice variants of CASP8. CASP-8b is the pro-apoptotic variant.	[286, 287]
CASP9	CASP-9a CASP-9b	LN-229 astrocytoma cells	CASP9a is the initiator caspase of the mitochondrial apoptotic pathway. CASP9b is the anti-apoptotic splice variant. Transient overexpression of CASP9b protects LN-229 astrocytoma cells from CD95 ligand-mediated apoptosis.	[288]

(continued)

Table 1 (continued)

Gene	Splice variants	Cancer type	Functional impact	References
FIR (FUSE-binding protein-interacting repressor)	sv-FIR	Primary colorectal cancers	Splice variant sv-FIR promotes tumor development by disabling FIR repression and inducing high levels of c-MYC to counteract apoptosis in colorectal cancer.	[57]
WT1 (Wilms tumor 1)	WT1(+KTS) WT1(-KTS)	Osteosarcoma nephroblastoma Wilms tumor, leukemia	In osteosarcoma cell lines expressing low levels of the wild-type transcript, inducible expression of WT1, particularly the (-KTS) isoform, triggers an initial G1 cell cycle arrest, followed by apoptosis. The WT1(-KTS) isoform appears to mediate transcriptional activation of genes implicated in cellular differentiation, possibly also repressing proliferation-associated genes. WT1(+KST) appears to regulate cell cycle and inhibits apoptosis.	[289, 290]
CK8 (Cytokeratin 8)	AS-CK8	Lung, non-small cell lung cancer cell lines and primary tumors	AS-CK8 lacks the caspase cleavage site. Cancer cells expressing this splice variant may have increased resistance to apoptosis.	[291]
Multidrug resistance				
MRP1	> > 20 splice variants	Ovarian tumor	Some of the splice variants confer resistance to doxorubicin.	[59]
M MAD2	MMAD2β	Human gastric adenocarcinoma cell line SGC7901	MAD2β can increase multidrug resistance in SGC7901 cells.	[292]
DNA excision/repair				
BRCA1	> than 12 splice variants	Breast and ovary	The nuclear localization signal is absent in some of the splice variants. Disruption of BRCA-1 pre-mRNA splicing patterns contributes to cell growth and development of breast and ovarian cancers.	[86, 293, 294]

(continued)

Table 1 (continued)

Gene	Splice variants	Cancer type	Functional impact	References
BRCA2	Δ12-BRCA2	Breast	Overexpression of the Δ12-BRCA2 splice variant is associated with steroid receptor-negative tumors.	[295]
XPC	XPC variant lacking exon 12	Xeroderma pigmentosum	This splice variant has diminished DNA repair function and may contribute to cancer susceptibility.	[296]
Miscellaneous				
Naf1	Naf1FL Naf1 $\alpha2$ Naf1 $\beta2$ Naf1 $\alpha3$ Naf1 $\beta3$ Naf1 $\alpha4$	Acute myeloid leukemia (AML) leukemia-lymphoma cell lines	Naf1 $\alpha2$ is the main transcript. Naf1FL and Naf1 $\alpha2$ have equal NF-κB inhibitory effects, while Naf1 $\alpha4$ is less effective. Naf1 $\alpha3$ has a dominant negative effect in AML patients.	[297]
IRF-1 (Interferon regulatory factor-1)	Variants lacking some combinations of exons 7, 8, and 9	Cervical cancer	Splice variants with deletions of functional domains leading to differential transcriptional activities.	[298]
SRA1 (Steroid receptor RNA Activator 1)	SRAP	Breast cancer cell lines	Decreased estrogen receptor activity in breast cancer cells suggesting an antagonistic role for SRAP.	[299]
Syk (Spleen tyrosine kinase)	Syk(S)	Breast	Expression of Syk(S) occurs frequently in primary breast tumors and may contribute to mammary tumor progression.	[300]
WNT2B	WNT2B2	Primary gastric cancer	WNT2B2 upregulation may lead to carcinogenesis through activation of the β-catenin-TCF signaling pathway.	[301]

(continued)

Table 1 (continued)

Gene	Splice variants	Cancer type	Functional impact	References
Met (Met tyrosine kinase receptor)	Met-SM	NIH3T3 mouse fibroblasts	Met-SM may contribute to development and progression of human cancer.	[302]
ER (Estrogen Receptor)	ERβ1 ER$\beta\Delta$125 ER$\beta\Delta$1256	MDA-MD-231 breast cancer cells	ER$\beta\Delta$1256 increases cell sensitivity toward lower concentrations of tamoxifen, ERβ1 and ER$\beta\Delta$125 weaken the growth-inhibitory effect of tamoxifen.	[303]

*Although many examples are provided, the list is not exhaustive and only selected references are included variants that either facilitate or inhibit cellular proliferation have been described [28]. The cell–cell adhesion glycoprotein CD44 whose expression is associated with the metastatic potential of cancer cells [29] is produced in more than 20 splicing isoforms. Isoforms that contain exon v6 induce metastasis in mammary and pancreatic carcinomas in rats [30], while inclusion of exon v10 modifies CD44 adhesion properties and contributes to cancer progression [31]. Integrins often interact with fibronectin, itself produced in various versions. The alternate EDB- and EDA-containing isoforms of fibronectin are involved in cell adhesion and spreading [32]. In breast and colon cancers, overexpression of RonD, the splice variant of the transmembrane receptor MSF (macrophage-stimulating factor) is overexpressed, which enhances the migratory properties of cancer cells [33]. Table 1 lists additional genes whose change in alternative splicing has been shown to affect cell adhesion properties and invasiveness.

2.3 Angiogenesis

Several splicing changes affect angiogenesis, most notably those of the vascular endothelial growth factor (VEGF) in which an alternative 3′ splice site causes an antiangiogenic form to be produced in normal tissues [34]. Recently, it was also shown that prostate tumors have reduced incorporation of exon 7. Experimental inhibition of exon 7 inclusion reduced the ability of transplanted cells to induce angiogenesis in mice [35]. Exon 7 incorporation is positively regulated by the RNA-binding protein T-STAR (also known as SLM-2) [36]. VEGF expression is itself affected by the alternative splicing products of the Estrogen receptor alpha and the cholecystokin-2/gastrin receptor (CCK_2 R) [37, 38]. Another relevant event is the removal of exon 3 of Survivin, which gives it a specific function in promoting angiogenesis [39].

2.4 Resistance to Apoptosis

Alternative splicing has a strong impact on the function of proteins implicated in apoptosis. A comprehensive inventory of isoforms derived by alternative splicing of apoptotic genes and a summary of their known functions appeared recently [40]. The functional consequences of alternative splicing have been demonstrated for the death receptor Fas, as well as the adaptor and regulatory proteins APAF1 and Survivin. The function of apoptotic mediators such as Bcl-x, Bfk, Mcl1, Bim and Bid, and several caspases were also shown to be modulated by alternative splicing [40]. The alternative splicing of these genes produces isoforms that often have different and sometimes opposing activities.

A close association with cancer is particularly well documented for the splicing variants of Bcl-x. Competing 5′ splice sites dictate the expression of the Bcl-x_L and Bcl-x_S isoforms, two proteins with antagonist regulatory functions [41]. Bcl-x_L is an anti-apoptotic protein that protects the integrity of mitochondria, and is overexpressed in many types of cancer cells [42–46]. On the other hand, the pro-apoptotic isoform Bcl-x_S can heterodimerize with Bcl-x_L to abrogate its anti-apoptotic activity [47]. Furthermore, Bcl-x_L overexpression is directly responsible for the resistance of cancer cells to stresses and chemotherapeutic drugs [41, 48–56].

Another example of a splicing event linked to apoptosis is FIR, a known inhibitor of MYC. In this case, a shorter splice isoform of FIR switches protein activity to facilitate the overexpression of MYC, inhibiting apoptosis [57]. The alternative splicing of protein kinase C delta (PKCδ) was also shown to produce an isoform that can protect human teratocarcinoma cells from apoptosis [58]. Other recent examples of splice isoforms affecting apoptosis are presented in Table 1.

2.5 Multidrug Resistance

Drug transporters defend cells against cytotoxic agents. Thus, alterations in their alternative splicing may alter the efficacy of anticancer agents. One major group of transporters are known as the multidrug resistance-associated proteins (MRP; ABCC gene family). Alternative splicing of many genes in this group creates functional variants, as is the case with MRP1 that produces splicing variants conferring resistance to doxorubicin in ovarian tumors [59]. Alternative splicing of MRP4, a drug-efflux pump mediating the efflux of nucleotide analogs, generates a non-functional protein via introduction of premature termination codons [60]. Differential expression of two mRNA isoforms of the ATP-binding cassette transporter gene ABCB 5 was reported in melanoma cells [61]. Several alternatively spliced P-glycoprotein transcripts have been found in multidrug-resistant cells and their expression correlates with drug resistance [62, 63]. Finally, BCRP (ABCG2) splice variants are differentially expressed in human drug-selected breast cancer cell lines [64].

The deregulated expression of dominant negative variants of p63 and p73 lacking the transactivation domain can inhibit the transactivation of target genes and apoptosis, thus contributing to chemoresistance [65]. A splice variant of the spindle checkpoint gene Mad2 abrogates mitotic arrest and adriamycin-induced apoptosis [66]. Finally, a MAP-kinase activating death domain (MADD) splice variant of the IG20 gene suppresses tumor cell survival and enhances susceptibility to apoptosis and anticancer drugs [67].

3 Alternative Splicing Control: Basic Principles

Before discussing specific examples of molecular alterations responsible for cancer-specific splicing patterns, it is important to review some key principles of splice site control and selection. Splice site selection is determined first by the sequence of splice sites. The sequence of constitutive splice sites that are used all the time usually matches the consensus CAG/GUGAGU, for a 5′ splice site («/» indicates the junction between exon and intron), and a polypyrimidine-rich tract followed by CAG/at the 3′ splice site (Fig. 2a). In contrast, alternative splice sites usually display various mismatches to the consensus sequence, which make them intrinsically weaker splice sites. This intrinsic weakness renders them amenable to modulation by control factors that may increase or decrease their use. Hence, the use of alternative splice sites is often influenced by the presence of nearby exonic or intronic auxiliary elements that promote or repress splicing. These sequence elements function by recruiting proteins that either directly modulate splice site recognition, affect the formation of specific splicing complexes or change the conformation of the pre-mRNA to promote the use of certain splice site combinations.

Direct modulation of splice site recognition is promoted by members of the SR family of proteins, which are frequently associated with stimulatory elements. However, other types of proteins with stimulatory activity have been identified (for example, CELF, hnRNP H, hnRNP L, TIA1, and TIAR) [68]. When these proteins are bound in the proximity of a splice site, they may interact with other components of the splicing machinery (U1 snRNP at the 5′ splice site or U2AF at the 3′ splice site) to improve their binding (Fig. 2b). Alternatively, some sequence elements located near splice sites may repress their use (Fig. 2c) by recruiting proteins that hinder the recognition or utilization of the adjacent splice sites.

In addition to the direct role of proteins recruited in the vicinity of a splice site, changes in the conformation of the pre-mRNA may also influence splicing decisions. These changes sometimes involve the formation of a secondary structure that blocks the utilization of a splice site [69]. In other cases, the changes are induced by an interaction between proteins bound at different locations on a pre-mRNA. Such spatial rearrangement can stimulate the use of a splice site located outside of the loop, and may simultaneously repress splice sites located inside that loop (Fig. 2d). Although this model was initially proposed to explain the mechanism of action of the hnRNP A1 protein in alternative splicing [70–72], it is also relevant to the mechanism of action of hnRNP H, and possibly hnRNP I/PTB and Nova-1 proteins [72–75]. hnRNP A1 may also counteract the activity of certain SR proteins through a different model which proposes that hnRNP A1 can nucleate and spread over regions of a pre-mRNA through cooperative RNA binding [76, 77].

Detailed investigations of selected alternative splicing events indicate that splice site selection is determined by a combination of several layers of positive and negative regulators. Thus, the frequency with which a given alternative splicing pattern is used will be determined by: (1) the intrinsic strength of each splice site involved, (2) the number, identity, and the position of control elements, and (3) the relative concentration and affinity of each RNA-binding protein to its respective binding site. The phosphorylation of specific SR and hnRNP proteins will also have an impact on splice site selection since this modification can affect their activity and cellular distribution [78].

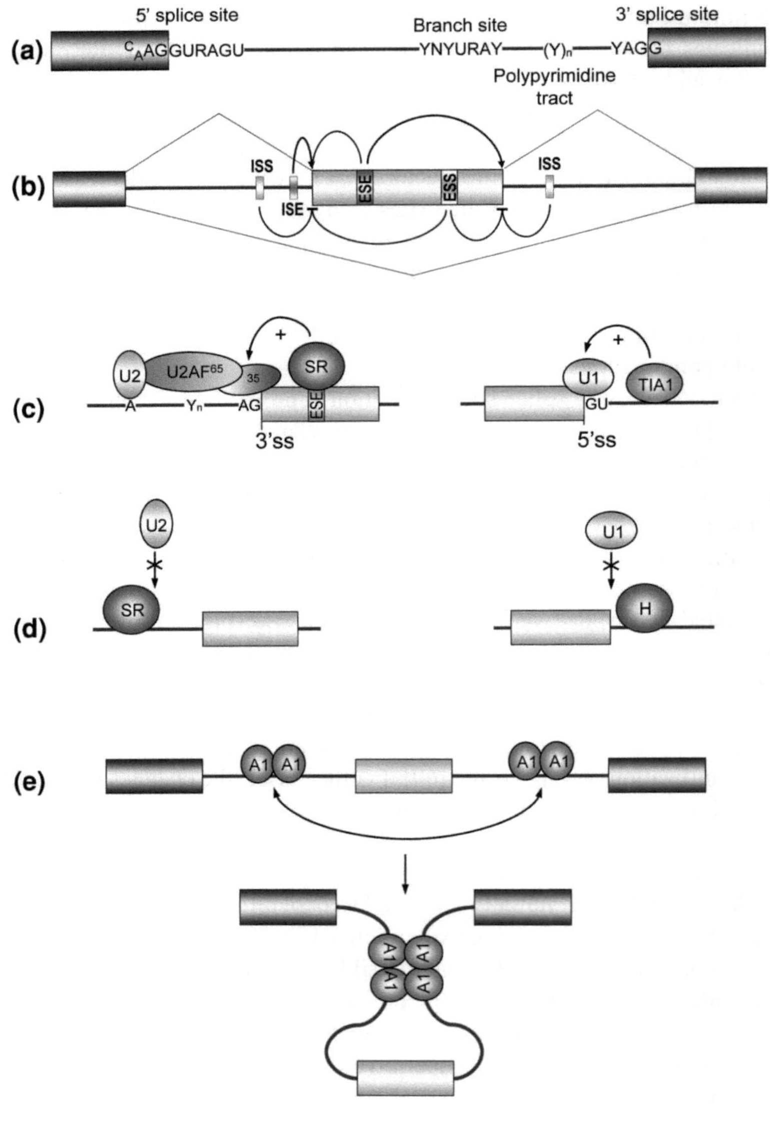

4 Molecular Basis for Splicing Alterations in Cancer

Different types of molecular perturbations can cause alterations in alternative splicing profiles. Point mutations at splice sites have been linked to numerous diseases and have been proposed to account for 15 % of human genetic diseases [2, 79]. This number is likely to be considerably larger since mutations in introns, which constitute the majority of the gene sequence, are rarely considered. A recent

◀**Fig. 2** Control of splice site selection. **a** Schematic representation of a splicing unit (*top*) and an alternative splicing unit (*bottom*). The consensus sequences of a 5′ splice site, a branch site and a 3′ splice site are shown. *R* purine, *Y* pyrimidine. Elements that control splicing decisions are shown and include positively acting exonic and intronic splicing enhancers (ESEs and ISEs, respectively), as well as negatively acting exonic and intronic splicing silencers (ESSs, ISSs, respectively). **b** Proteins bound to exonic or intronic enhancers can recruit or stabilize the binding of splicing factors to the 3′ (*left*) or 5′ (*right*) splice site. In the illustrated examples, an SR protein bound to an ESE enhances U2AF and U2 snRNP binding to the 3′ splice site/branch site region [102, 217], while binding of TIA1 to ISE can stimulate recognition of an adjacent upstream 5′ splice site by the U1 snRNP [126]. **c** Splicing inhibition. Steric interference caused by the presence of a protein bound in the proximity of a splice site impedes its recognition. The SR and hnRNP H proteins can, respectively, inhibit the binding of the U2 and U1 snRNPs [218], [219]. **d** Change in pre-mRNA conformation can be promoted by an interaction between hnRNP A1 proteins bound to introns flanking an alternative exon, provoking repression of the looped out exon, and stimulation of splicing between the distal pair of exons [72]

study suggests that as much as 60 % of the point mutations that cause genetic diseases affect splicing decisions [80]. Thus, we can anticipate that several cancer-related genes sustain mutations at splice sites or in regions bound by proteins that control the selection of splice sites. Exonic mutations that create a stop codon can also affect the function of a splicing control element, thereby modifying splicing profiles [81]. In other cases, missense mutations, again through changes in splicing, may have a more profound impact on protein structure than the predicted change in amino acids caused by the mutations. Finally, even mutations that are considered to be neutral because they do not change amino acids can have an impact on alternative splicing [2, 3]. The following sections present some examples of mutations (Fig. 3) and changes in the expression of splicing factors (Fig. 4) that affect the splicing of cancer-associated genes.

4.1 Mutations at Splice Sites and in Auxiliary Elements

According to the Cancer Genome Project of the Welcome Trust Sanger Institute (http://www.sanger.ac.uk/genetics/CGP/Census/), about 363 human genes have mutations that have been associated with cancer; 90 % of these genes have somatic mutations, approximately 20 % show germline mutations that predispose to cancer, and 10 % show both somatic and germline mutations. Specifically, 42 of these 363 genes have sustained mutations that affect splicing. Splicing mutations are the most prevalent type of mutations found in the NF1 gene, which is implicated in neurofibromatosis, the most common form of autosomal dominant cancer in humans [82]. Mutations in the splice sites of NF2 are used as markers to grade the severity of the disease [83].

Similarly, approximately 30 mutations affecting the splice sites of p53 have been reported in different cancers [84]. Another interesting example concerns the tumor suppressor gene APC, where two mutations have been closely associated with the development of familial adenomatous polyposis [85]. One of these mutations creates a splice site that promotes the deletion of one nucleotide resulting in the production of a truncated APC protein. Other mutations that weaken or create new splice sites in different genes associated with cancers are listed in Fig. 3. This list includes well-known genes such BRCA1, BRCA2, CDKN2, PTEN, KIT, ATM, and XPC.

Mutations in *cis*-acting splicing regulatory elements can also modify the relative abundance of splicing variants or induce the utilization of new splice sites. For example, a mutation of an exonic element in the BRCA1 gene reduces the binding of ASF/SF2, thereby increasing the exclusion of exon 18 [86]. Many mutations that affect splicing control elements have been described in the BRCA1 gene [87]. A polymorphism in the intron upstream of exon 2 in KLF6 creates a binding site for SRp40 that activates cryptic sites in exon 2 [88]. This mutation is associated with an increased risk of prostate cancer. The altered KLF6 proteins may counteract the tumor-suppressor activity of the wild-type protein. Intronic and exonic mutations in the cadherin CDH17 gene that do not directly affect the splice junctions have been proposed to interfere with splicing decisions [89]. Other examples of this type of mutation have been reported in NF1, APC, and MLH1 genes (Fig. 3).

The diversity of splicing control elements suggests that most intronic or exonic mutations that were initially considered silent mutations may in fact have an important impact on constitutive and alternative splicing. For the same reasons, a large subset of single nucleotide polymorphisms (SNPs) found within the human population may modulate alternative splicing. For example, a SNP in an SRp40 binding site in the APC gene correlates with exon omission and attenuated familial adenomatous polyposis [90]. These differences may predispose some individuals to develop certain types of cancers, while other polymorphisms may increase their resistance. Consistent with this view, a recent study has identified a high frequency of alternative splicing in microsatellite regions linked with human longevity or resistance to anticancer treatments [91].

4.2 Alterations in the Activity of Splicing Proteins

While many *cis*-acting mutations have been shown to affect splicing, the majority of alterations in alternative splicing profiles appear to proceed from changes in the expression or activity of splicing factors [4]. Because a proof for the direct contribution of such changes to cancer is not always available, only experimentally proven cases will be discussed below.

4.2.1 Chromosomal Translocations

In some cancers, as in Ewing's sarcomas, chromosomal translocations affect the genes EWS and TLS (FUS or hnRNP P2) that encode RNA-binding proteins. The interaction of these proteins with splicing factors such as SF1, U1C, YB-1 and some SR proteins may explain why their translocation has an impact on splicing control [92–95]. Translocations between these genes and transcription factors of the ETS family result in the production of chimeric proteins with strong transcriptional activity and oncogenic properties, as for example EWS-FLI1,

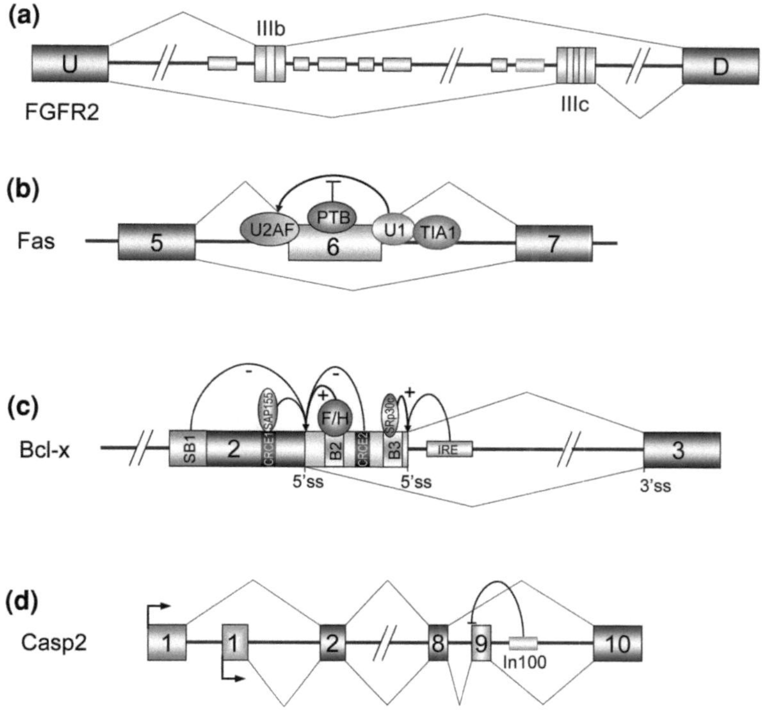

Fig. 3 Alternative splicing of selected cancer-related genes (see main text for details)

EWS-NOR1, and TLS-ERG [96]. The failure of the hybrid proteins EWS-FLI1 and TLS-ERG to recruit the YB-1 and SR proteins may compromise their role in splicing [95, 97]. The interaction of EWS-FLI1 and TLS-ERG with transcriptionally active form of RNA polymerase II [94, 95, 98] may affect the cotranscriptional selection of splice sites. EWS-NOR1 can interact with the snRNP protein U1C. EWS-NOR1 can also enhance the use of a distal 5′ splice site in a reporter pre-mRNA more efficiently than the EWS protein alone [99]. In leukemia, the well-known Bcr-Abl translocation has been associated with splicing defects in SLP65, Bruton's tyrosine kinase, Pyk2 and Ikaros. However, the mechanism responsible for these alterations may be indirect since Bcr-Abl enhances the expression of SRPK1, a kinase that modulates the activity of SR proteins [100].

4.2.2 Alterations in the Expression and Localization of Splicing Control Factors

Viral transformation was first associated with the upregulation and increased activity of SR proteins [101], and this change affected fibronectin pre-mRNA splicing [102]. The first case of a deregulation in the expression of hnRNP and SR proteins in cancer cells was observed in colon adenocarcinomas [103]. Since then, alterations in the expression of a variety of RNA-binding proteins have been

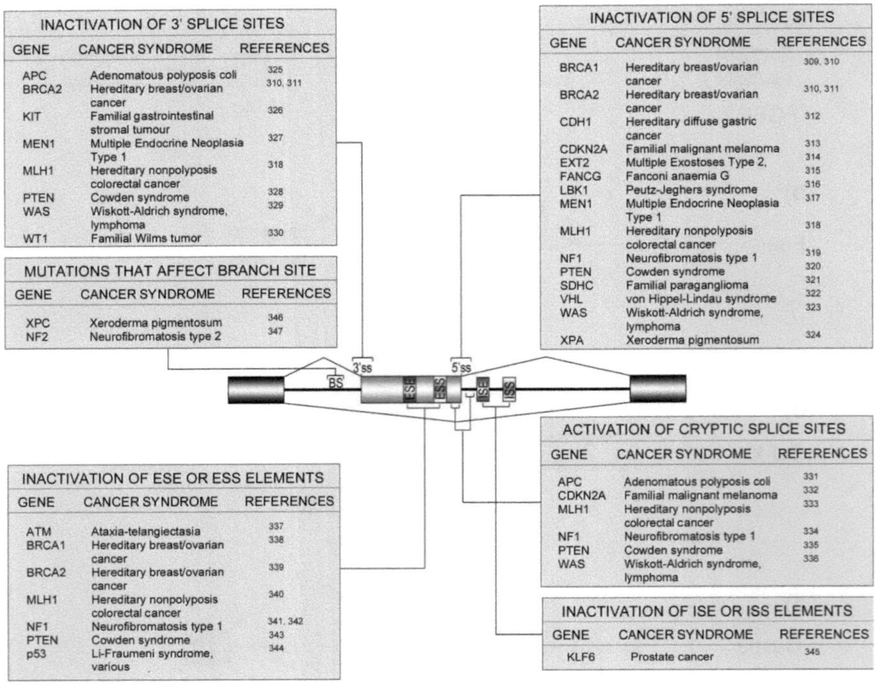

Fig. 4 Specific examples of mutations reported to affect alternative splicing in cancer. Mutations are organized according to their impact on the inactivation or activation of splice sites by directly changing the structure of the splicing signals or control elements. The name of the gene that is affected, the type of cancer in which it was reported, and relevant references are given

reported in different types of cancers [104] (see Table 2). For example, expression of the SR protein ASF/SF2 is upregulated in many types of cancers and can elicit the transformation of immortal rodent fibroblasts [105]. Notably, ASF/SF2 shifts the alternative splicing of three pre-mRNAs: BIN1 produces an isoform that lacks tumor–suppressor activity; a MNK2 kinase variant can phosphorylate eiF4E in a MAP kinase-independent manner; the S6K1 kinase is spliced to produce an oncogenic isoform [105]. Since ASF/SF2 overexpression in breast cancer has been linked to cell motility through the production of RonD [33], ASF/SF2 may contribute to early and late steps of carcinogenesis.

While over expression of SR proteins has been linked to cancer, downregulation and altered phosphorylation are relevant to apoptosis, a process that is often defective in cancer cells. A reduction in ASF/SF2 can induce apoptosis. Genomic DNA fragmentation is blocked because the drop in ASF/SF2 changes the alternative splicing profile of the ICAD nuclease to favor the expression of the inactive isoform [106]. Similarly, induction of the apoptotic pathway through activation of the death receptor Fas dephosphorylates SR proteins [107]. Fas and the anticancer drug gemcitabine increase the levels of ceramide that activates protein phosphatase 1 (PP1), which in turn can act on SR proteins. Since ceramide

Table 2 Altered expression of splicing factors associated with a functional impact in cell growth

Splicing factor	Cancer type	Functional impact	References
SR proteins	Colon adenocarcinomas	mRNA levels of different SR proteins are usually lower in tumor samples compared to nonpathological tissues surrounding the tumor. This reduction is more drastic in patients showing an important alteration in CD44 splicing and may be related to the development of metastases	[103]
Tra2β1	Breast	A significant induction of Tra2β1 is found in invasive breast cancer. Given the role Tra2β1 in the alternative splicing of CD44, Tra2β1 expression may affect tumor progression and metastasis	[123]
SRp55	Breast	Higher expression of SRp55 protein is associated with an altered pattern of CD44 variants incorporating exon v7	[304]
SC35 and ASF/SF2	Ovarian	SC35 and ASF/SF2 are induced in ovarian cancer tissues. Their altered expression may be linked with changes in the alternative splicing of CD44	[117]
SF2/ASF	Breast, colon	SF2/ASF promotes the production of the RonD isoform to regulate cell motility and locomotion. Increased SF2/ASF expression is also associated with the redistribution of β-catenin, reorganization of cytoskeleton, and downregulation of E-cadherin. SF2/ASF may play a role in regulating malignant transformation by inducing a RonD-mediated epithelial to mesenchymal transition. SF2/ASF is upregulated in various tumors. SF2/ASF controls the alternative splicing of tumor suppressor BIN1 and the kinases MNK2 and S6K1 favoring splicing of BIN1 isoforms that lack tumor-suppressor activity. Thus the splicing factor SF2/ASF can act as an oncoprotein. Knockdown of ASF/SF2 promotes apoptosis	[33] [105] [106]
SRm160	Various	Upon Ras activation, overexpression of SRm160 stimulates expression of the CD44 isoforms that contain exon v5. Such isoforms correlate with enhanced malignancy and invasiveness	[122]

(continued)

Table 2 (continued)

Splicing factor	Cancer type	Functional impact	References
SRPK1 (Serine-arginine protein kinase 1)	Breast, colon, dysplastic and neoplastic pancreatic ductal cells	SRPK1 is overexpressed in breast and colon cancers and its expression increases with tumor grade levels. Knockdown of SRPK1 in breast and colon cancer cell lines increases the gemcitabine and cisplatin-induced apoptotic response	[174]
PTB (hnRNP I)	Glioblastomas	The expression of PTB in malignant glioblastomas is increased relative to glial cells. This overexpression correlates with increased skipping of the FGFR1α exon	[115]
PTB and SRp20	Ovarian	Both PTB and SRp20 are overexpressed in most ovarian tumors. This overexpression correlates with the increased number of splice variants of MRP1	[59]
hnRNP A1/A2	Various	The expression of hnRNP A1/A2 proteins is elevated in a variety of cancers, whereas A1/A2 expression is lower in normal tissues. Knockdown of hnRNP A1/A2 proteins induces apoptosis of cancer cell lines but not mortal cell lines. hnRNP A1 has been implicated in the alternative splicing of CD44 and Bcl-x	[120], [305–308]
SRPK1 (Serine-arginine protein kinase 1)	Breast, colon, dysplastic and neoplastic pancreatic ductal cells	SRPK1 is overexpressed in breast and colon cancers and its expression increases with tumor grade levels. Knockdown of SRPK1 in breast and colon cancer cell lines increases the gemcitabine and cisplatin-induced apoptotic response	[174]

*Only selected examples are listed

promotes a shift toward the production of the pro-apoptotic Bcl-x_S protein, a reduction in phosphorylation of SR proteins may elicit apoptosis.

An increase in the levels of hnRNP I/PTB and SRp20 in ovarian cancers that are resistant to doxorubicin correlates with the overexpression of some isoforms of the multidrug resistance protein MRP1 [59]. Moreover, PTB knockdown suppresses growth and invasiveness [108]. Overexpression of the alternative splicing factor SPF45 is often observed in tumors and may confer resistance to chemotherapeutic agents [109].

Components of the constitutive splicing machinery may also be subject to differential regulation in tumors. The branchpoint binding protein SF1 is down-regulated in mouse intestinal tumorigenesis. Expression of SF1 is regulated by β-catenin and it affects alternative splicing of several genes including WISP1, FGFR3 and the Estrogen receptor-beta [110]. In pancreatic tumors, the expression of U2AF35 (part of the other main protein complex that recognizes 3′ splice sites) is also often repressed. This situation promotes the synthesis of a constitutively active isoform of the CCK-B receptor and a resulting stimulation of cellular proliferation [111]. The breast cancer-associated scaffold attachment factor SAFB1 interacts with a plethora of splicing factors and affects splicing [112].

In general, however, while several studies have reported increased expression of specific RNA-binding proteins in cancer tissues, the functional impact of these differences in the alternative splicing of important genes in cancer remains poorly documented. A few of the most important cases where this link has been established are presented below.

FGFRs. Approximately 10 distinct elements control the alternative splicing of the mutually exclusive IIIb and IIIc exons in FGFR2 (Fig. 4a). Fox-2 and hnRNP I/PTB proteins have been implicated in the activity of some of these controlling elements [113, 114]. hnRNP I/PTB also controls the alternative splicing of FGFR1. Interestingly, the high levels of hnRNP I/PTB in glioblastomas may promote the exclusion of exon α, thereby improving its affinity for the ligand [115].

*CD*44. An increase in the expression of some SR proteins is associated with the progression from the pre-neoplastic to the metastatic status of mammary tumors [103, 116]. This observation correlates with modifications in the alternative splicing of the cell-surface glycoprotein CD44 in human mammary tumors [103]. In ovarian cancers, an increase in the expression of SR proteins and their hyper-phosphorylated forms has also been observed [117]. In addition, exon v9 of CD44 contains a stimulatory element that can be bound by low molecular weight SR proteins [118].

Sam68 and hnRNP A1 also contribute to the alternative splicing of CD44 by controlling the inclusion of exon v5 [119, 120]. A protein of the same family as Sam68, T-STAR (SLM2), can also bind to the v5 exon to promote its inclusion and this is antagonized by other RNA-binding proteins such as SRp30c, hnRNP G, and SAF-B, as well as by SIAH-1, a ubiquitin ligase and candidate tumor suppressor [121]. The inclusion of exon v5 is stimulated by the phosphorylation of Sam68 following activation of the Ras signaling pathway. This stimulation requires the participation of the splicing co-activator SRm160, which interacts with Sam68

[122]. As demonstrated in a recent study, the binding of Tra2β to exon v4 of CD44 and its synergic action with the nucleic acid-binding protein YB-1 enhance the inclusion of both exons v4 and v5 [123].

Interestingly, overexpression of Brm, a component of the SWI/SNF chromatin remodeling complex can promote the inclusion of the v5–v9 exons through a process that requires Sam68 [124].

Ron. The binding of the SR protein ASF/SF2 to a sequence of exon 12 on the pre-mRNA of Ron, a tyrosine kinase transmembrane receptor, improves the utilization of its 3′ splice site and enhances the exclusion of the immediate upstream exon 11. Upregulation of ASF/SF2 in cancer cells is associated with enhanced exon 11 skipping and generation of RonD, an isoform that improves the motility and invasive properties of these cells. RonD is upregulated in metastatic breast and colon cancers [33, 125].

Fas. Alternative splicing of the pre-mRNA encoding the cell death receptor Fas generates two isoforms through inclusion or skipping of exon 6. The membrane-bound long isoform activates the extrinsic apoptotic pathway, while the soluble short isoform that lacks the transmembrane domain is an anti-apoptotic factor. The production of the long isoform is facilitated by TIA1 and TIAR that bind to a U-rich sequence situated immediately downstream of the 5′ splice site of alternative exon 6. These proteins stimulate the binding of the U1 snRNP at this 5′ splice site (Fig. 4b) [126]. In contrast, the exclusion of exon 6 is enhanced by the binding of hnRNP I/PTB to exon 6 which interferes with the communication between the downstream U1 snRNP bound to the 5′ splice site and U2AF bound to the upstream 3′ splice site [127].

Bcl-x. The alternative use of two 5′ splice sites produces the pro- and anti-apoptotic isoforms of Bcl-x (Fig. 4c). Several regulatory elements have been identified in the regions flanking these splice sites. Intronic regulatory elements (IRE) may repress the use of the 5′ splice site of Bcl-x_L following induction by IL-6 and GM-CSF, or treatment with TPA [128]. In addition, two exonic regions known as CRCE1 and CRCE2 mediate the pro-apoptotic effect conferred by ceramide on the splicing of Bcl-x [129]. Given that the U2 snRNP-associated protein SAP155 binds to CRCE1 and that its genetic depletion by RNA interference also promotes Bcl-x_S usage, the signaling pathway activated by ceramide possibly prevents SAP155 binding. More recently, a role for Sam68 has also been uncovered [130]. Although the *cis*-acting element mediating this function is currently unknown, Sam68 appears to interact with hnRNP A1 to elicit a splicing shift toward Bcl-x_S. Three other regions have been identified as important for controlling the use of the alternative 5′ splice sites. One of them (B2) is specifically bound by hnRNP F/H proteins and is required to enforce the use of Bcl-x_S 5′ splice site [131]. The B3 region is bound by SRp30c and enforces Bcl-x_L usage [132]. Finally, a region (SB1) upstream of the Bcl-x_S 5′ splice site distinct from CRCE1 represses the use of the 5′ splice site of Bcl-x_S. This SB1-dependent splicing repression is lifted by drugs that inactivate protein kinase C, as well as by a variety of anticancer agents [133, 134]. The pathways that control this aspect of Bcl-x_S splicing vary considerably between different cancer cell lines.

Caspase 2. Members of the SR and hnRNP family of proteins participate in the alternative splicing control of caspase 2 [135]. Overexpressing SR proteins enhances the exclusion of exon 9 to favor the production of the pro-apoptotic isoform Casp2L. In contrast, overexpressing hnRNP A1 stimulates the inclusion of exon 9 and the production of the anti-apoptotic isoform Casp2S [136]. The intronic sequence In100 is a control element modulating the alternative splicing of caspase 2 (Fig. 4d). This element is bound by hnRNP I/PTB and it prevents splicing between exons 9 and 10 through formation of a nonproductive complex with splicing factors recruited at the In100 site [137].

4.2.3 Other Perturbations that Impact Alternative Splicing

As discussed above, cancer cells can accumulate genetic changes that directly affect the splicing machinery or splicing regulatory elements in pre-mRNAs to deregulate alternative splicing patterns. In addition, at least four other molecular processes may affect the production of splicing variants to impact on carcinogenesis. These include transcription, RNA editing, NMD, and signal transduction events.

Transcription

Simple overexpression of pre-mRNAs may contribute to deregulated alternative splicing. For overexpressed pre-mRNAs, there might not be enough available control factors to modulate their splicing. In addition, the sequestration of splicing factors by this pre-mRNA may affect the splicing of other pre-mRNAs, similar to the situation occurring when triplet repeat expansion in the 3′ untranslated region of the DMPK pre-mRNA sequesters MBNL with an impact on the alternative splicing of cardiac troponin T, tau, insulin receptor, ClC-1, and myotubularin-related 1 pre-mRNAs [138, 139].

The mechanistic coupling of RNA synthesis by RNA polymerase II to alternative splice site choice has been documented [140, 141]. Both enhancer and core promoter elements can modulate the alternative splicing of their nascent pre-mRNA [142, 143]. Promoter identity can control alternative splicing through the differential recruitment of transcription factors and cofactors, such as Brm [124], CoAA [144] and Spi-1 [145], or by recruitment of specific splicing factors, such as SRp20 [146]. Ultimately, promoter-specific transcription complexes can dictate alternative splice site choice by altering the rate of elongation and/or the processivity of RNA polymerase II [147, 148], or through physical interactions with the splicing machinery. Consequently, factors that modify the status of chromatin that change the intrinsic speed of the transcriptional complex or that modify its sensitivity to pausing sites can potentially affect alternative splicing.

In addition to the impact of different complexes at a single promoter on alternative splicing, there is now convincing evidence for the impact of multiple promoters of a single gene on alternative splicing. For Bcl-x [149] and caspase-2 [150], the choice of alternative promoters can define the ratio of splice variant expression. The literature now contains a growing list of genes that contain alternative promoters [151]. In fact, a recent bioinformatics analysis estimated that 52 % of human genes contain alternative promoters [152]. In this context, oncogenic alterations of transcription factors, as well as genetic or epigenetic changes in promoter regions could influence the alternative splicing patterns in tumor cells. We already know that there must be considerable tissue- and cancer-specific variations in the combinatorial assemblies at promoters. What remains to be discovered is the extent of the contribution of these transcriptional aspects to global patterns of alternative splicing in cancer.

RNA Editing

RNA editing is a process that directly modifies specific adenosine residues into inosines [153]. RNA editing can influence the secondary structure of specific pre-mRNAs in preparation for splicing. In some types of tumors, editing defects can affect the alternative splicing of the PTPN6 phosphatase and glutamate receptor pre-mRNAs [154, 155]. Because the contribution of RNA editing to the alternative splicing of cancer-related genes has not been investigated systematically, it is likely that more examples of this type exist.

NMD

NMD is a surveillance process that eliminates mRNA molecules containing a stop codon localized more than 50 nucleotides upstream of exon/exon junction [156, 157]. Therefore, NMD can potentially neutralize the impact of mutations that create new termination codons [157, 158]. While NMD can affect the accumulation of some splicing variants, its widespread contribution in controlling the expression of splicing isoforms is unlikely [15] but controversial [159]. Interestingly, the non-productive isoforms of splicing factors that are generated from the alternative splicing of exons enriched in ultra conserved sequences form a distinct class of NMD-regulated transcripts [17, 19].

It is possible but yet undocumented that changes in the expression or activity of factors involved in regulation of the NMD may promote the accumulation of the mutated or aberrantly spliced transcripts and therefore may contribute to cancer. Although the number of examples supporting a role for NMD in cancer remains small [160, 161], this pathway appears to contribute to the elimination of mRNA encoding proteins involved in drug-resistance [60]. Such alterations in the NMD pathway may contribute to tumorigenesis.

Signal Transduction

Cell signaling impacts alternative splicing [162, 163] and a typical means by which such changes can be mediated is by the phosphorylation of SR proteins, which causes them to accumulate in different subcellular compartments [164]. The upregulation of PKA and the $MKK_{3/6}$/p38 signaling pathway results in the cytoplasmic localization of hnRNP I/PTB and hnRNP A1, respectively [165, 166]. Another splicing factor displaying this behavior is KSRP, which is implicated in the inclusion a specific exon in the c-src mRNA in neurons [167]. KSRP accumulates in the nucleus when neuroblastoma cells are induced to differentiate [167]. Therefore, the altered subcellular localization of splicing factors via their post-translational modification can potentially play a role in the deregulation of splicing in cancer cells. The impact of splicing factor localization on the cancer phenotype is likely underappreciated, as documenting changes in localization is considerably more laborious than determining changes in total expression levels of the mRNA or protein.

The interface between signal transduction and splice site selection is just beginning to be explored. The Ras/PI 3-kinase/AKT pathway is often activated in human cancer [168]. This pathway can modulate the activity of SR proteins to affect the alternative splicing of fibronectin and PKC βII [169, 170]. The Ras-dependent signaling pathway is also implicated in the alternative splicing of CD44 [171]. The intricate interplay between alternative splicing and cell signaling is illustrated by the fact that just as signaling affects alternative splicing, so alternative splicing can affect signaling. For example, the inclusion of exon v6 in CD44 promoted by Ras helps to sustain late Ras signaling [172]. The SR protein kinase SRPK1 is overexpressed in many types of cancers and its downregulation increases the sensitivity of cells to anticancer drugs [173], and MAP2 K is alternatively spliced in response to activation of SRPK1 [174]. Another recent example of a link between signaling and splicing control involves the Notch3 signaling pathway which regulates the splicing of Ikaros in leukemia by inducing the RNA-binding protein HuD [175–177]. The deregulated expression of CDK12 and cyclin L1/L2 can also affect alternative splicing decisions [178].

Thus, it would not be too surprising if cancer-specific alterations in signaling pathways impact the production of isoforms that contribute to neoplastic transformation. However, the contribution of signal transduction events to splicing decisions that are relevant to cancer remains to be more fully investigated.

Arginine methylation of splicing factors also affects their localization and activity [179, 180]. Recently, the arginine methylase CARM1 was shown to control splicing decisions [181]. Although cancer-specific defects in the arginine methylation of splicing factors are yet to be reported, important contributions of this pathway to various aspects of cell growth can be anticipated.

5 Outlooks and Challenges

5.1 Global Detection of Splicing Variation in Cancer

The existence of cancer-specific signatures made up of individual alternative splicing events was initially investigated by using large-scale compilation of cDNAs and expressed-sequences tags (ESTs). Computational approaches revealed considerable differences between the alternative splicing patterns of normal and cancer prostate tissues [182, 183]. Genome-wide profiling of splicing events became possible with the development of DNA oligonucleotide microarrays. Using this technology, one of the first observations was that the genes displaying tissue-specific alternative splicing were largely different from the genes presenting tissue-specific differences in steady-state expression levels [184]. Indeed, a quarter of the genes that showed alternative splicing between normal and cancerous prostate had no detectable change in overall gene expression level [185]. A similar conclusion was obtained when mining for differences in expression profiles and the detection of splicing isoforms between melanoma and melanocytes [186]. Overall, the classification of tumors was improved when alternative splicing was considered, strongly arguing in favor of mining the wealth of alternative splicing diversity for the purpose of developing a complementary disease-specific signature that could have diagnostic and prognostic value.

Splicing-sensitive arrays were generated using limited sets of alternative splice junction probes and used to detect splicing changes in cancer tissues. For example, changes in splicing profiles and the abundance of splicing factors in Hodgkin lymphoma was observed using an array that measured mRNA levels and 100 splicing events [187]. More recently, a similar design was used to compare alternative splicing of 64 genes in breast cancer cell lines and xenografts [188]. In this case, four genes were found to be differentially spliced between breast cancer and normal cell lines and four other tumor-associated genes were spliced differently according to cell culture conditions.

A new technique called DASL was developed to measure the expression of cancer-related splice isoforms. This technique combines targeted microarray and PCR techniques and treats splicing isoforms as separate genes. DASL therefore estimates changes in global gene expression level, as a normal microarray does, while providing additional information on the ratio of splice isoforms variants [189]. Recently, this approach has been used for the analysis of 1,500 different splice variants from 364 genes in six prostate tumor cell lines and 22 prostate tumors [185, 190]. Fourteen genes had different isoforms whose expression in normal tissues inversely correlated with their expression in tumor samples, implying a likely switch in alternative splicing.

Companies have also designed microarrays for cancer biomarker discovery using known alternatively spliced junction probes identified through bioinformatics mining of EST libraries. The Jivan cancer-specific splice variant array covers 524 putative cancer-specific splices although this has been largely superseded by their total splice form microarray that includes 193,000 specific splice junctions. ExonHit also has pathway-specific microarrays and a 'genome-wide' alternative splice junction microarray. The other approach to splicing discovery is to print probes for every exon:exon junction and deduce alternative splicing patterns from the relative junction expression patterns. The first large-scale splicing microarrays using this approach covered about half of the known exon:exon junctions in the human transcriptome and monitored splicing globally in multiple normal and cancer cell lines [191]. Affymetrix now produces a Human Exon GeneChip microarray that detects over 1,000,000 different human exons. This was used to compare splicing between ten matched normal tumor colon cancer pairs and nine high confidence differences were confirmed by RT-PCR [192].

One drawback of most current global approaches is that they rely on previously documented splicing events and are therefore not designed to discover novel splicing events. Because our current collection of existing splicing events is likely incomplete, biased, and poorly validated, there is a need to incorporate strategies that can identify novel splicing events and technologies that can accurately validate the quantitative differences detected between samples. Current microarray technologies may be superseded in the future by high-throughput sequencing technologies of single molecules [193]. However, although all the above approaches are designed to improve the annotation and assessment of alternative splicing events, they all fail to provide a description of the complete structure of splice isoforms. Indeed, pre-mRNA often sustains multiple alternative splicing events, sometimes involving regions that are far apart. Given that splicing decisions taken in one region can affect the splicing outcome of an apparently distinct unit [194], we cannot assume that all combinations of potential isoforms are represented in the mRNA population. The only currently reliable way to obtain this information remains through cDNA cloning and large-scale projects in this direction would provide a useful complement to current high-throughput mapping efforts directed at specific alternative splicing units.

5.2 Depleting Specific Splice Isoforms

We have seen that mutations in splicing elements of key genes and expression defects of splicing control factors can contribute to neoplastic transformation. The alterations in the splicing profiles observed in tumors may lead to the production of novel isoforms. In other cases, the isoforms may correspond to molecules that are normally expressed in other cell types or at other stages of development. Most frequently, splicing alterations will involve differences in the relative abundance of isoforms already expressed in the normal tissue. Although several of these alterations may have a neutral impact, other splicing alterations may confer growth advantages to cancer cells. For example, the signaling pathways that inhibit cell proliferation or induce cell death may be neutralized leading to cell propagation and invasion. Considering the enormous potential for diversity emanating from alternative splicing, the number of isoforms that are known to affect the growth of cancer cells is most probably vastly underestimated. More extensive annotation of the function of different isoforms is a priority that represents a challenge both in terms of commitment and methodology.

To help with the goal of attributing function to splice variants, the RNA interference (RNAi) technology represents a useful approach because it can be used to reduce the expression of specific isoforms. Although this approach has been used successfully in *Drosophila* cells [195], it is yet to be used in a systematic manner in human cells. If RNA interference-based approaches turn out to promote transcriptional silencing in addition to RNA degradation [196, 197], depletion of specific mRNA isoforms may only be possible with siRNAs targeting exon-exon junctions. This caveat could seriously compromise the use of RNA interference as a tool to assess isoform function.

5.3 Reprogramming Alternative Splicing

A different approach aims at reprogramming alternative splicing decisions. The spectacular physiological improvement obtained by reprogramming the Duchenne muscular dystrophy gene in a mouse model [198] supports applying this strategy to cancer. The original version of the approach employs a complementary oligonucleotide to cover the targeted splice site (Fig. 5a). By blocking the 5′ splice site of the anti-apoptotic Bcl-x_L with 2′-O-methyl oligonucleotides, Mercatante et al. [199]

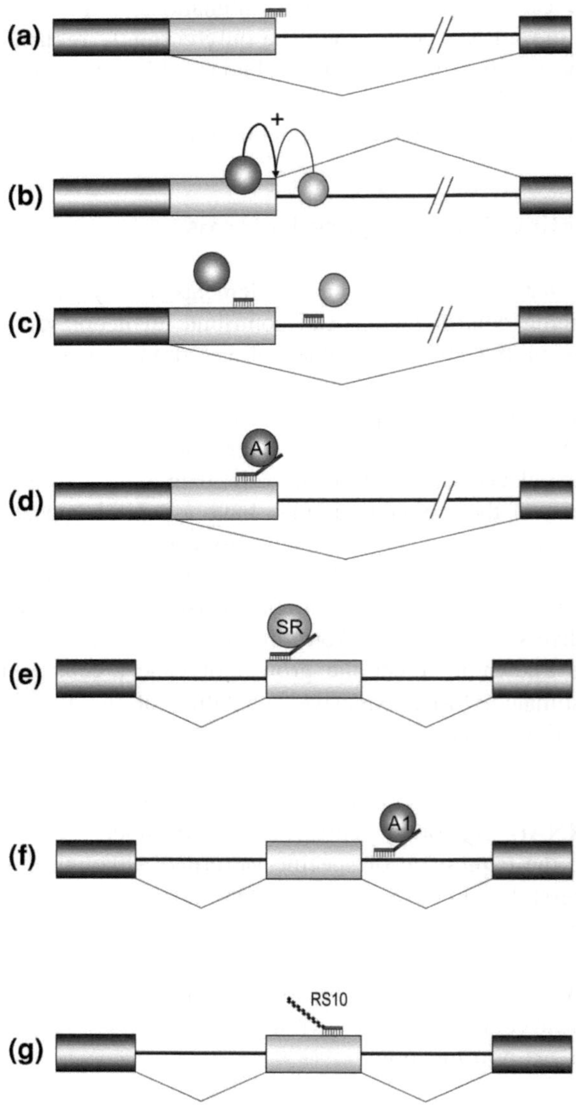

◀**Fig. 5** Reprogramming of alternative splicing through use of oligonucleotides. **a** An oligonucleotide blocking a splice site favors the use of an alternative site. **b** Oligonucleotides complementary to exonic or intronic controlling elements can prevent the binding of control factors. If these elements are ESEs and ISEs as shown, the oligos will stimulate splicing to an alternative site. **c** A complex between hnRNP A1 protein and the tail of an oligonucleotide partially complementary to an exonic sequence can provoke steric interference to reduce the use of a splice site and favor alternative splice site selection. **d** When the tail of the oligo contains a sequence of high affinity for a SR protein, splicing to the adjacent site can be stimulated. **e** If the hnRNP A1 binding tail is contained in an oligo complementary to an intron region near the 5′ splice site, splicing stimulation can occur. **f** A PNA (*peptide-nucleic acid*) portion covalently linked to an RNA sequence complementary to an exon can stimulate exon inclusion when the PNA tail contains repetitions of the dipeptide arginine-serine to mimic the RS domain of SR proteins

could decrease the concentrations of the Bcl-x_L isoform and increase the level of the corresponding pro-apoptotic Bcl-x_S isoform. This change in the splicing profile of Bcl-x increased the sensitivity of cells to chemotherapeutic agents and even induced apoptosis in some cell lines [200]. Similar approaches have been successfully applied on the FGFR1 and the MYC pre-mRNAs [201, 202].

An alternative strategy involves using antisense oligonucleotides that target splicing control elements (Fig. 5b). An oligonucleotide complementary to a sequence upstream of 5′ splice site of Bcl-x_L strongly repressed the use of this site [203] probably because its hybridization neutralizes a positive controlling element [131]. In a similar way, inactivating intronic repressor elements can also be used to modulate alternative splicing [202, 204]. Modification of the oligonucleotide with a non-hybridizing tail that contains one or several binding sites for a protein produces a bifunctional oligonucleotide that can recruit factors to a specific region on the pre-mRNA. For example, binding of hnRNP A1 to the tail of a bifunctional oligonucleotide sterically interferes with the efficient utilization of a neighboring 5′ splice site (Fig. 5c) [205]. The architecture of the tail can be modified to provide binding sites for other factors [206]. The general concept is flexible and changing the identity of the recruited protein or modifying the hybridization site can be used to stimulate splicing (Fig. 5d and e) [72, 207]. A PNA (peptide-nucleic acid) version has also been used with success. In this case, the tail is made of alternating serine and arginine amino acids that mimic SR proteins in their ability to promote exon inclusion (Fig. 5f) [208, 209]. The above approaches can be used to document the functions of different splice isoforms and therefore help to define new therapeutic targets. The development of oligonucleotides whose chemistries are compatible with human use may offer new therapeutic means for anticancer treatment. Although *trans*-acting non-coding nucleic acid molecules to reprogram splicing have been used by researchers for many years, only recently did we realize that this molecular strategy is used normally by cells to modulate splicing decisions. A snoRNA was recently shown to shift the splicing of a serotonin receptor [210]. Likewise, microRNAs (miRNAs) have very recently been shown to regulate alternative splicing during muscle differentiation [211, 212]. Given that miRNA expression is often altered in cancer cells [213], it is likely that additional examples of misregulation of splicing through miRNAs will be found in cancer-associated genes.

Another interesting approach consists in modifying the expression or activity of proteins that affect alternative splicing. This strategy has potential value given that the inhibition of the SRPK1 kinase through RNA interference reduces cellular proliferation and increases apoptosis in cells derived from pancreatic tumors [173, 174]. A more classic pharmacological approach consists in screening libraries for chemical compounds to identify small antagonist molecules with therapeutic value. An application of this strategy has resulted in the discovery of compounds that inhibit other kinases specific for SR proteins and that affect alternative splicing [214, 215]. Recently, screening assays have uncovered molecules that directly target SR proteins and that preferentially inhibit splicing events required for HIV replication [216]. These encouraging results justify that similar approaches be attempted with other regulatory splicing factors.

6 Conclusions

Cancer can arise from alterations in a variety of cellular pathways including signal transduction, cell cycle, and apoptosis. Alternative splicing is an important process that participates in the complex regulation of these cancer-related pathways. Despite incomplete information, it is becoming increasingly evident that defects in alternative splicing imposed by mutations or changes in the levels of splicing factors can generate isoforms whose activities contribute to the initiation and progression of cancer. Given current efforts at documenting the function of splice variants and at cataloguing cancer-specific splicing alterations, we can expect that the role of alternative splicing in cancer will provide many novel anticancer targets. In the meantime, the results of different approaches aimed at reprogramming splice site usage will pave the way for novel therapeutic strategies against cancer.

References

1. Caceres JF, Kornblihtt AR (2002) Alternative splicing: multiple control mechanisms and involvement in human disease. Trends Genet 18(4):186–193
2. Cartegni L, Chew SL, Krainer AR (2002) Listening to silence and understanding nonsense: exonic mutations that affect splicing. Nat Rev Genet 3(4):285–298
3. Pagani F, Baralle FE (2004) Genomic variants in exons and introns: identifying the splicing spoilers. Nat Rev Genet 5(5):389–396
4. Brinkman BM (2004) Splice variants as cancer biomarkers. Clin Biochem 37(7):584–594
5. Venables JP (2006) Unbalanced alternative splicing and its significance in cancer. BioEssays 28(4):378–386
6. Srebrow A, Kornblihtt AR (2006) The connection between splicing and cancer. J Cell Sci 119(Pt 13):2635–2641
7. Revil T, Shkreta L, Chabot B (2006) Pre-mRNA alternative splicing in cancer: functional impact, molecular mechanisms and therapeutic perspectives. Bull Cancer 93(9):909–919
8. Venables JP (ed) (2006) Alternative splicing in cancer. Transworld Res Network
9. Pajares MJ, Ezponda T, Catena R, Calvo A, Pio R, Montuenga LM (2007) Alternative splicing: an emerging topic in molecular and clinical oncology. Lancet Oncol 8(4):349–357
10. Skotheim RI, Nees M (2007) Alternative splicing in cancer: noise, functional, or systematic? Int J Biochem Cell Biol 39(7–8):1432–1449

11. Forch P, Valcarcel J (2003) Splicing regulation in Drosophila sex determination. Prog Mol Subcell Biol 31:127–151
12. Peterson ML (1994) Regulated immunoglobulin (Ig) RNA processing does not require specific cis-acting sequences: non-Ig RNA can be alternatively processed in B cells and plasma cells. Mol Cell Biol 14(12):7891–7898
13. Lou H, Gagel RF (1998) Alternative RNA processing–its role in regulating expression of calcitonin/calcitonin gene-related peptide. J Endocrinol 156(3):401–405
14. Black DL (1998) Splicing in the inner ear: a familiar tune, but what are the instruments? Neuron 20(2):165–168
15. Pan Q, Saltzman AL, Kim YK et al (2006) Quantitative microarray profiling provides evidence against widespread coupling of alternative splicing with nonsense-mediated mRNA decay to control gene expression. Genes Dev 20(2):153–158
16. Wollerton MC, Gooding C, Wagner EJ, Garcia-Blanco MA, Smith CW (2004) Autoregulation of polypyrimidine tract binding protein by alternative splicing leading to nonsense-mediated decay. Mol Cell 13(1):91–100
17. Ni JZ, Grate L, Donohue JP et al (2007) Ultraconserved elements are associated with homeostatic control of splicing regulators by alternative splicing and nonsense-mediated decay. Genes Dev 21(6):708–718
18. Sureau A, Gattoni R, Dooghe Y, Stevenin J, Soret J (2001) SC35 autoregulates its expression by promoting splicing events that destabilize its mRNAs. EMBO J 20(7):1785–1796
19. Lareau LF, Inada M, Green RE, Wengrod JC, Brenner SE (2007) Unproductive splicing of SR genes associated with highly conserved and ultraconserved DNA elements. Nature 446(7138):926–929
20. Tress ML, Martelli PL, Frankish A et al (2007) The implications of alternative splicing in the ENCODE protein complement. Proc Natl Acad Sci U S A 104(13):5495–5500
21. Carstens RP, Eaton JV, Krigman HR, Walther PJ, Garcia-Blanco MA (1997) Alternative splicing of fibroblast growth factor receptor 2 (FGF-R2) in human prostate cancer. Oncogene 15(25):3059–3065
22. Moffa AB, Ethier SP (2007) Differential signal transduction of alternatively spliced FGFR2 variants expressed in human mammary epithelial cells. J Cell Physiol 210(3):720–731
23. Oltean S, Sorg BS, Albrecht T et al (2006) Alternative inclusion of fibroblast growth factor receptor 2 exon IIIc in dunning prostate tumors reveals unexpected epithelial mesenchymal plasticity. Proc Natl Acad Sci U S A 103(38):14116–14121
24. Bourdon JC, Fernandes K, Murray-Zmijewski F et al (2005) p53 isoforms can regulate p53 transcriptional activity. Genes Dev 19(18):2122–2137
25. Ozaki T, Nakagawara A (2005) p73, a sophisticated p53 family member in the cancer world. Cancer Sci 96(11):729–737
26. Bartel F, Taubert H, Harris LC (2002) Alternative and aberrant splicing of MDM2 mRNA in human cancer. Cancer Cell 2(1):9–15
27. Fridman JS, Hernando E, Hemann MT, de Stanchina E, Cordon-Cardo C, Lowe SW (2003) Tumor promotion by Mdm2 splice variants unable to bind p53. Cancer Res 63(18):5703–5706
28. Lovecchio M, Maiorano E, Vacca RA et al (2003) beta 1C integrin expression in human endometrial proliferative diseases. Am J Pathol 163(6):2543–2553
29. Hsieh HF, Yu JC, Ho LI, Chiu SC, Harn HJ (1999) Molecular studies into the role of CD44 variants in metastasis in gastric cancer. Mol Pathol 52(1):25–28
30. Wallach SB, Friedmann A, Naor D (2000) The CD44 receptor of the mouse LB T-cell lymphoma: analysis of the isoform repertoire and ligand binding properties by reverse-transcriptase polymerase chain reaction and antisense oligonucleotides. Cancer Detect Prev 24(1):33–45
31. Miyake H, Eto H, Arakawa S, Kamidono S, Hara I (2002) Over expression of CD44V8-10 in urinary exfoliated cells as an independent prognostic predictor in patients with urothelial cancer. J Urol 167(3):1282–1287

32. Hashimoto-Uoshima M, Yan YZ, Schneider G, Aukhil I (1997) The alternatively spliced domains EIIIB and EIIIA of human fibronectin affect cell adhesion and spreading. J Cell Sci 110(Pt 18):2271–2280
33. Ghigna C, Giordano S, Shen H et al (2005) Cell motility is controlled by SF2/ASF through alternative splicing of the ron protooncogene. Mol Cell 20(6):881–890
34. Ladomery MR, Harper SJ, Bates DO (2007) Alternative splicing in angiogenesis: the vascular endothelial growth factor paradigm. Cancer Lett 249(2):133–142
35. Catena R, Muniz-Medina V, Moralejo B et al (2007) Increased expression of VEGF(121)/VEGF(165–189) ratio results in a significant enhancement of human prostate tumor angiogenesis. Int J Cancer 120(10):2096–2109
36. Cohen CD, Doran PP, Blattner SM et al (2005) Sam68-like mammalian protein 2, identified by digital differential display as expressed by podocytes, is induced in proteinuria and involved in splice site selection of vascular endothelial growth factor. J Am Soc Nephrol 16(7):1958–1965
37. Chao C, Goluszko E, Lee YT et al (2007) Constitutively active CCK2 receptor splice variant increases src-dependent HIF-1 alpha expression and tumor growth. Oncogene 26(7):1013–1019
38. Koduri S, Goldhar AS, Vonderhaar BK (2006) Activation of vascular endothelial growth factor (VEGF) by the ER-alpha variant, ERDelta3. Breast Cancer Res Treat 95(1):37–43
39. Caldas H, Fangusaro JR, Boue DR, Holloway MP, Altura RA (2007) Dissecting the role of endothelial SURVIVIN deltaEx3 in angiogenesis. Blood 109(4):1479–1489
40. Schwerk C, Schulze-Osthoff K (2005) Regulation of apoptosis by alternative pre-mRNA splicing. Mol Cell 19(1):1–13
41. Minn AJ, Boise LH, Thompson CB (1996) Bcl-x(S) anatagonizes the protective effects of Bcl-x(L). J Biol Chem 271(11):6306–6312
42. Tu Y, Renner S, Xu F et al (1998) BCL-X expression in multiple myeloma: possible indicator of chemoresistance. Cancer Res 58(2):256–262
43. Takehara T, Liu X, Fujimoto J, Friedman SL, Takahashi H (2001) Expression and role of Bcl-xL in human hepatocellular carcinomas. Hepatology 34(1):55–61
44. Olopade OI, Adeyanju MO, Safa AR et al (1997) Overexpression of BCL-x protein in primary breast cancer is associated with high tumor grade and nodal metastases. Cancer J Sci Am 3(4):230–237
45. Yang CC, Lin HP, Chen CS, Yang YT, Tseng PH, Rangnekar VM (2003) Bcl-xL mediates a survival mechanism independent of the phosphoinositide 3-kinase/Akt pathway in prostate cancer cells. J Biol Chem 278(28):25872–25878
46. Wincewicz A, Sulkowska M, Koda M, Kanczuga-Koda L, Witkowska E, Sulkowski S (2007) Significant coexpression of GLUT-1, Bcl-xL, and bax in colorectal cancer. Ann N Y Acad Sci 1095:53–61
47. Chang BS, Kelekar A, Harris MH, Harlan JE, Fesik SW, Thompson CB (1999) The BH3 domain of Bcl-x(S) is required for inhibition of the antiapoptotic function of Bcl-x(L). Mol Cell Biol 19(10):6673–6681
48. Dole MG, Jasty R, Cooper MJ, Thompson CB, Nunez G, Castle VP (1995) Bcl-xL is expressed in neuroblastoma cells and modulates chemotherapy-induced apoptosis. Cancer Res 55(12):2576–2582
49. Simonian PL, Grillot DA, Nunez G (1997) Bcl-2 and Bcl-XL can differentially block chemotherapy-induced cell death. Blood 90(3):1208–1216
50. Lebedeva I, Rando R, Ojwang J, Cossum P, Stein CA (2000) Bcl-xL in prostate cancer cells: effects of overexpression and down-regulation on chemosensitivity. Cancer Res 60(21):6052–6060
51. Williams J, Lucas PC, Griffith KA et al (2005) Expression of Bcl-xL in ovarian carcinoma is associated with chemoresistance and recurrent disease. Gynecol Oncol 96(2):287–295
52. Cho HJ, Kim JK, Kim KD et al (2006) Upregulation of Bcl-2 is associated with cisplatin-resistance via inhibition of bax translocation in human bladder cancer cells. Cancer Lett 237(1):56–66

53. Vilenchik M, Raffo AJ, Benimetskaya L, Shames D, Stein CA (2002) Antisense RNA down-regulation of bcl-xL expression in prostate cancer cells leads to diminished rates of cellular proliferation and resistance to cytotoxic chemotherapeutic agents. Cancer Res 62(7):2175–2183
54. Zhu H, Guo W, Zhang L et al (2005) Bcl-XL small interfering RNA suppresses the proliferation of 5-fluorouracil-resistant human colon cancer cells. Mol Cancer Ther 4(3):451–456
55. Konishi T, Sasaki S, Watanabe T, Kitayama J, Nagawa H (2006) Overexpression of hRFI inhibits 5-fluorouracil-induced apoptosis in colorectal cancer cells via activation of NF-kappaB and upregulation of BCL-2 and BCL-XL. Oncogene 25(22):3160–3169
56. Wang P, Song JH, Song DK, Zhang J, Hao C (2006) Role of death receptor and mitochondrial pathways in conventional chemotherapy drug induction of apoptosis. Cell Signal 18(9):1528–1535
57. Matsushita K, Tomonaga T, Shimada H et al (2006) An essential role of alternative splicing of c-myc suppressor FUSE-binding protein-interacting repressor in carcinogenesis. Cancer Res 66(3):1409–1417
58. Patel NA, Song SS, Cooper DR (2006) PKCdelta alternatively spliced isoforms modulate cellular apoptosis in retinoic acid-induced differentiation of human NT2 cells and mouse embryonic stem cells. Gene Expr 13(2):73–84
59. He X, Ee PL, Coon JS, Beck WT (2004) Alternative splicing of the multidrug resistance protein 1/ATP binding cassette transporter subfamily gene in ovarian cancer creates functional splice variants and is associated with increased expression of the splicing factors PTB and SRp20. Clin Cancer Res 10(14):4652–4660
60. Lamba JK, Adachi M, Sun D et al (2003) Nonsense mediated decay downregulates conserved alternatively spliced ABCC4 transcripts bearing nonsense codons. Hum Mol Genet 12(2):99–109
61. Chen KG, Szakacs G, Annereau JP et al (2005) Principal expression of two mRNA isoforms (ABCB 5alpha and ABCB 5beta) of the ATP-binding cassette transporter gene ABCB 5 in melanoma cells and melanocytes. Pigment Cell Res 18(2):102–112
62. Devine SE, Hussain A, Davide JP, Melera PW (1991) Full length and alternatively spliced pgp1 transcripts in multidrug-resistant chinese hamster lung cells. J Biol Chem 266(7):4545–4555
63. Ma JF, Grant G, Staelens B, Howard DL, Melera PW (1999) In vitro translation of a 2.3-kb splicing variant of the hamster pgp1 gene whose presence in transfectants is associated with decreased drug resistance. Cancer Chemother Pharmacol 43(1):19–28
64. Nakanishi T, Shiozawa K, Hassel BA, Ross DD (2006) Complex interaction of BCRP/ ABCG2 and imatinib in BCR-ABL-expressing cells: BCRP-mediated resistance to imatinib is attenuated by imatinib-induced reduction of BCRP expression. Blood 108(2):678–684
65. Muller M, Schleithoff ES, Stremmel W, Melino G, Krammer PH, Schilling T (2006) One, two, three-p53, p63, p73 and chemosensitivity. Drug Resist Updat 9(6):288–306
66. Yin F, Du Y, Hu W et al (2006) Mad2beta, an alternative variant of Mad2 reducing mitotic arrest and apoptosis induced by adriamycin in gastric cancer cells. Life Sci 78(12):1277–1286
67. Efimova EV, Al-Zoubi AM, Martinez O et al (2004) IG20, in contrast to DENN-SV, (MADD splice variants) suppresses tumor cell survival, and enhances their susceptibility to apoptosis and cancer drugs. Oncogene 23(5):1076–1087
68. Black DL (2003) Mechanisms of alternative pre-messenger RNA splicing. Annu Rev Biochem 72:291–336
69. Blanchette M, Chabot B (1997) A highly stable duplex structure sequesters the 5′ splice site region of hnRNP A1 alternative exon 7B. RNA 3(4):405–419
70. Blanchette M, Chabot B (1999) Modulation of exon skipping by high-affinity hnRNP A1-binding sites and by intron elements that repress splice site utilization. EMBO J 18(7):1939–1952
71. Nasim FU, Hutchison S, Cordeau M, Chabot B (2002) High-affinity hnRNP A1 binding sites and duplex-forming inverted repeats have similar effects on 5′ splice site selection in support of a common looping out and repression mechanism. RNA 8(8):1078–1089
72. Martinez-Contreras R, Fisette JF, Nasim FU, Madden R, Cordeau M, Chabot B (2006) Intronic binding sites for hnRNP A/B and hnRNP F/H proteins stimulate pre-mRNA splicing. PLoS Biol 4(2):e21

73. Wagner EJ, Garcia-Blanco MA (2001) Polypyrimidine tract binding protein antagonizes exon definition. Mol Cell Biol 21(10):3281–3288
74. Amir-Ahmady B, Boutz PL, Markovtsov V, Phillips ML, Black DL (2005) Exon repression by polypyrimidine tract binding protein. RNA 11(5):699–716
75. Ule J, Stefani G, Mele A et al (2006) An RNA map predicting Nova-dependent splicing regulation. Nature 444(7119):580–586
76. Domsic JK, Wang Y, Mayeda A, Krainer AR, Stoltzfus CM (2003) Human immunodeficiency virus type 1 hnRNP A/B-dependent exonic splicing silencer ESSV antagonizes binding of U2AF65 to viral polypyrimidine tracts. Mol Cell Biol 23(23):8762–8772
77. Zhu J, Mayeda A, Krainer AR (2001) Exon identity established through differential antagonism between exonic splicing silencer-bound hnRNP A1 and enhancer-bound SR proteins. Mol Cell 8(6):1351–1361
78. Soret J, Gabut M, Tazi J (2006) SR proteins as potential targets for therapy. Prog Mol Subcell Biol 44:65–87
79. Krawczak M, Reiss J, Cooper DN (1992) The mutational spectrum of single base-pair substitutions in mRNA splice junctions of human genes: causes and consequences. Hum Genet 90(1–2):41–54
80. Lopez-Bigas N, Blencowe BJ, Ouzounis CA (2006) Highly consistent patterns for inherited human diseases at the molecular level. Bioinformatics 22(3):269–277
81. Disset A, Bourgeois CF, Benmalek N, Claustres M, Stevenin J, Tuffery-Giraud S (2006) An exon skipping-associated nonsense mutation in the dystrophin gene uncovers a complex interplay between multiple antagonistic splicing elements. Hum Mol Genet 15(6):999–1013
82. Serra E, Ars E, Ravella A et al (2001) Somatic NF1 mutational spectrum in benign neurofibromas: mRNA splice defects are common among point mutations. Hum Genet 108(5):416–429
83. Baser ME, Kuramoto L, Woods R et al (2005) The location of constitutional neurofibromatosis 2 (NF2) splice site mutations is associated with the severity of NF2. J Med Genet 42(7):540–546
84. Holmila R, Fouquet C, Cadranel J, Zalcman G, Soussi T (2003) Splice mutations in the p53 gene: case report and review of the literature. Hum Mutat 21(1):101–102
85. Neklason DW, Solomon CH, Dalton AL, Kuwada SK, Burt RW (2004) Intron 4 mutation in APC gene results in splice defect and attenuated FAP phenotype. Fam Cancer 3(1):35–40
86. Liu HX, Cartegni L, Zhang MQ, Krainer AR (2001) A mechanism for exon skipping caused by nonsense or missense mutations in BRCA1 and other genes. Nat Genet 27(1):55–58
87. Yang Y, Swaminathan S, Martin BK, Sharan SK (2003) Aberrant splicing induced by missense mutations in BRCA1: clues from a humanized mouse model. Hum Mol Genet 12(17):2121–2131
88. Narla G, DiFeo A, Yao S et al (2005) Targeted inhibition of the KLF6 splice variant, KLF6 SV1, suppresses prostate cancer cell growth and spread. Cancer Res 65(13):5761–5768
89. Wang XQ, Luk JM, Leung PP, Wong BW, Stanbridge EJ, Fan ST (2005) Alternative mRNA splicing of liver intestine-cadherin in hepatocellular carcinoma. Clin Cancer Res 11(2 Pt 1):483–489
90. Venesio T, Balsamo A, Sfiligoi C et al (2007) Constitutional high expression of an APC mRNA isoform in a subset of attenuated familial adenomatous polyposis patients. J Mol Med 85(3):301–308
91. Zhuo D, Madden R, Elela SA, Chabot B (2007) Modern origin of numerous alternatively spliced human introns from tandem arrays. Proc Natl Acad Sci U S A 104(3):882–886
92. Hallier M, Lerga A, Barnache S, Tavitian A, Moreau-Gachelin F (1998) The transcription factor Spi-1/PU.1 interacts with the potential splicing factor TLS. J Biol Chem 273(9):4838–4842
93. Knoop LL, Baker SJ (2000) The splicing factor U1C represses EWS/FLI-mediated transactivation. J Biol Chem 275(32):24865–24871
94. Yang L, Embree LJ, Hickstein DD (2000) TLS-ERG leukemia fusion protein inhibits RNA splicing mediated by serine-arginine proteins. Mol Cell Biol 20(10):3345–3354
95. Chansky HA, Hu M, Hickstein DD, Yang L (2001) Oncogenic TLS/ERG and EWS/Fli-1 fusion proteins inhibit RNA splicing mediated by YB-1 protein. Cancer Res 61(9):3586–3590
96. Janknecht R (2005) EWS-ETS oncoproteins: the linchpins of Ewing tumors. Gene 363:1–14

97. Knoop LL, Baker SJ (2001) EWS/FLI alters 5′-splice site selection. J Biol Chem 276(25):22317–22322
98. Yang L, Chansky HA, Hickstein DD (2000) EWS. Fli-1 fusion protein interacts with hyperphosphorylated RNA polymerase II and interferes with serine-arginine protein-mediated RNA splicing. J Biol Chem 275(48):37612–37618
99. Ohkura N, Yaguchi H, Tsukada T, Yamaguchi K (2002) The EWS/NOR1 fusion gene product gains a novel activity affecting pre-mRNA splicing. J Biol Chem 277(1):535–543
100. Salesse S, Dylla SJ, Verfaillie CM (2004) p210BCR/ABL-induced alteration of pre-mRNA splicing in primary human CD34 + hematopoietic progenitor cells. Leukemia 18(4):727–733
101. Chabot B, Frappier D, La Branche H (1992) Differential ASF/SF2 activity in extracts from normal WI38 and transformed WI38VA13 cells. Nucleic Acids Res 20(19):5197–5204
102. Lavigueur A, La Branche H, Kornblihtt AR, Chabot B (1993) A splicing enhancer in the human fibronectin alternate ED1 exon interacts with SR proteins and stimulates U2 snRNP binding. Genes Dev 7((12A)):2405–2417
103. Ghigna C, Moroni M, Porta C, Riva S, Biamonti G (1998) Altered expression of heterogenous nuclear ribonucleoproteins and SR factors in human colon adenocarcinomas. Cancer Res 58(24):5818–5824
104. Pino I, Pio R, Toledo G et al (2003) Altered patterns of expression of members of the heterogeneous nuclear ribonucleoprotein (hnRNP) family in lung cancer. Lung Cancer 41(2):131–143
105. Karni R, de Stanchina E, Lowe SW, Sinha R, Mu D, Krainer AR (2007) The gene encoding the splicing factor SF2/ASF is a proto-oncogene. Nat Struct Mol Biol 14(3):185–193
106. Li X, Wang J, Manley JL (2005) Loss of splicing factor ASF/SF2 induces G2 cell cycle arrest and apoptosis, but inhibits internucleosomal DNA fragmentation. Genes Dev 19(22):2705–2714
107. Chalfant CE, Ogretmen B, Galadari S, Kroesen BJ, Pettus BJ, Hannun YA (2001) FAS activation induces dephosphorylation of SR proteins; dependence on the de novo generation of ceramide and activation of protein phosphatase 1. J Biol Chem 276(48):44848–44855
108. He X, Pool M, Darcy KM et al (2007) Knockdown of polypyrimidine tract-binding protein suppresses ovarian tumor cell growth and invasiveness in vitro. Oncogene 26(34):4961–4968
109. Perry WL 3rd, Shepard RL, Sampath J et al (2005) Human splicing factor SPF45 (RBM17) confers broad multidrug resistance to anticancer drugs when overexpressed–a phenotype partially reversed by selective estrogen receptor modulators. Cancer Res 65(15):6593–6600
110. Shitashige M, Naishiro Y, Idogawa M et al (2007) Involvement of splicing factor-1 in beta-catenin/T-cell factor-4-mediated gene transactivation and pre-mRNA splicing. Gastroenterology 132(3):1039–1054
111. Ding WQ, Kuntz SM, Miller LJ (2002) A misspliced form of the cholecystokinin-B/gastrin receptor in pancreatic carcinoma: role of reduced sellular U2AF35 and a suboptimal 3′-splicing site leading to retention of the fourth intron. Cancer Res 62(3):947–952
112. Sergeant KA, Bourgeois CF, Dalgliesh C, Venables JP, Stevenin J, Elliott DJ (2007) Alternative RNA splicing complexes containing the scaffold attachment factor SAFB2. J Cell Sci 120(Pt 2):309–319
113. Le Guiner C, Plet A, Galiana D, Gesnel MC, Del Gatto-Konczak F, Breathnach R (2001) Polypyrimidine tract-binding protein represses splicing of a fibroblast growth factor receptor-2 gene alternative exon through exon sequences. J Biol Chem 276(47):43677–43687
114. Baraniak AP, Chen JR, Garcia-Blanco MA (2006) Fox-2 mediates epithelial cell-specific fibroblast growth factor receptor 2 exon choice. Mol Cell Biol 26(4):1209–1222
115. Jin W, McCutcheon IE, Fuller GN, Huang ES, Cote GJ (2000) Fibroblast growth factor receptor-1 alpha-exon exclusion and polypyrimidine tract-binding protein in glioblastoma multiforme tumors. Cancer Res 60(5):1221–1224
116. Stickeler E, Kittrell F, Medina D, Berget SM (1999) Stage-specific changes in SR splicing factors and alternative splicing in mammary tumorigenesis. Oncogene 18(24):3574–3582
117. Fischer DC, Noack K, Runnebaum IB et al (2004) Expression of splicing factors in human ovarian cancer. Oncol Rep 11(5):1085–1090
118. Galiana-Arnoux D, Lejeune F, Gesnel MC, Stevenin J, Breathnach R, Del Gatto-Konczak F (2003) The CD44 alternative v9 exon contains a splicing enhancer responsive to the SR proteins 9G8, ASF/SF2, and SRp20. J Biol Chem 278(35):32943–32953

119. Matter N, Herrlich P, Konig H (2002) Signal-dependent regulation of splicing via phosphorylation of Sam68. Nature 420(6916):691–695
120. Matter N, Marx M, Weg-Remers S, Ponta H, Herrlich P, Konig H (2000) Heterogeneous ribonucleoprotein A1 is part of an exon-specific splice-silencing complex controlled by oncogenic signaling pathways. J Biol Chem 275(45):35353–35360
121. Venables JP, Dalgliesh C, Paronetto MP et al (2004) SIAH1 targets the alternative splicing factor T-STAR for degradation by the proteasome. Hum Mol Genet 13(14):1525–1534
122. Cheng C, Sharp PA (2006) Regulation of CD44 alternative splicing by SRm160 and its potential role in tumor cell invasion. Mol Cell Biol 26(1):362–370
123. Watermann DO, Tang Y, Zur Hausen A, Jager M, Stamm S, Stickeler E (2006) Splicing factor Tra2-beta1 is specifically induced in breast cancer and regulates alternative splicing of the CD44 gene. Cancer Res 66(9):4774–4780
124. Batsche E, Yaniv M, Muchardt C (2006) The human SWI/SNF subunit Brm is a regulator of alternative splicing. Nat Struct Mol Biol 13(1):22–29
125. Zhou YQ, He C, Chen YQ, Wang D, Wang MH (2003) Altered expression of the RON receptor tyrosine kinase in primary human colorectal adenocarcinomas: generation of different splicing RON variants and their oncogenic potential. Oncogene 22(2):186–197
126. Forch P, Puig O, Martinez C, Seraphin B, Valcarcel J (2002) The splicing regulator TIA-1 interacts with U1-C to promote U1 snRNP recruitment to 5′ splice sites. EMBO J 21(24):6882–6892
127. Izquierdo JM, Majos N, Bonnal S et al (2005) Regulation of Fas alternative splicing by antagonistic effects of TIA-1 and PTB on exon definition. Mol Cell 19(4):475–484
128. Li CY, Chu JY, Yu JK et al (2004) Regulation of alternative splicing of Bcl-x by IL-6 GM-CSF and TPA. Cell Res 14(6):473–479
129. Massiello A, Salas A, Pinkerman RL, Roddy P, Roesser JR, Chalfant CE (2004) Identification of two RNA cis-elements that function to regulate the 5′ splice site selection of Bcl-x pre-mRNA in response to ceramide. J Biol Chem 279(16):15799–15804
130. Paronetto MP, Achsel T, Massiello A, Chalfant CE, Sette C (2007) The RNA-binding protein Sam68 modulates the alternative splicing of Bcl-x. J Cell Biol 176(7):929–939
131. Garneau D, Revil T, Fisette JF, Chabot B (2005) Heterogeneous nuclear ribonucleoprotein F/H proteins modulate the alternative splicing of the apoptotic mediator Bcl-x. J Biol Chem 280(24):22641–22650
132. Cloutier P, Toutant J, Shkreta L, Goekjian S, Revil T, Chabot B (2008) Antagonistic effects of the SRp30c protein and cryptic 5′ splice sites on the alternative splicing of the apoptotic regulator Bcl-x. J Biol Chem 283(31):21315–21324
133. Revil T, Toutant J, Shkreta L, Garneau D, Cloutier P, Chabot B (2007) Protein kinase C-dependent control of Bcl-x alternative splicing. Mol Cell Biol 27(24):8431–8441
134. Shkreta L, Froehlich U, Paquet ER, Toutant J, Elela SA, Chabot B (2008) Anticancer drugs affect the alternative splicing of Bcl-x and other human apoptotic genes. Mol Cancer Ther 7(6):1398–1409
135. Wu JY, Tang H, Havlioglu N (2003) Alternative pre-mRNA splicing and regulation of programmed cell death. Prog Mol Subcell Biol 31:153–185
136. Jiang ZH, Zhang WJ, Rao Y, Wu JY (1998) Regulation of Ich-1 pre-mRNA alternative splicing and apoptosis by mammalian splicing factors. Proc Natl Acad Sci U S A 95(16):9155–9160
137. Cote J, Dupuis S, Jiang Z, Wu JY (2001) Caspase-2 pre-mRNA alternative splicing: Identification of an intronic element containing a decoy 3′ acceptor site. Proc Natl Acad Sci U S A 98(3):938–943
138. Faustino NA, Cooper TA (2003) Pre-mRNA splicing and human disease. Genes Dev 17(4):419–437
139. Ho TH, Charlet BN, Poulos MG, Singh G, Swanson MS, Cooper TA (2004) Muscleblind proteins regulate alternative splicing. EMBO J 23(15):3103–3112
140. Auboeuf D, Batsche E, Dutertre M, Muchardt C, O'Malley BW (2007) Coregulators: transducing signal from transcription to alternative splicing. Trends Endocrinol Metab 18(3):122–129

141. Kornblihtt AR (2005) Promoter usage and alternative splicing. Curr Opin Cell Biol 17(3):262–268
142. Cramer P, Pesce CG, Baralle FE, Kornblihtt AR (1997) Functional association between promoter structure and transcript alternative splicing. Proc Natl Acad Sci U S A 94(21):11456–11460
143. Gendra E, Colgan DF, Meany B, Konarska MM (2007) A sequence motif in the SV40 early core promoter affects alternative splicing of transcribed mRNA. J Biol Chem 282(16):11648–11657
144. Auboeuf D, Dowhan DH, Li X et al (2004) CoAA, a nuclear receptor coactivator protein at the interface of transcriptional coactivation and RNA splicing. Mol Cell Biol 24(1):442–453
145. Guillouf C, Gallais I, Moreau-Gachelin F (2006) Spi-1/PU.1 oncoprotein affects splicing decisions in a promoter binding-dependent manner. J Biol Chem 281(28):19145–19155
146. de la Mata M, Kornblihtt AR (2006) RNA polymerase II C-terminal domain mediates regulation of alternative splicing by SRp20. Nat Struct Mol Biol 13(11):973–980
147. de la Mata M, Alonso CR, Kadener S et al (2003) A slow RNA polymerase II affects alternative splicing in vivo. Mol Cell 12(2):525–532
148. Nogues G, Kadener S, Cramer P et al (2003) Control of alternative pre-mRNA splicing by RNA Pol II elongation: faster is not always better. IUBMB Life 55(4–5):235–241
149. Pecci A, Viegas LR, Baranao JL, Beato M (2001) Promoter choice influences alternative splicing and determines the balance of isoforms expressed from the mouse bcl-X gene. J Biol Chem 276(24):21062–21069
150. Logette E, Wotawa A, Solier S, Desoche L, Solary E, Corcos L (2003) The human caspase-2 gene: alternative promoters, pre-mRNA splicing and AUG usage direct isoform-specific expression. Oncogene 22(6):935–946
151. Landry JR, Mager DL, Wilhelm BT (2003) Complex controls: the role of alternative promoters in mammalian genomes. Trends Genet 19(11):640–648
152. Kimura K, Wakamatsu A, Suzuki Y et al (2006) Diversification of transcriptional modulation: large-scale identification and characterization of putative alternative promoters of human genes. Genome Res 16(1):55–65
153. Bass BL (2002) RNA editing by adenosine deaminases that act on RNA. Annu Rev Biochem 71:817–846
154. Beghini A, Ripamonti CB, Peterlongo P et al (2000) RNA hyperediting and alternative splicing of hematopoietic cell phosphatase (PTPN6) gene in acute myeloid leukemia. Hum Mol Genet 9(15):2297–2304
155. Maas S, Patt S, Schrey M, Rich A (2001) Underediting of glutamate receptor GluR-B mRNA in malignant gliomas. Proc Natl Acad Sci U S A 98(25):14687–14692
156. Weischenfeldt J, Lykke-Andersen J, Porse B (2005) Messenger RNA surveillance: neutralizing natural nonsense. Curr Biol 15(14):R559–R562
157. Rossi MR, Hawthorn L, Platt J, Burkhardt T, Cowell JK, Ionov Y (2005) Identification of inactivating mutations in the JAK1, SYNJ2, and CLPTM1 genes in prostate cancer cells using inhibition of nonsense-mediated decay and microarray analysis. Cancer Genet Cytogenet 161(2):97–103
158. Ware MD, DeSilva D, Sinilnikova OM, Stoppa-Lyonnet D, Tavtigian SV, Mazoyer S (2006) Does nonsense-mediated mRNA decay explain the ovarian cancer cluster region of the BRCA2 gene? Oncogene 25(2):323–328
159. Green RE, Lewis BP, Hillman RT et al (2003) Widespread predicted nonsense-mediated mRNA decay of alternatively-spliced transcripts of human normal and disease genes. Bioinformatics 19(Suppl 1):i118–i121
160. El-Bchiri J, Buhard O, Penard-Lacronique V, Thomas G, Hamelin R, Duval A (2005) Differential nonsense mediated decay of mutated mRNAs in mismatch repair deficient colorectal cancers. Hum Mol Genet 14(16):2435–2442
161. De Rosa M, Morelli G, Cesaro E et al (2007) Alternative splicing and nonsense-mediated mRNA decay in the regulation of a new adenomatous polyposis coli transcript. Gene 395(1–2):8–14
162. Tarn WY (2007) Cellular signals modulate alternative splicing. J Biomed Sci 14(4):517–522
163. Blaustein M, Pelisch F, Srebrow A (2007) Signals, pathways and splicing regulation. Int J Biochem Cell Biol 39(11):2031–2048

164. Ding JH, Zhong XY, Hagopian JC et al (2006) Regulated cellular partitioning of SR protein-specific kinases in mammalian cells. Mol Biol Cell 17(2):876–885
165. Xie J, Lee JA, Kress TL, Mowry KL, Black DL (2003) Protein kinase A phosphorylation modulates transport of the polypyrimidine tract-binding protein. Proc Natl Acad Sci U S A 100(15):8776–8781
166. Allemand E, Guil S, Myers M, Moscat J, Caceres JF, Krainer AR (2005) Regulation of heterogenous nuclear ribonucleoprotein A1 transport by phosphorylation in cells stressed by osmotic shock. Proc Natl Acad Sci U S A 102(10):3605–3610
167. Hall MP, Huang S, Black DL (2004) Differentiation-induced colocalization of the KH-type splicing regulatory protein with polypyrimidine tract binding protein and the c-src pre-mRNA. Mol Biol Cell 15(2):774–786
168. Scheid MP, Woodgett JR (2001) PKB/AKT: functional insights from genetic models. Nat Rev Mol Cell Biol 2(10):760–768
169. Blaustein M, Pelisch F, Coso OA, Bissell MJ, Kornblihtt AR, Srebrow A (2004) Mammary epithelial-mesenchymal interaction regulates fibronectin alternative splicing via phosphatidylinositol 3-kinase. J Biol Chem 279(20):21029–21037
170. Patel NA, Kaneko S, Apostolatos HS et al (2005) Molecular and genetic studies imply Akt-mediated signaling promotes protein kinase CbetaII alternative splicing via phosphorylation of serine/arginine-rich splicing factor SRp40. J Biol Chem 280(14):14302–14309
171. Konig H, Ponta H, Herrlich P (1998) Coupling of signal transduction to alternative pre-mRNA splicing by a composite splice regulator. EMBO J 17(10):2904–2913
172. Cheng C, Yaffe MB, Sharp PA (2006) A positive feedback loop couples Ras activation and CD44 alternative splicing. Genes Dev 20(13):1715–1720
173. Hayes GM, Carrigan PE, Beck AM, Miller LJ (2006) Targeting the RNA splicing machinery as a novel treatment strategy for pancreatic carcinoma. Cancer Res 66(7):3819–3827
174. Hayes GM, Carrigan PE, Miller LJ (2007) Serine-arginine protein kinase 1 overexpression is associated with tumorigenic imbalance in mitogen-activated protein kinase pathways in breast, colonic, and pancreatic carcinomas. Cancer Res 67(5):2072–2080
175. Bellavia D, Mecarozzi M, Campese AF et al (2007) Notch3 and the Notch3-upregulated RNA-binding protein HuD regulate Ikaros alternative splicing. EMBO J 26(6):1670–1680
176. Shin C, Manley JL (2004) Cell signalling and the control of pre-mRNA splicing. Nat Rev Mol Cell Biol 5(9):727–738
177. Blaustein M, Pelisch F, Tanos T et al (2005) Concerted regulation of nuclear and cytoplasmic activities of SR proteins by AKT. Nat Struct Mol Biol 12(12):1037–1044
178. Chen HH, Wang YC, Fann MJ (2006) Identification and characterization of the CDK12/cyclin L1 complex involved in alternative splicing regulation. Mol Cell Biol 26(7):2736–2745
179. Shen EC, Henry MF, Weiss VH, Valentini SR, Silver PA, Lee MS (1998) Arginine methylation facilitates the nuclear export of hnRNP proteins. Genes Dev 12(5):679–691
180. Yu MC, Bachand F, McBride AE, Komili S, Casolari JM, Silver PA (2004) Arginine methyltransferase affects interactions and recruitment of mRNA processing and export factors. Genes Dev 18(16):2024–2035
181. Ohkura N, Takahashi M, Yaguchi H, Nagamura Y, Tsukada T (2005) Coactivator-associated arginine methyltransferase 1, CARM1, affects pre-mRNA splicing in an isoform-specific manner. J Biol Chem 280(32):28927–28935
182. Hui L, Zhang X, Wu X et al (2004) Identification of alternatively spliced mRNA variants related to cancers by genome-wide ESTs alignment. Oncogene 23(17):3013–3023
183. Xu Q, Lee C (2003) Discovery of novel splice forms and functional analysis of cancer-specific alternative splicing in human expressed sequences. Nucleic Acids Res 31(19):5635–5643
184. Pan Q, Shai O, Misquitta C et al (2004) Revealing global regulatory features of mammalian alternative splicing using a quantitative microarray platform. Mol Cell 16(6):929–941
185. Zhang C, Li HR, Fan JB et al (2006) Profiling alternatively spliced mRNA isoforms for prostate cancer classification. BMC Bioinformatics 7:202
186. Watahiki A, Waki K, Hayatsu N et al (2004) Libraries enriched for alternatively spliced exons reveal splicing patterns in melanocytes and melanomas. Nat Methods 1(3):233–239

187. Relogio A, Ben-Dov C, Baum M et al (2005) Alternative splicing microarrays reveal functional expression of neuron-specific regulators in Hodgkin lymphoma cells. J Biol Chem 280(6):4779–4784
188. Li C, Kato M, Shiue L, Shively JE, Ares M Jr, Lin RJ (2006) Cell type and culture condition-dependent alternative splicing in human breast cancer cells revealed by splicing-sensitive microarrays. Cancer Res 66(4):1990–1999
189. Yeakley JM, Fan JB, Doucet D et al (2002) Profiling alternative splicing on fiber-optic arrays. Nat Biotechnol 20(4):353–358
190. Li HR, Wang-Rodriguez J, Nair TM et al (2006) Two-dimensional transcriptome profiling: identification of messenger RNA isoform signatures in prostate cancer from archived paraffin-embedded cancer specimens. Cancer Res 66(8):4079–4088
191. Johnson JM, Castle J, Garrett-Engele P et al (2003) Genome-wide survey of human alternative pre-mRNA splicing with exon junction microarrays. Science 302(5653):2141–2144
192. Gardina PJ, Clark TA, Shimada B et al (2006) Alternative splicing and differential gene expression in colon cancer detected by a whole genome exon array. BMC Genomics 7:325
193. Margulies M, Egholm M, Altman WE et al (2005) Genome sequencing in microfabricated high-density picolitre reactors. Nature 437(7057):376–380
194. Fededa JP, Petrillo E, Gelfand MS et al (2005) A polar mechanism coordinates different regions of alternative splicing within a single gene. Mol Cell 19(3):393–404
195. Celotto AM, Graveley BR (2002) Exon-specific RNAi: a tool for dissecting the functional relevance of alternative splicing. RNA 8(6):718–724
196. Morris KV, Chan SW, Jacobsen SE, Looney DJ (2004) Small interfering RNA-induced transcriptional gene silencing in human cells. Science 305(5688):1289–1292
197. Kim DH, Villeneuve LM, Morris KV, Rossi JJ (2006) Argonaute-1 directs siRNA-mediated transcriptional gene silencing in human cells. Nat Struct Mol Biol 13(9):793–797
198. Goyenvalle A, Vulin A, Fougerousse F et al (2004) Rescue of dystrophic muscle through U7 snRNA-mediated exon skipping. Science 306(5702):1796–1799
199. Mercatante DR, Bortner CD, Cidlowski JA, Kole R (2001) Modification of alternative splicing of Bcl-x pre-mRNA in prostate and breast cancer cells. Analysis of apoptosis and cell death. J Biol Chem 276(19):16411–16417
200. Mercatante DR, Mohler JL, Kole R (2002) Cellular response to an antisense-mediated shift of Bcl-x pre-mRNA splicing and antineoplastic agents. J Biol Chem 277(51):49374–49382
201. Giles RV, Spiller DG, Clark RE, Tidd DM (1999) Antisense morpholino oligonucleotide analog induces missplicing of C-myc mRNA. Antisense Nucleic Acid Drug Dev 9(2):213–220
202. Bruno IG, Jin W, Cote GJ (2004) Correction of aberrant FGFR1 alternative RNA splicing through targeting of intronic regulatory elements. Hum Mol Genet 13(20):2409–2420
203. Taylor JK, Zhang QQ, Wyatt JR, Dean NM (1999) Induction of endogenous Bcl-xS through the control of Bcl-x pre-mRNA splicing by antisense oligonucleotides. Nat Biotechnol 17(11):1097–1100
204. Singh NK, Singh NN, Androphy EJ, Singh RN (2006) Splicing of a critical exon of human survival motor neuron is regulated by a unique silencer element located in the last intron. Mol Cell Biol 26(4):1333–1346
205. Villemaire J, Dion I, Elela SA, Chabot B (2003) Reprogramming alternative pre-messenger RNA splicing through the use of protein-binding antisense oligonucleotides. J Biol Chem 278(50):50031–50039
206. Gendron D, Carriero S, Garneau D et al (2006) Modulation of 5′ splice site selection using tailed oligonucleotides carrying splicing signals. BMC Biotechnol 6:5
207. Skordis LA, Dunckley MG, Yue B, Eperon IC, Muntoni F (2003) Bifunctional antisense oligonucleotides provide a trans-acting splicing enhancer that stimulates SMN2 gene expression in patient fibroblasts. Proc Natl Acad Sci U S A 100(7):4114–4119
208. Cartegni L, Krainer AR (2003) Correction of disease-associated exon skipping by synthetic exon-specific activators. Nat Struct Biol 10(2):120–125
209. Wilusz JE, Devanney SC, Caputi M (2005) Chimeric peptide nucleic acid compounds modulate splicing of the bcl-x gene in vitro and in vivo. Nucleic Acids Res 33(20):6547–6554

210. Kishore S, Stamm S (2006) The snoRNA HBII-52 regulates alternative splicing of the serotonin receptor 2C. Science 311(5758):230–232
211. Bland CS, Cooper TA (2007) Micromanaging alternative splicing during muscle differentiation. Dev Cell 12(2):171–172
212. Boutz PL, Chawla G, Stoilov P, Black DL (2007) MicroRNAs regulate the expression of the alternative splicing factor nPTB during muscle development. Genes Dev 21(1):71–84
213. Calin GA, Croce CM (2006) MicroRNA-cancer connection: the beginning of a new tale. Cancer Res 66(15):7390–7394
214. Muraki M, Ohkawara B, Hosoya T et al (2004) Manipulation of alternative splicing by a newly developed inhibitor of Clks. J Biol Chem 279(23):24246–24254
215. Pilch B, Allemand E, Facompre M et al (2001) Specific inhibition of serine- and arginine-rich splicing factors phosphorylation, spliceosome assembly, and splicing by the antitumor drug NB-506. Cancer Res 61(18):6876–6884
216. Soret J, Bakkour N, Maire S et al (2005) Selective modification of alternative splicing by indole derivatives that target serine-arginine-rich protein splicing factors. Proc Natl Acad Sci U S A 102(24):8764–8769
217. Wang Z, Hoffmann HM, Grabowski PJ (1995) Intrinsic U2AF binding is modulated by exon enhancer signals in parallel with changes in splicing activity. RNA 1(1):21–35
218. Kanopka A, Muhlemann O, Akusjarvi G (1996) Inhibition by SR proteins of splicing of a regulated adenovirus pre-mRNA. Nature 381(6582):535–538
219. Caputi M, Zahler AM (2002) SR proteins and hnRNP H regulate the splicing of the HIV-1 tev-specific exon 6D. EMBO J 21(4):845–855
220. Vickers SM, Huang ZQ, MacMillan-Crow L, Greendorfer JS, Thompson JA (2002) Ligand activation of alternatively spliced fibroblast growth factor receptor-1 modulates pancreatic adenocarcinoma cell malignancy. J Gastrointest Surg 6(4):546–553
221. Jang JH (2005) Reciprocal relationship in gene expression between FGFR1 and FGFR3: implication for tumorigenesis. Oncogene 24(5):945–948
222. Kornmann M, Ishiwata T, Matsuda K et al (2002) IIIc isoform of fibroblast growth factor receptor 1 is overexpressed in human pancreatic cancer and enhances tumorigenicity of hamster ductal cells. Gastroenterology 123(1):301–313
223. Sturla LM, Merrick AE, Burchill SA (2003) FGFR3IIIS: a novel soluble FGFR3 spliced variant that modulates growth is frequently expressed in tumour cells. Br J Cancer 89(7):1276–1284
224. Jang JH, Shin KH, Park YJ, Lee RJ, McKeehan WL, Park JG (2000) Novel transcripts of fibroblast growth factor receptor 3 reveal aberrant splicing and activation of cryptic splice sequences in colorectal cancer. Cancer Res 60(15):4049–4052
225. Takaishi S, Sawada M, Morita Y, Seno H, Fukuzawa H, Chiba T (2000) Identification of a novel alternative splicing of human FGF receptor 4: soluble-form splice variant expressed in human gastrointestinal epithelial cells. Biochem Biophys Res Commun 267(2):658–662
226. Leong CO, Vidnovic N, DeYoung MP, Sgroi D, Ellisen LW (2007) The p63/p73 network mediates chemosensitivity to cisplatin in a biologically defined subset of primary breast cancers. J Clin Invest 117(5):1370–1380
227. Nyman U, Sobczak-Pluta A, Vlachos P, Perlmann T, Zhivotovsky B, Joseph B (2005) Full-length p73alpha represses drug-induced apoptosis in small cell lung carcinoma cells. J Biol Chem 280(40):34159–34169
228. Watson IR, Blanch A, Lin DC, Ohh M, Irwin MS (2006) Mdm2-mediated NEDD8 modification of TAp73 regulates its transactivation function. J Biol Chem 281(45):34096–34103
229. Steinman HA, Burstein E, Lengner C et al (2004) An alternative splice form of Mdm2 induces p53-independent cell growth and tumorigenesis. J Biol Chem 279(6):4877–4886
230. Chandler DS, Singh RK, Caldwell LC, Bitler JL, Lozano G (2006) Genotoxic stress Induces coordinately regulated alternative splicing of the p53 modulators MDM2 and MDM4. Cancer Res 66(19):9502–9508
231. Bartel F, Schulz J, Bohnke A et al (2005) Significance of HDMX-S (or MDM4) mRNA splice variant overexpression and HDMX gene amplification on primary soft tissue sarcoma prognosis. Int J Cancer 117(3):469–475

232. Giglio S, Mancini F, Gentiletti F et al (2005) Identification of an aberrantly spliced form of HDMX in human tumors: a new mechanism for HDM2 stabilization. Cancer Res 65(21):9687–9694
233. Agrawal S, Eng C (2006) Differential expression of novel naturally occurring splice variants of PTEN and their functional consequences in Cowden syndrome and sporadic breast cancer. Hum Mol Genet 15(5):777–787
234. Colgin LM, Wilkinson C, Englezou A, Kilian A, Robinson MO, Reddel RR (2000) The hTERTalpha splice variant is a dominant negative inhibitor of telomerase activity. Neoplasia 2(5):426–432
235. Burd CJ, Petre CE, Morey LM et al (2006) Cyclin D1b variant influences prostate cancer growth through aberrant androgen receptor regulation. Proc Natl Acad Sci U S A 103(7):2190–2195
236. Knudsen KE, Diehl JA, Haiman CA, Knudsen ES (2006) Cyclin D1: polymorphism, aberrant splicing and cancer risk. Oncogene 25(11):1620–1628
237. Leung YK, Lau KM, Mobley J, Jiang Z, Ho SM (2005) Overexpression of cytochrome P450 1A1 and its novel spliced variant in ovarian cancer cells: alternative subcellular enzyme compartmentation may contribute to carcinogenesis. Cancer Res 65(9):3726–3734
238. Yu Y, Jiang X, Schoch BS, Carroll RS, Black PM, Johnson MD (2007) Aberrant splicing of cyclin-dependent kinase-associated protein phosphatase KAP increases proliferation and migration in glioblastoma. Cancer Res 67(1):130–138
239. Di Modugno F, DeMonte L, Balsamo M et al (2007) Molecular cloning of hMena (ENAH) and its splice variant hMena +11a: epidermal growth factor increases their expression and stimulates hMena +11a phosphorylation in breast cancer cell lines. Cancer Res 67(6):2657–2665
240. Carson DJ, Santoro IM, Groden J (2004) Isoforms of the APC tumor suppressor and their ability to inhibit cell growth and tumorigenicity. Oncogene 23(42):7144–7148
241. Kawasaki Y, Sato R, Akiyama T (2003) Mutated APC and Asef are involved in the migration of colorectal tumour cells. Nat Cell Biol 5(3):211–215
242. Cooper DL, Dougherty GJ (1995) To metastasize or not? Selection of CD44 splice sites. Nat Med 1(7):635–637
243. Scotlandi K, Zuntini M, Manara MC, et al. (2007) CD99 isoforms dictate opposite functions in tumour malignancy and metastases by activating or repressing c-Src kinase activity. Oncogene 26(46):6604–6618
244. Byun HJ, Hong IK, Kim E et al (2006) A splice variant of CD99 increases motility and MMP-9 expression of human breast cancer cells through the AKT-, ERK-, and JNK-dependent AP-1 activation signaling pathways. J Biol Chem 281(46):34833–34847
245. Oyama F, Hirohashi S, Sakamoto M, Titani K, Sekiguchi K (1993) Coordinate oncodevelopmental modulation of alternative splicing of fibronectin pre-messenger RNA at ED-A, ED-B, and CS1 regions in human liver tumors. Cancer Res 53(9):2005–2011
246. Khan ZA, Chan BM, Uniyal S et al (2005) EDB fibronectin and angiogenesis: a novel mechanistic pathway. Angiogenesis 8(3):183–196
247. Wang L, Lin SH, Wu WG et al (2000) C-CAM1, a candidate tumor suppressor gene, is abnormally expressed in primary lung cancers. Clin Cancer Res 6(8):2988–2993
248. Luo W, Wood CG, Earley K, Hung MC, Lin SH (1997) Suppression of tumorigenicity of breast cancer cells by an epithelial cell adhesion molecule (C-CAM1): the adhesion and growth suppression are mediated by different domains. Oncogene 14(14):1697–1704
249. DiFeo A, Narla G, Hirshfeld J et al (2006) Roles of KLF6 and KLF6-SV1 in ovarian cancer progression and intraperitoneal dissemination. Clin Cancer Res 12(12):3730–3739
250. Camacho-Vanegas O, Narla G, Teixeira MS, et al. (2007) Functional inactivation of the KLF6 tumor suppressor gene by loss of heterozygosity and increased alternative splicing in glioblastoma. Int J Cancer 121(6):1390–1395
251. Esufali S, Charames GS, Pethe VV, Buongiorno P, Bapat B (2007) Activation of tumor-specific splice variant Rac1b by dishevelled promotes canonical Wnt signaling and decreased adhesion of colorectal cancer cells. Cancer Res 67(6):2469–2479
252. Matos P, Jordan P (2006) Rac1, but not Rac1B, stimulates RelB-mediated gene transcription in colorectal cancer cells. J Biol Chem 281(19):13724–13732

253. Takafuji V, Forgues M, Unsworth E, Goldsmith P, Wang XW (2007) An osteopontin fragment is essential for tumor cell invasion in hepatocellular carcinoma. Oncogene 26(44):6361–6371
254. Aigner A, Juhl H, Malerczyk C, Tkybusch A, Benz CC, Czubayko F (2001) Expression of a truncated 100 kDa HER2 splice variant acts as an endogenous inhibitor of tumour cell proliferation. Oncogene 20(17):2101–2111
255. Woolard J, Wang WY, Bevan HS et al (2004) VEGF165b, an inhibitory vascular endothelial growth factor splice variant: mechanism of action, in vivo effect on angiogenesis and endogenous protein expression. Cancer Res 64(21):7822–7835
256. Lokeshwar VB, Estrella V, Lopez L et al (2006) HYAL1-v1, an alternatively spliced variant of HYAL1 hyaluronidase: a negative regulator of bladder cancer. Cancer Res 66(23):11219–11227
257. van Nimwegen MJ, Verkoeijen S, van Buren L, Burg D, van de Water B (2005) Requirement for focal adhesion kinase in the early phase of mammary adenocarcinoma lung metastasis formation. Cancer Res 65(11):4698–4706
258. Song SW, Fuller GN, Zheng H, Zhang W (2005) Inactivation of the invasion inhibitory gene IIp45 by alternative splicing in gliomas. Cancer Res 65(9):3562–3567
259. Luther T, Kotzsch M, Meye A et al (2003) Identification of a novel urokinase receptor splice variant and its prognostic relevance in breast cancer. Thromb Haemost 89(4):705–717
260. Midis GP, Shen Y, Owen-Schaub LB (1996) Elevated soluble Fas (sFas) levels in nonhematopoietic human malignancy. Cancer Res 56(17):3870–3874
261. Ugurel S, Rappl G, Tilgen W, Reinhold U (2001) Increased soluble CD95 (sFas/CD95) serum level correlates with poor prognosis in melanoma patients. Clin Cancer Res 7(5):1282–1286
262. Ueno T, Toi M, Tominaga T (1999) Circulating soluble Fas concentration in breast cancer patients. Clin Cancer Res 5(11):3529–3533
263. Nonomura N, Nishimura K, Ono Y et al (2000) Soluble Fas in serum from patients with renal cell carcinoma. Urology 55(1):151–155
264. Benedict MA, Hu Y, Inohara N, Nunez G (2000) Expression and functional analysis of Apaf-1 isoforms. Extra Wd-40 repeat is required for cytochrome c binding and regulated activation of procaspase-9. J Biol Chem 275(12):8461–8468
265. Ogawa T, Shiga K, Hashimoto S, Kobayashi T, Horii A, Furukawa T (2003) APAF-1-ALT, a novel alternative splicing form of APAF-1, potentially causes impeded ability of undergoing DNA damage-induced apoptosis in the LNCaP human prostate cancer cell line. Biochem Biophys Res Commun 306(2):537–543
266. Li F (2005) Role of survivin and its splice variants in tumorigenesis. Br J Cancer 92(2):212–216
267. Krieg A, Mahotka C, Krieg T et al (2002) Expression of different survivin variants in gastric carcinomas: first clues to a role of survivin-2B in tumour progression. Br J Cancer 86(5):737–743
268. Vegran F, Boidot R, Oudin C, Riedinger JM, Lizard-Nacol S (2005) Distinct expression of Survivin splice variants in breast carcinomas. Int J Oncol 27(4):1151–1157
269. Tsujimoto Y, Croce CM (1986) Analysis of the structure, transcripts, and protein products of bcl-2, the gene involved in human follicular lymphoma. Proc Natl Acad Sci U S A 83(14):5214–5218
270. Tanaka S, Saito K, Reed JC (1993) Structure-function analysis of the Bcl-2 oncoprotein. Addition of a heterologous transmembrane domain to portions of the Bcl-2 beta protein restores function as a regulator of cell survival. J Biol Chem 268(15):10920–10926
271. Boise LH, Gonzalez-Garcia M, Postema CE et al (1993) bcl-x, a bcl-2-related gene that functions as a dominant regulator of apoptotic cell death. Cell 74(4):597–608
272. Marone M, Scambia G, Mozzetti S et al (1998) bcl-2, bax, bcl-XL, and bcl-XS expression in normal and neoplastic ovarian tissues. Clin Cancer Res 4(2):517–524
273. Wu J, Shao ZM, Shen ZZ et al (2000) Significance of apoptosis and apoptotic-related proteins, Bcl-2, and Bax in primary breast cancer. Breast J 6(1):44–52

274. Schmitt E, Paquet C, Beauchemin M, Dever-Bertrand J, Bertrand R (2000) Characterization of Bax-sigma, a cell death-inducing isoform of Bax. Biochem Biophys Res Commun 270(3):868–879
275. Shi B, Triebe D, Kajiji S, Iwata KK, Bruskin A, Mahajna J (1999) Identification and characterization of baxepsilon, a novel bax variant missing the BH2 and the transmembrane domains. Biochem Biophys Res Commun 254(3):779–785
276. Chang DW, Xing Z, Pan Y et al (2002) c-FLIP(L) is a dual function regulator for caspase-8 activation and CD95-mediated apoptosis. EMBO J 21(14):3704–3714
277. Longley DB, Wilson TR, McEwan M et al (2006) c-FLIP inhibits chemotherapy-induced colorectal cancer cell death. Oncogene 25(6):838–848
278. Mulherkar N, Ramaswamy M, Mordi DC, Prabhakar BS (2006) MADD/DENN splice variant of the IG20 gene is necessary and sufficient for cancer cell survival. Oncogene 25(47):6252–6261
279. Bae J, Leo CP, Hsu SY, Hsueh AJ (2000) MCL-1S, a splicing variant of the antiapoptotic BCL-2 family member MCL-1, encodes a proapoptotic protein possessing only the BH3 domain. J Biol Chem 275(33):25255–25261
280. Liu JW, Chandra D, Tang SH, Chopra D, Tang DG (2002) Identification and characterization of Bimgamma, a novel proapoptotic BH3-only splice variant of Bim. Cancer Res 62(10):2976–2981
281. Yamaguchi T, Okada T, Takeuchi K et al (2003) Enhancement of thymidine kinase-mediated killing of malignant glioma by BimS, a BH3-only cell death activator. Gene Ther 10(5):375–385
282. Abrams MT, Robertson NM, Yoon K, Wickstrom E (2004) Inhibition of glucocorticoid-induced apoptosis by targeting the major splice variants of BIM mRNA with small interfering RNA and short hairpin RNA. J Biol Chem 279(53):55809–55817
283. Wang L, Miura M, Bergeron L, Zhu H, Yuan J (1994) Ich-1, an Ice/ced-3-related gene, encodes both positive and negative regulators of programmed cell death. Cell 78(5):739–750
284. Droin N, Beauchemin M, Solary E, Bertrand R (2000) Identification of a caspase-2 isoform that behaves as an endogenous inhibitor of the caspase cascade. Cancer Res 60(24):7039–7047
285. Vegran F, Boidot R, Oudin C, Riedinger JM, Bonnetain F, Lizard-Nacol S (2006) Overexpression of caspase-3 s splice variant in locally advanced breast carcinoma is associated with poor response to neoadjuvant chemotherapy. Clin Cancer Res 12(19):5794–5800
286. Muzio M, Chinnaiyan AM, Kischkel FC et al (1996) FLICE, a novel FADD-homologous ICE/CED-3-like protease, is recruited to the CD95 (Fas/APO-1) death–inducing signaling complex. Cell 85(6):817–827
287. Himeji D, Horiuchi T, Tsukamoto H, Hayashi K, Watanabe T, Harada M (2002) Characterization of caspase-8L: a novel isoform of caspase-8 that behaves as an inhibitor of the caspase cascade. Blood 99(11):4070–4078
288. Waltereit R, Weller M (2002) The role of caspases 9 and 9-short (9S) in death ligand- and drug-induced apoptosis in human astrocytoma cells. Brain Res Mol Brain Res 106(1–2):42–49
289. Lee SB, Haber DA (2001) Wilms tumor and the WT1 gene. Exp Cell Res 264(1):74–99
290. Richard DJ, Schumacher V, Royer-Pokora B, Roberts SG (2001) Par4 is a coactivator for a splice isoform-specific transcriptional activation domain in WT1. Genes Dev 15(3):328–339
291. Tojo Y, Bandoh S, Fujita J et al (2003) Aberrant messenger RNA splicing of the cytokeratin 8 in lung cancer. Lung Cancer 42(2):153–161
292. Yin F, Hu WH, Qiao TD, Fan DM (2004) Multidrug resistant effect of alternative splicing form of MAD2 gene-MAD2beta on human gastric cancer cell. Zhonghua Zhong Liu Za Zhi 26(4):201–204
293. Lixia M, Zhijian C, Chao S, Chaojiang G, Congyi Z (2007) Alternative splicing of breast cancer associated gene BRCA1 from breast cancer cell line. J Biochem Mol Biol 40(1):15–21
294. Orban TI, Olah E (2003) Emerging roles of BRCA1 alternative splicing. Mol Pathol 56(4):191–197
295. Bieche I, Lidereau R (1999) Increased level of exon 12 alternatively spliced BRCA2 transcripts in tumor breast tissue compared with normal tissue. Cancer Res 59(11):2546–2550

296. Khan SG, Muniz-Medina V, Shahlavi T et al (2002) The human XPC DNA repair gene: arrangement, splice site information content and influence of a single nucleotide polymorphism in a splice acceptor site on alternative splicing and function. Nucleic Acids Res 30(16):3624–3631
297. Shiote Y, Ouchida M, Jitsumori Y et al (2006) Multiple splicing variants of Naf1/ABIN-1 transcripts and their alterations in hematopoietic tumors. Int J Mol Med 18(5):917–923
298. Lee EJ, Jo M, Park J, Zhang W, Lee JH (2006) Alternative splicing variants of IRF-1 lacking exons 7, 8, and 9 in cervical cancer. Biochem Biophys Res Commun 347(4):882–888
299. Hube F, Guo J, Chooniedass-Kothari S et al (2006) Alternative splicing of the first intron of the steroid receptor RNA activator (SRA) participates in the generation of coding and noncoding RNA isoforms in breast cancer cell lines. DNA Cell Biol 25(7):418–428
300. Wang L, Duke L, Zhang PS et al (2003) Alternative splicing disrupts a nuclear localization signal in spleen tyrosine kinase that is required for invasion suppression in breast cancer. Cancer Res 63(15):4724–4730
301. Katoh M, Kirikoshi H, Terasaki H, Shiokawa K (2001) WNT2B2 mRNA, up-regulated in primary gastric cancer, is a positive regulator of the WNT- beta-catenin-TCF signaling pathway. Biochem Biophys Res Commun 289(5):1093–1098
302. Lee JH, Gao CF, Lee CC, Kim MD (2006) Vande Woude GF. An alternatively spliced form of Met receptor is tumorigenic. Exp Mol Med 38(5):565–573
303. Treeck O, Pfeiler G, Horn F et al (2007) Novel estrogen receptor beta transcript variants identified in human breast cancer cells affect cell growth and apoptosis of COS-1 cells. Mol Cell Endocrinol 264(1–2):50–60
304. Pind MT, Watson PH (2003) SR protein expression and CD44 splicing pattern in human breast tumours. Breast Cancer Res Treat 79(1):75–82
305. Patry C, Bouchard L, Labrecque P et al (2003) Small interfering RNA-mediated reduction in heterogeneous nuclear ribonucleoparticule A1/A2 proteins induces apoptosis in human cancer cells but not in normal mortal cell lines. Cancer Res 63(22):7679–7688
306. Zhou J, Nong L, Wloch M, Cantor A, Mulshine JL, Tockman MS (2001) Expression of early lung cancer detection marker: hnRNP-A2/B1 and its relation to microsatellite alteration in non-small cell lung cancer. Lung Cancer 34(3):341–350
307. Zech VF, Dlaska M, Tzankov A, Hilbe W (2006) Prognostic and diagnostic relevance of hnRNP A2/B1, hnRNP B1 and S100 A2 in non-small cell lung cancer. Cancer Detect Prev 30(5):395–402
308. Hiraki A, Murakami T, Aoe K et al (2006) Heterogeneous nuclear ribonucleoprotein B1 expression in malignant mesothelioma. Cancer Sci 97(11):1175–1181
309. Brose MS, Volpe P, Paul K et al (2004) Characterization of two novel BRCA1 germ-line mutations involving splice donor sites. Genet Test 8(2):133–138
310. Chen X, Truong TT, Weaver J et al (2006) Intronic alterations in BRCA1 and BRCA2: effect on mRNA splicing fidelity and expression. Hum Mutat 27(5):427–435
311. Bonatti F, Pepe C, Tancredi M et al (2006) RNA-based analysis of BRCA1 and BRCA2 gene alterations. Cancer Genet Cytogenet 170(2):93–101
312. Humar B, Toro T, Graziano F et al (2002) Novel germline CDH1 mutations in hereditary diffuse gastric cancer families. Hum Mutat 19(5):518–525
313. Loo JC, Liu L, Hao A et al (2003) Germline splicing mutations of CDKN2A predispose to melanoma. Oncogene 22(41):6387–6394
314. Wolf M, Hemminki A, Kivioja A et al (1998) A novel splice site mutation of the EXT2 gene in a finnish hereditary multiple exostoses family. Mutations in brief no. 197. Online. Hum Mutat 12(5):362
315. Tamary H, Dgany O, Toledano H et al (2004) Molecular characterization of three novel Fanconi anemia mutations in Israeli Arabs. Eur J Haematol 72(5):330–335
316. Hastings ML, Resta N, Traum D, Stella A, Guanti G, Krainer AR (2005) An LKB1 AT-AC intron mutation causes Peutz-Jeghers syndrome via splicing at noncanonical cryptic splice sites. Nat Struct Mol Biol 12(1):54–59
317. Turner JJ, Leotlela PD, Pannett AA et al (2002) Frequent occurrence of an intron 4 mutation in multiple endocrine neoplasia type 1. J Clin Endocrinol Metab 87(6):2688–2693

318. Baehring J, Sutter C, Kadmon M, Doeberitz MV, Gebert J (2006) A 'nonsense' mutation leads to aberrant splicing of hMLH1 in a German hereditary non-polyposis colorectal cancer family. Fam Cancer 5(2):195–199
319. Nemoto H, Tate G, Schirinzi A et al (2006) Novel NF1 gene mutation in a Japanese patient with neurofibromatosis type 1 and a gastrointestinal stromal tumor. J Gastroenterol 41(4):378–382
320. Reifenberger J, Rauch L, Beckmann MW, Megahed M, Ruzicka T, Reifenberger G (2003) Cowden's disease: clinical and molecular genetic findings in a patient with a novel PTEN germline mutation. Br J Dermatol 148(5):1040–1046
321. Niemann S, Muller U, Engelhardt D, Lohse P (2003) Autosomal dominant malignant and catecholamine-producing paraganglioma caused by a splice donor site mutation in SDHC. Hum Genet 113(1):92–94
322. Martella M, Salviati L, Casarin A et al (2006) Molecular analysis of two uncharacterized sequence variants of the VHL gene. J Hum Genet 51(11):964–968
323. Abu-Amero KK, Owaidah TM, Al Jefri A, Al-Ghonaium A, Fawaz IM, Al-Hamed MH (2004) A novel splice site mutation in the WAS gene causes Wiskott-Aldrich syndrome in two siblings of a Saudi family. Blood Coagul Fibrinolysis 15(7):599–603
324. Tanioka M, Budiyant A, Ueda T et al (2005) A novel XPA gene mutation and its functional analysis in a Japanese patient with xeroderma pigmentosum group A. J Invest Dermatol 125(2):244–246
325. Spirio L, Green J, Robertson J et al (1999) The identical 5′ splice-site acceptor mutation in five attenuated APC families from Newfoundland demonstrates a founder effect. Hum Genet 105(5):388–398
326. Chen LL, Sabripour M, Wu EF, Prieto VG, Fuller GN, Frazier ML (2005) A mutation-created novel intra-exonic pre-mRNA splice site causes constitutive activation of KIT in human gastrointestinal stromal tumors. Oncogene 24(26):4271–4280
327. Tala HP, Carvajal CA, Gonzalez AA et al (2006) New splicing mutation of MEN1 gene affecting the translocation of menin to the nucleus. J Endocrinol Invest 29(10):888–893
328. Martinez R, Schackert HK, von Kannen S, Lichter P, Joos S, Schackert G (2003) Independent molecular development of metachronous glioblastomas with extended intervening recurrence-free interval. Brain Pathol 13(4):598–607
329. Ariga T, Yamada M, Pudua FR, Sakiyama Y (1996) Detection of a novel splice-site mutation that results in skipping exon 3 of the WASP gene in a patient with Wiskott-Aldrich syndrome. Biochim Biophys Acta 1317(3):158–160
330. Kanemoto K, Ishikura K, Ariyasu D et al (2007) WT1 intron 9 splice acceptor site mutation in a 46, XY male with focal segmental glomerulosclerosis. Pediatr Nephrol 22(3):454–458
331. Aceto G, Cristina Curia M, Veschi S et al (2005) Mutations of APC and MYH in unrelated Italian patients with adenomatous polyposis coli. Hum Mutat 26(4):394
332. Rutter JL, Goldstein AM, Davila MR, Tucker MA, Struewing JP (2003) CDKN2A point mutations D153spl(c.457G > T) and IVS2 + 1G > T result in aberrant splice products affecting both p16INK4a and p14ARF. Oncogene 22(28):4444–4448
333. Pagenstecher C, Wehner M, Friedl W et al (2006) Aberrant splicing in MLH1 and MSH2 due to exonic and intronic variants. Hum Genet 119(1–2):9–22
334. Raponi M, Upadhyaya M, Baralle D (2006) Functional splicing assay shows a pathogenic intronic mutation in neurofibromatosis type 1 (NF1) due to intronic sequence exonization. Hum Mutat 27(3):294–295
335. Trojan J, Plotz G, Brieger A et al (2001) Activation of a cryptic splice site of PTEN and loss of heterozygosity in benign skin lesions in Cowden disease. J Invest Dermatol 117(6):1650–1653
336. Andreu N, Carreras C, Prieto F, Estivill X, Volpini V, Fillat C (2003) Identification and characterization of a novel splice-site mutation in a patient with Wiskott-Aldrich syndrome. J Hum Genet 48(11):590–593
337. Heikkinen K, Mansikka V, Karppinen SM, Rapakko K, Winqvist R (2005) Mutation analysis of the ATR gene in breast and ovarian cancer families. Breast Cancer Res 7(4):R495–R501

338. Mazoyer S, Puget N, Perrin-Vidoz L, Lynch HT, Serova-Sinilnikova OM, Lenoir GM (1998) A BRCA1 nonsense mutation causes exon skipping. Am J Hum Genet 62(3):713–715
339. Fackenthal JD, Cartegni L, Krainer AR, Olopade OI (2002) BRCA2 T2722R is a deleterious allele that causes exon skipping. Am J Hum Genet 71(3):625–631
340. McVety S, Li L, Gordon PH, Chong G, Foulkes WD (2006) Disruption of an exon splicing enhancer in exon 3 of MLH1 is the cause of HNPCC in a Quebec family. J Med Genet 43(2):153–156
341. Baralle M, Skoko N, Knezevich A et al (2006) NF1 mRNA biogenesis: effect of the genomic milieu in splicing regulation of the NF1 exon 37 region. FEBS Lett 580(18):4449–4456
342. Bottillo I, De Luca A, Schirinzi A et al (2007) Functional analysis of splicing mutations in exon 7 of NF1 gene. BMC Med Genet 8:4
343. Suphapeetiporn K, Kongkam P, Tantivatana J, Sinthuwiwat T, Tongkobpetch S, Shotelersuk V (2006) PTEN c.511C > T nonsense mutation in a BRRS family disrupts a potential exonic splicing enhancer and causes exon skipping. Jpn J Clin Oncol 36(12):814–821
344. Gorlov IP, Gorlova OY, Frazier ML, Amos CI (2004) Missense mutations in cancer suppressor gene TP53 are colocalized with exonic splicing enhancers (ESEs). Mutat Res 554(1–2):175–183
345. Narla G, Difeo A, Reeves HL et al (2005) A germline DNA polymorphism enhances alternative splicing of the KLF6 tumor suppressor gene and is associated with increased prostate cancer risk. Cancer Res 65(4):1213–1222
346. Khan SG, Metin A, Gozukara E et al (2004) Two essential splice lariat branchpoint sequences in one intron in a xeroderma pigmentosum DNA repair gene: mutations result in reduced XPC mRNA levels that correlate with cancer risk. Hum Mol Genet 13(3):343–352
347. De Klein A, Riegman PH, Bijlsma EK et al (1998) A G– > A transition creates a branch point sequence and activation of a cryptic exon, resulting in the hereditary disorder neurofibromatosis 2. Hum Mol Genet 7(3):393–398

Alternative Splicing of Tumor Suppressors and Oncogenes

Claudia Ghigna, Silvano Riva and Giuseppe Biamonti

Abstract

Alternative splicing is a fundamental mechanism to modulate gene expression programs in response to different growth and environmental stimuli. There is now ample evidence that alternative splicing errors, caused by mutations in *cis*-acting elements and defects and/or imbalances in *trans*-acting factors, may be causatively associated to cancer progression. Recent work indicates the existence of an intricate network of interactions between alternative splicing events and signal transduction pathways. In this network, splicing factors occupy a central position and appear to function both as targets and effectors of regulatory circuits. Thus, a change in their activity deeply affects alternative splicing profiles and hence the cell behavior. Here, we discuss a number of cases that exemplify the involvement of deregulated alternative splicing in tumor progression.

Keywords

Alternative splicing and cell membrane proteins · Alternative splicing and cell invasiveness · Alternative splicing and EMT · Alternative splicing and signal transduction

Contents

C. Ghigna · S. Riva · G. Biamonti (✉)
Istituto di Genetica Molecolare, Consiglio Nazionale delle Ricerche,
Pavia 27100, Italy
e-mail: biamonti@igm.cnr.it

J. Y. Wu (ed.), *RNA and Cancer*, Cancer Treatment and Research,
DOI: 10.1007/978-3-642-31659-3_4,

1 Introduction

Extensive duplications within the genome followed by a variety of modifications of the genetic information account for the complexity of proteomes in prokaryotes and lower eukaryotes. However, during evolution the number of genes stopped growing in parallel with the complexity of the proteome and evolution of metazoan is marked by new mechanisms to generate protein diversity. Thus, the human genome contains only 20,000–25,000 genes (International Human genome Sequencing Consortium, 2004)—twice as many as in the fly—while the proteome might number more than several hundred thousand of protein species [1]. This discrepancy in number between genes and proteins leads to a better appreciation of alternative splicing as the source of the proteome complexity.

The term "alternative splicing" describes any situation in which a single primary transcript can be spliced in more than one pattern to generate multiple, distinct, mature RNAs [2]. There are remarkable examples of hundreds and even thousands of functionally divergent mRNAs and proteins being produced from a single gene. The *Drosophila DSCAM* gene is both a fascinating example of the subtle structural changes that can be introduced in a protein and an extraordinary demonstration of the number of proteins that can be generated from a single gene through alternative splicing (if all combinations of alternatively spliced exons were used the *DSCAM* gene would produce 38.016 different DSCAM proteins!) [3].

It has been estimated that more than 90 % of human genes encode for transcripts that undergo alternative splicing, which underscores a major role of this mechanism in the regulation of the gene expression [4, 5]. Indeed, appropriate spatio-temporal generation of splicing variants is required for organism development, to define cell identity, and for cell adaptation to environmental cues. Although the molecular details are still to be deciphered, it is likely that proper alternative splicing depends on extensive regulation networks similar to the ones that ensure transcriptional control.

We can distinguish two types of exons (Fig. 1). Most exons are constitutive which means that they are always spliced and included in the mature mRNA. On the contrary, a regulated exon is sometimes included and sometimes excluded from the mRNA and is called a cassette exon. In certain cases, multiple cassette exons are mutually exclusive, i.e. the mature mRNA always contains only one of

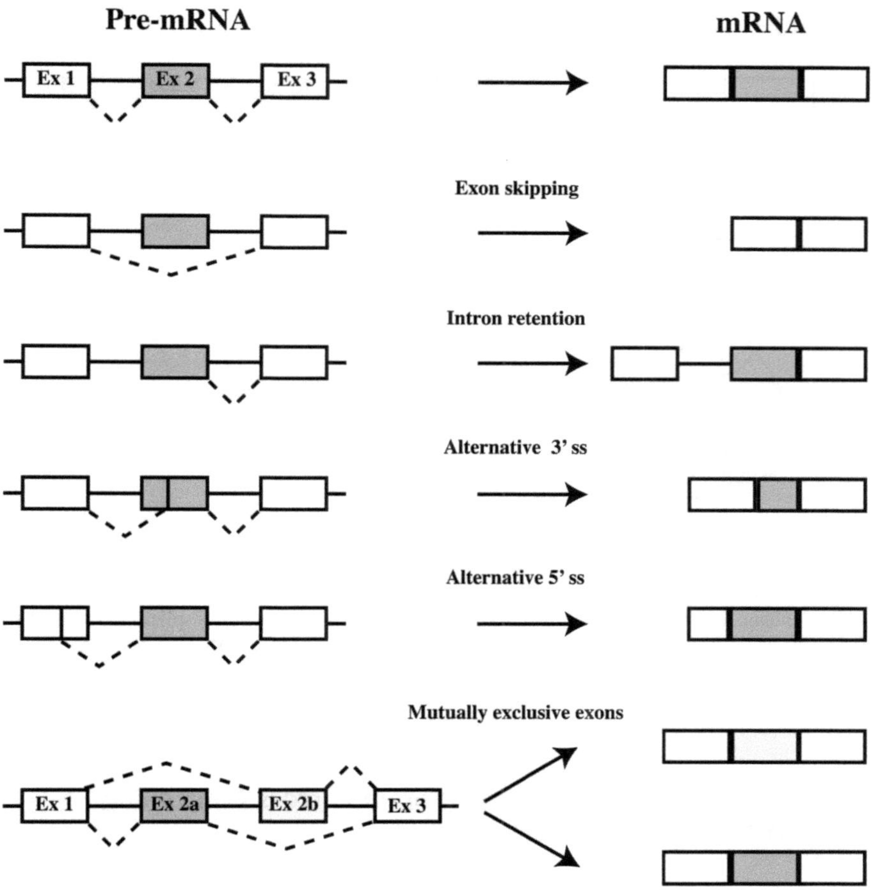

Fig. 1 Different types of alternative splicing. Alternatively spliced mRNAs result from exon skipping, intron retention, usage of alternative 5′- (donor) or 3′- (acceptor) sites, and from selection of mutually exclusive exons. At the protein level, alternative splicing drastically affects the amino acid sequence by deletion or insertion of domains, frame-shifts, or stop codons. Alternative splicing in non-coding regions of the mature mRNA might impact on translation and mRNA stability

several possible exon choices. In rare cases, a whole intron is removed or retained to give two different messenger RNAs. Alternative 5′ or 3′ splice sites can result in exons of different size. Additionally, alternative splicing of transcripts initiated at different transcription start sites leads to mature mRNAs with different first exons. The 3′ terminal exons can also vary by coupling alternative splicing with alternative polyadenylation. To understand the mechanisms that control alternative splicing is a major task of future studies.

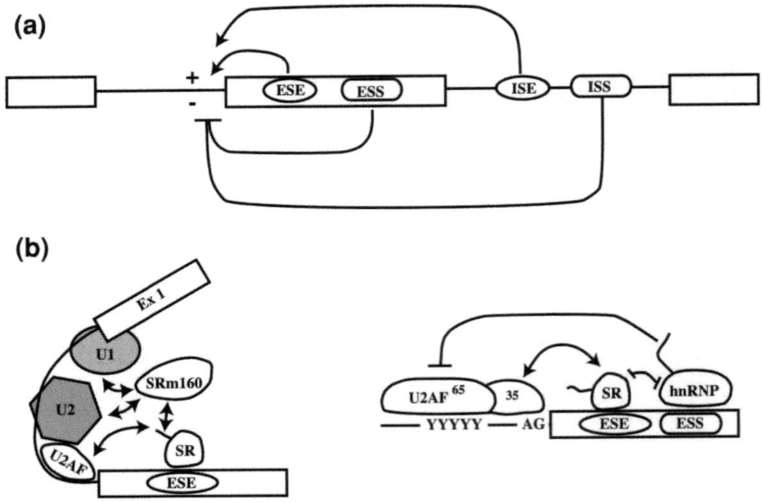

Fig. 2 *Cis-* and *trans-*acting elements that control alternative splicing. **a** Alternatively spliced exons are usually characterized by weak splice sites. Recognition of these sites depends on splicing regulatory elements: exonic splicing enhancers (*ESE*) and silencers (*ESS*) and intronic splicing enhancers (*ISE*) and silencers (*ISS*). **b** ESE elements are bound by splicing factors of the SR family. Via interactions with proteins of the splicing apparatus, the RS domain of SR factors promotes the assembly of the spliceosome on the upstream exon. In addition, SR proteins can counteract the inhibitory activity of hnRNP proteins bound to ESS elements

1.1 Sequence Elements and Protein Factors Controlling Alternative Splicing

The mechanisms of splice site selection in constitutive and alternative splicing appear to be closely connected, since components of the spicing machinery that are essential for splicing of constitutive exons are also implicated in the regulation of alternatively spliced sequences [2]. From a mechanistic standpoint, the different types of alternative splicing can be simply viewed as a problem of splice site recognition by the splicing machinery, the spliceosome: the decision as to whether a particular exon, or exon region, is included in the final mRNA molecule mainly depends on the recognition and utilization of the splice sites that flank the exon.

Alternative exons are often characterized by short and degenerate splice sites whose recognition by the spliceosome is modulated by a number of auxiliary cis-acting elements, referred to as enhancers and silencers of splicing that respectively promote and inhibit exon recognition. These regulatory elements are frequently clustered on the pre-mRNA [6] and can be found both within exons (ESEs, Exonic Splicing Enhancers and ESSs Exonic Splicing Silencers) and introns (ISEs, Intronic Splicing Enhancer, ISSs, Intronic Splicing Silencers) [7] (Fig. 2a). The best-characterized splicing enhancers are typically purine-rich. A variety of RNA-binding assay and in vitro and in vivo selection (SELEX) experiments have shown that these sequences function by providing binding sites for serine-arginine (SR) proteins, a family of essential splicing factors highly conserved in metazoans [8, 9]. All members of this family share a modular structure consisting of one or two copies of an RNA-recognition motif (RRM) followed by a C-terminal domain rich in alternating serine and arginine residues (the RS domain) [10]. The RRMs determine the RNA-binding specificity, whereas the RS domain mediates protein–protein interactions that are essential for the recruitment of the splicing apparatus and for pairing of 5′- and 3′-splice sites [11–13] (Fig. 2b). In addition, RS domains are targets of phosphorylation events that influence the activity [14] and the sub-cellular localization of SR proteins [15]. A number of SR-specific kinases, including the SR protein kinases SRPK1 and 2 [15, 16] topoisomerase I [17] and the cdc-like kinase CLK/Sty [18], has been identified. The role of these kinases is still poorly understood; however, in some cases they appear to control different properties of splicing factors. Thus, for instance, phosphorylation by cytoplasmic SRPK1, is required for nuclear import [15] and the successive accumulation in nuclear speckles of shuttling SR proteins. Thereafter, phosphorylation by CLK/Sty kinase controls mobilization from nuclear speckles to sites of pre-mRNA splicing in the nucleoplasm.

Several models have been proposed for the function of ESEs and SR proteins. According to one of these models, upon binding to an ESE, SR proteins promote exon definition by directly recruiting the splicing machinery through specific protein–protein interactions mediated by the RS domain [19–21] (Fig. 2b). Another model predicts that the main function of ESE-bound SR proteins is to antagonize the negative effect on splicing of an inhibitory protein that is bound to a juxtaposed silencer element (ESS) [22]. These models of splicing enhancement are not necessarily mutually exclusive, as they might reflect different requirements in the context of different exons. Splicing silencers identified to date appear remarkably diverse. They may act as binding sites for factors that block access of the splicing machinery to a splice site. Among the proteins interacting with silencers there are heterogeneous nuclear ribonucleoproteins (hnRNP), a group of RNA-binding proteins that share the ability to interact with nascent pre-mRNAs. Similar to SR factors, hnRNP proteins have a modular structure. They contain at least one of three different RNA-binding domains: RRMs, KH-(hnRNP K homology) domain, and RGG domain (a protein region rich in Arg-Gly-Gly repetitions). These domains provide a certain level of RNA-binding specificity. HnRNPs also contain the so-called “auxiliary” domains, very different in sequence, that control the sub-cellular localization and the interaction with other proteins. RNA-binding specificity and protein–protein interactions contribute to the assembly of the ribonucleoprotein complexes that are the substrates for the ensuing splicing reaction. Two hnRNP proteins, hnRNP A1 and hnRNP I (better known as polypyrimidine tract-binding protein or PTB) have been characterized in detail as mediators of silencer activity [22].

Only in few cases alternatively spliced exons are controlled by tissue-specific splicing regulators. An example is provided by the Nova-1 and Nova-2 proteins [23] that are expressed almost exclusively in neurons of the central nervous system, where they control alternative splicing of genes involved in the regulation of synapse activity. The vast majority of alternative splicing events, on the contrary, appear to be controlled by the relative abundance and/or activity of widely expressed antagonistic SR factors and hnRNP proteins through a combinatorial mechanism, with multiple positive and negative factors and sequence elements influencing the final outcome of the splicing reaction. This is exemplified by antagonistic SF2/ASF, an SR factor, and hnRNP A1 proteins: high levels of SF2/ASF induce exon inclusion whereas high levels of hnRNP A1 promote exon skipping [22, 24]. Recent studies indicate that signaling pathways may control in splicing decisions by affecting the sub-cellular distribution and/or activity of splicing regulators [25, 26]. Many SR factors and hnRNP proteins continuously and rapidly shuttle between the nucleus and the cytoplasm [27], which unveils a cytoplasmic function of these proteins, as for instance in mRNA translation. Several stress treatments perturb the nucleo-cytoplasmic distribution of some splicing regulators. For instance, osmotic stress leads to cytoplasmic accumulation of hnRNP A1 while a number of splicing regulators, including SF2/ASF, is sequestered in nuclear stress bodies after treatments that activate the heat shock response [25, 26]. This opens the exciting possibility that stressing conditions, as for instance those in the tumor microenvironment may influence the splicing profile of a number of genes thus affecting cell identity.

The complexity of the regulatory pathways underlying alternative splicing makes their molecular characterization a really challenging task. So far, only a few systems of regulated splice site choice have been genetically or biochemically dissected, and many regulatory proteins and sequence elements are as yet to be identified.

2 Alternative Splicing and Cancer

The idea that alternative splicing plays a prominent role in the modulating diverse and even antagonistic cell functions has recently gained momentum due to a surge in careful examination of gene transcripts. Indeed, the generation of protein isoforms through alternative splicing enables fine-tuning of critical cellular processes such as proliferation, differentiation, apoptosis, migration, and survival to stressing conditions. It is not unexpected, therefore, that the alteration of the normal splicing profile of critical genes can be causatively linked to inherited and acquired genetic diseases. There are several examples of hereditary genetic disorders associated with defects in the splicing profile of specific genes. These include, among others, spinal muscular atrophy, myotonic dystrophy, retinitis pigmentosa, Frasier syndrome, atypical cystic fibrosis, and certain neurodegenerative diseases [28, 29]. It has been calculated that 15–50 % of point mutations that cause hereditary diseases alter pre-mRNA processing by affecting canonical 5′ and 3′ splice sites, branch sites, or polyadenylation signals [30, 31]. In some cases, mutations affect splicing regulatory elements (enhancers and silencer) and prevent the interaction with splicing regulators (hnRNPs and SR factors) thus changing pre-mRNA processing. Indeed, the analysis of a database of 50 single-base substitutions that cause exon skipping in human genes showed that more than 50 % of these substitutions, which include missense, nonsense, and translationally silent mutations, disrupted at least one target motif for SR proteins in ESEs [32]. Notably, premature stop codons introduced as a consequence of splicing defects, far from resulting in the synthesis of shorter nonfunctional proteins, target the mRNA to degradation by the nonsense-mediated decay pathway (NMD) [33]. As a consequence no protein at all is synthesized by the cell. In the last few years, a link has emerged between cancer development and inappropriate alternative splicing [22, 29]. The transition from normal cell growth to neoplasia and subsequently to malignancy is a multistep selection process that affects important cell features. Recent progress in molecular and cell biology indicate that altered splicing profiles of critical genes may impact on all the major aspects of cancer cell biology including cell cycle control, activation of signal transduction pathways, the ability to survive to stressful conditions that elicit apoptosis, activation of gene expression programs involved in angiogenesis, cell motility, and invasive phenotypes associated with metastatic spreading of the tumor. A good example is the tumor-suppressor *BRCA*1 gene. Germline mutations in this gene are well-known markers of predisposition to breast and ovarian cancers. A nonsense mutation in exon 18 was the first one that was shown to affect splicing by disrupting an ESE element and inducing exon skipping [34]. Since then, panoply of mutations that presumably affect splicing enhancers and silencers has been described in *BRCA*1. An in silico approach using the program ESEfinder [35] has identified 23 highly conserved ESEs in the 22 exons of the *BRCA*1 gene. About 60 % of these ESEs are predicted to be affected by sequence variants reported in the Breast Cancer Information Core [36]. Similar observations have been done with a number of tumor-associated genes such as *p*53, *APC, FHIT* and *LKB*1, *cyclin D* and *p*16 *arf*. However, all these cases, and many others that are continuously described, represent an extension of the concept according to which cancer progression is due to a number of stable genetic mutations that perturb the structure, the function or the abundance of critical proteins. In this sense, splicing defects can be viewed as one of routes through which gene mutations cause tumorigenesis. More interesting from our point of view, is the observation, reported by many studies over the last 20 years that a number of alternative splicing events that distinguish the cancerous cell from its normal counterpart do not result from mutations in the affected gene. This implies that the splicing defect is due to an alteration in the expression and/or activity of splicing regulators [22, 29]. Indeed, changes in the repertoire of SR factors and hnRNP proteins frequently occur in tumors and are accompanied by alterations in the ratio between alternative splicing products, a typical signature of cancerous cells with predictable effects on cellular behavior [37–41]. As a matter of fact, cancerous cell lines show a high level of alternative splicing events that are not conserved between human and mouse and are not expressed in normal tissues [42] strengthening the idea that a change in the level of splicing regulators in cancer cells may severely impact on gene expression programs. From this viewpoint, splicing regulators can be considered as true oncoproteins and tumor suppressors depending on their antagonistic functions on splice site selection.

Also post-translational modifications of splicing regulators may be relevant for tumor progression. Thus, SRPK1 is over-expressed in breast and colonic tumors and the level of this kinase increases in parallel with the tumor grade [43]. Interestingly, RNAi-mediated down-regulation of SRPK1 in breast and colon tumor cell lines promotes cell apoptosis and makes the cell more sensitive to chemotherapeutic intervention [43]. This suggests that SRPK1 inhibitors may be effective either as stand-alone anti-tumor drugs or in combination with conventional chemotherapeutic regimens.

2.1 Alternative Splicing and Apoptosis

Apoptosis or programmed cell death is essential for proper development and for maintenance of cellular homeostasis in multicellular organisms. Consequently, abnormalities in this crucial physiological process impact on important human pathologies among which autoimmune disorders, degenerative diseases, and cancer. An increasing body of data indicates a role of alternative splicing in controlling programmed cell death [44] and, in a way, the choice between cell life and death. Indeed, for a number of critical genes, alternative splicing determines the choice between proteins isoforms with distinct and even opposing functions in the apoptotic cascade. This is thoroughly discussed by Schwerk and Schulze-Osthoff [44]. Here we will focus on two genes, *caspase*-9 and *Bcl-X*, that very well illustrate the link between external stimuli and splice site choice. These two examples point to alternative splicing as a potent gene expression regulator that is involved in the ability of the cells to cope with stressful conditions originating from environmental changes. Alternative splicing of exon of the *caspase*-9 gene leads to the production of two proteins: a long caspase-9a isoform, which is a post-mitochondrial initiator of the apoptotic cascade, and a short caspase-9b protein that lacks the catalytic domain and acts as a dominant-negative inhibitor of apoptosis possibly by interfering with the formation of the functional "apoptosome complex" with Apaf1 [45]. Bcl-X is a member of the *Bcl*II family that directs mitochondrial breakdown during apoptosis. Alternative 5′ splice sites within exon 2 are involved in the production of two protein isoforms: a long antiapoptotic form (Bcl-XL) and a short apoptosis-promoting protein (Bcl-XS) [46]. Several RNA processing factors including Sam68, the SR factor SF2/ASF, hnRNP F/H proteins, and SAP155 contribute in controlling the choice between the two alternative 5′-splice sites. For instance, Sam68 over-expression induces the production of pro-apoptotic Bcl-XS and this effect is reverted upon Sam68 phosphorylation [47]. On the other hand, hnRNP F/H proteins [48] promote the usage of the *Bcl-XS*-5′ splice site by binding to a G-rich stretch immediately downstream of this site [49]. All these RNA processing factors are necessary to modulate *Bcl-X* splicing in response to different extra-cellular factors including interleukin-6, granulocyte–macrophage colony stimulating factor (GM-CSF), TPA [50], and ceramide. The lipid ceramide is a mediator/regulator of apoptosis, and promotes the expression of the pro-apoptotic splicing variants Bcl-XS and caspase-9a with the concomitant loss in the anti-apoptotic isoforms Bcl-XL and caspase-9b. In the case of *Bcl-X*, the choice between the two alternative 5′-splice sites is controlled by a ceramide responsive element (CRCE 1) within exon 2 [51] and bound by SAP155 [51]. Down-regulation of SAP155 by RNA interference increases the production of Bcl-XS and mimics the effect of exogenous ceramide on the activation of the *Bcl-XS* 5′ splice site. Ceramide acts by modulating the phosphorylation status of SR proteins in a phosphatase-1 (PP1)-dependent manner [51]. Several studies have demonstrated a role for PP1 in regulating alternative splicing and spliceosomal targets for PP1 have been described [52–54]. One of these is the SR factor SF2/ASF which is a major regulator both of *caspase*-9 and of *Bcl-X* pre-mRNAs processing [55].

The ratio of caspase-9 and Bcl-X splice variants has a direct relevance in the cell sensitivity to a wide variety of apoptotic agents and may have significance in drugs resistance and chemotherapeutic sensitivity. Consequently, the possibility to modulate the production of the different isoforms via pharmaceutical manipulation of alternative splicing may open up new therapeutic avenues for the treatment of cancer.

2.2 Alternative Splicing and Cell Membrane Proteins

Recently, the link between alternative splicing and tumor development has started to emerge from the study of cell surface proteins and their molecular partners, most of which can control invasive growth and formation of metastases. Since cancer-related splice variants can provide unique biomarkers for diagnosis and treatment of cancer, alternative splicing of these molecules has been thoroughly investigated. Below we report a few relevant examples.

*CD*44 is the main receptor for hyaluronan, which is the major component of extracellular matrix (ECM). Alternative splicing of *CD*44 pre-mRNA responds to alterations in the ECM that influence cell growth, survival, and differentiation. Moreover, it is critical for organ development, neuronal axon guidance, immune functions, haematopoiesis, and tumor development. The coding region of the *CD*44 gene consists of 21 constitutive exons and contains a block of 10 consecutive variant exons (v1–v10) that are subjected to extensive alternative splicing leading to the production of several isoforms [56]. The physiological relevance of these isoforms is poorly understood. However, a large number of studies indicate that specific CD44 splicing variants, which include exon v5 and or v6, are mainly found in proliferating cells and tumors, and their expression often correlates with enhanced malignancy and invasiveness [57]. For example, isoforms including exon v6 (CD44v6) are bad prognostic markers of gastric cancer. By means of antibodies specifically directed against the v6 peptide, it has been shown that CD44v6 isoforms are frequently up-regulated in squamous cell carcinomas and in a proportion of adenocarcinomas of different origin [58]. These results paved the way to the development of new therapeutic tools and radiolabeled anti-v6 antibodies are in clinical trials for the treatment of head and neck cancers [59].

Recent findings indicate that changes in the epigenome enhance the probability of the transformed cell to metastasise. While a genetic mutation initiates the cancer, the epigenetic change would be necessary to promote cancer progression. Importantly, epigenetic reorganization of the chromatin structure and histone modifications can also modulate specific alternative splicing decisions. This has been shown for the *CD*44 gene where the information stored in the histones bound to variant exons is conveyed via HP1γ to the splicing factors and mediates the association of nascent pre-mRNA with chromatin [60].

The gene of the fibroblast growth factor receptor (FGFR1) is characterized by alternative splicing of a single exon encoding an Ig-like loop in the extracellular domain. The FGFR1-β isoform, which originates from skipping of this exon, has a higher affinity for fibroblast growth factors [61] and its increased expression correlates with cancer in the pancreas, and in brain, and with poor prognosis in breast tumors [62, 63]. Moreover, contrary to the full-length protein, FGFR1-β promotes tumor formation in nude mice [61]. The ratio between the two isoforms is controlled by two RNA processing factors: SRp55 and the polypyrimidine tract-binding protein (PTB). Splicing regulator SRp55 binds to a 69-nucleotide exonic splicing enhancer (ESE), which is required for alpha-exon inclusion [64]. On the other hand, PTB, also known as hnRNP I, directly binds to a sequence upstream of the α-exon and when overexpressed promotes exon skipping and production of FGFR1-β. Thus, the up-regulation of PTB observed in brain tumors may be causatively linked to the deregulated splicing profile of FGFR1 [65]. This provides a further example of the link between the altered levels of specific RNA-binding proteins and the appearance of the cancerous phenotype, which supports the idea that RNA processing factors may be true oncoproteins. Antisense oligos directed either against the PTB mRNA or complementary to the PTB binding site upstream of α-exon can reduce the FGFR1-β/FGFR1-α ratio and restore FGFR1 splicing in cell cultures [66]. Interestingly, splicing restoration causes an up-regulation of caspases 3 and 7, which, ultimately, may be a mechanism for splicing-related gene therapy [66].

The *TrkA*/*NTRK*1 (neurotrophin receptor tropomyosin-related kinase A) gene encodes the receptor of nerve growth factor (NGF). TrkA is a tumor-suppressing trans-membrane receptor that is mutated to constitutively active forms in many cancers. A constitutively active isoform, called TrkAIII, is generated through alternative splicing events that promote skipping of exons 6, 7, and 9. This isoform lacks the regulatory immunoglobulin-like domains located in the extracellular region of the receptor and its expression is restricted to undifferentiated early neural progenitors, to human neuroblastomas (NBs), and to a subset of other neural crest-derived tumors. Interestingly, the production of TrkAIII is stimulated by hypoxia, which suggests the possibility that stressing conditions may ultimately lead to the expression of an isoform that increases cell survival. Indeed, TrkAIII over-expression confers to the cells the ability to form tumors, to resist apoptosis, and to stimulate angiogenesis. This is due to the ability to TrkAIII to activate the

PI3K/AKT signaling pathway and to upregulate the vascular endothelial growth factor (VEGF) [67].

The fibroblast growth factor receptor 3 (FGFR3) is involved in tumor suppression and maintenance of the differentiated state. Various alternative splicing events leading to frame-shifts around the third immunoglobulin loop are expressed at high levels in colorectal cancer [68].

*KAI*1/*CD*82 is a transmembrane glycoprotein that suppresses the formation of metastases. A variant lacking the 28 amino acids encoded by exon 7 fails to localize to the cell membrane and its expression in gastric cancer tumors associated with short survival time [69].

The cell adhesion molecule *C-CAM*1, also called *CEACAM*1, has two major isoforms, L-form *C-CAM*1 and S-form *C-CAM*1, which are produced through alternative splicing of exon 7 (53 bp). Skipping of this exon dramatically affects the length of the protein, since it generates a frame shift that leads to a premature stop codon in exon 8. As a result, S-form *C-CAM*1 lacks the 73-amino acid cytoplasmic domain that is implicated in insulin receptor signaling. Interestingly, expression of S-form *C-CAM*1 increases during lung tumorigenesis [70].

*Integrin β*1*C* differs from *integrin* 1*A* for the inclusion of an alternative exon that changes the cytoplasmic tail of the protein. The 1C form inhibits cell proliferation and is down-regulated in endometrial cancers [71].

The expression of the anti-apoptotic protein *survivin* is grossly elevated in many cancers, while the surviving 2B splice variant has a growth-inhibitory effect and is lost in late-stage breast [72] and colonic cancers [73].

The proteins listed above lay at the starting point of signal transduction cascades that, as detailed below, may influence the activity of splicing regulators. Thus, expression of alternatively spliced variants of cell surface proteins may have a strong impact on the splicing profile of several additional genes. On the other hand, activation of signal transduction pathways in response to external stimuli may affect the splicing profile of cell membrane proteins. This could lead to a self-sustained loop characterized by a mutual influence between cell membrane proteins and signal transduction pathways with important effects on the cell identity.

2.3 Alternative Splicing and Cell Invasiveness

There are several examples of alternative splicing events that control the expression of genes involved in cell motility and invasion, a pre-requisite for the formation of cancer metastases.

This is the case of specific alternative splicing variants of the *androgen* and *estrogen receptors* that are involved in mammary carcinomas [74, 75]. Interestingly, an isoform of estrogen receptor alpha due to skipping of exon 3 (delta3ER) is a more potent activator of VEGF than the wild-type receptor, linking this variant to angiogenesis of breast tumors [76].

*Rac*1 is a member of the Ras superfamily of small GTPases involved in signal transduction pathways that induce the formation of lamellipodia, stimulate cell proliferation, and activate the JNK/SAPK protein kinase cascade [77]. The splice variant Rac1b, which is generated by inclusion of a 57-nucleotide cassette exon, has been shown to lead to anchorage-independent cell growth. Interestingly, expression of Rac1b increases in colorectal tumors at various stages of neoplastic process, as compared to adjacent normal tissues [78]. Alternative splicing of *Rac*1 is controlled by matrix metallo proteases (MMPs). MMPs are up-regulated in nearly all cancers [79] and play a major role in modulating cell–cell and cell-substratum adhesion, in promoting tumor cell proliferation, invasion, angiogenesis, and metastases [80]. In particular, MMP-3 can cause epithelial-mesenchymal transition (EMT) and malignant transformation in cultured cells, and genomically unstable mammary carcinomas in transgenic mice. Exposure of mouse mammary epithelial cells to MMP-3 induces the expression of Rac1b, which causes an increase in cellular reactive oxygen species (ROS) by stimulating the release of mitochondrial superoxide into the cytoplasm. This leads to genomic instability [80] and can drive tumorigenesis. Interestingly, splicing factor SF2/ASF has been recently linked to genomic instability [81]. Depletion of SF2/ASF from the cells, results in the formation of RNA:DNA structures (R-loops), in which nascent pre-mRNAs form stable hybrids with the template DNA strand. These structures lead to increased DNA damage that in turn activates cell cycle checkpoints, DNA repair systems, and apoptosis. These findings open the exciting possibility that transcription and subsequent RNA processing not only cooperate to guarantee efficient production of mature mRNAs but also to assume genome integrity.

Genomic amplification and high-level overexpression of the fibroblast growth factor receptor 2 (FGFR2) are frequently observed in breast cancer. Two of the several FGFR2 variants so far described are relevant for tumor progression and originate from the mutually exclusive use of exon IIIb in epithelia and exon IIIc in mesenchyme. The choice of exon IIIc in mesenchymal cells, which involves activation of this exon and repression of exon IIIb, depends on several factors among which PTB [82]. Selection of the epithelial cell-specific exon is controlled by (U)GCAUG elements, which are bound by Fox protein family members. Interestingly, Fox-2 isoforms are differentially expressed in IIIb+ cells in comparison to IIIc+ cells. Fox-2 is critical for the IIIc-to-IIIb switch observed in cells grown to overconfluency that show molecular and morphological changes consistent with a mesenchymal-to-epithelial transition [83]. By means of minigene constructs that use the GFP reporter protein to visualize alternative splicing of FGFR2, it has been possible to follow splicing decision during prostate tumor progression in rats. These experiments revealed unexpected EMTs in primary tumors. These transitions were observed more frequently where tumor cells were in contact with stroma, among lung micrometastases, in the organ parenchyma, and immediately adjacent to blood vessels [84]. Recently, it has been reported that the expression of FGFR2-IIIb is also controlled by two epithelial cell-type-specific RNA-binding proteins, called epithelial splicing regulatory proteins 1 and 2 (ESRP1 and ESRP2) [85]. By regulating alternative pattern of *CD*44, p120-Catenin (*CTNND*1) and hMena (*ENAH*), ESRP1 and ESRP2 are coordinators of an cell-type-specific post-transcriptional program that accompany the EMT (or its reversal MET) process.

Antibody-based targeted delivery of bioactive agents to sites of tumor is an attractive therapeutic strategy for cancer treatment. The most promising target for this strategy is *fibronectin*, which is a secreted extracellular molecule and a key determinant for control of proliferation, cell migration, cell invasiveness, and metastatic behavior of tumor cells. Several fibronectin isoforms are produced through alternative splicing [86]. One of these, the EDB isoform, is generated through inclusion of the type III repeat extra domain B (EDB) exon, which encodes 91 amino acids sequence perfectly conserved in mouse, rat, rabbit, dog, monkey, and man. The EDB variant is specifically expressed in embryos and is essentially undetectable in healthy adults. However, EDB-containing fibronectin is abundant in many aggressive solid tumors, and displays either predominantly vascular or diffuse stromal patterns of expression, depending on the tumor type [87–89]. Antibodies against the EDB isoform allow a more accurate diagnosis of high-grade astrocytomas [90], and clinical trials have now started to use anti-EDB antibodies to target radioactive iodine to colorectal and lung tumors [91, 92]. Inclusion of the *EDB* exon is regulated by a purine-rich splicing-enhancer whose activity is controlled by the SRp40 protein [93]. Interestingly, overexpression of this splicing factor occurs in mouse mammary tumors [38].

Recently, we have used the *Ron* proto-oncogene as a model to investigate the relationship between alternative splicing and tumor progression. Ron, the human receptor for the macrophage-stimulating protein (MSP), is a heterodimeric protein (p185-Ron) composed of α and β subunits both deriving from the processing of a common precursor (Fig. 3). Binding to MSP stimulates the intrinsic tyrosine kinase activity of Ron and results in phosphorylation of its docking site for multiple transducer and adaptor proteins leading to the activation of signaling cascades. Ron is a member of the scatter factor receptor family, which includes Met, the hepatocyte growth factor (HGF) receptor. In addition to promoting cell growth and protection from apoptosis, these factors control cell dissociation, motility, and invasion of extracellular matrices, a process known as "invasive growth" or "scattering" [94]. Invasive growth is physiologically relevant during development, organogenesis, and tissue regeneration. However, it can also mediate invasiveness of epithelial cancer. The splicing profile of the *Ron* gene is frequently altered in cancer cells with the production of different isoforms: ΔRon (skipping of exon 11), RonΔ160 (skipping of exons 5 and 6) and RonΔ165 (skipping of exons 5, 6 and 11) [95, 96]. Over-expression of any of these isoforms increases cell motility (scatter-like activity). However, only RonΔ160 or RonΔ155 are able to induce focus formation, sustained anchorage-independent growth, and the ability to form metastatic tumors in mice [96]. This oncogenic potential is channeled through the P3K-AKT pathway [97]. Also Met transcripts undergo alternative splicing and an isoform, called Met-SM, originates from skipping of exon 14 which encodes a 47 amino acid segment in the juxtamembrane domain. This isoform has been recently shown to play an important role in development and progression of human cancer [98].

We have studied in detail the alternative splicing of exon 11 that is involved in the production the constitutively active ΔRon, (Fig. 3). The choice between

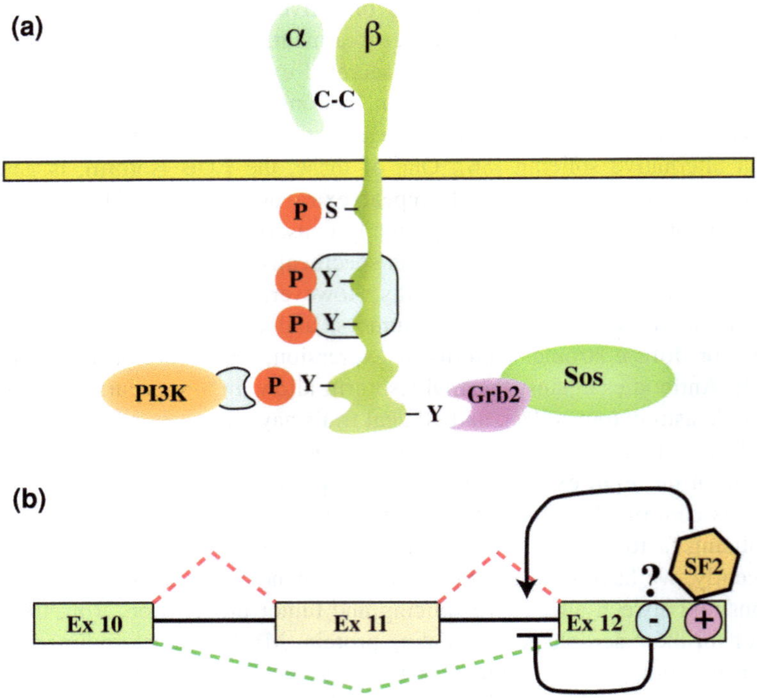

Fig. 3 Schematic representation of the Ron receptor. **a** Ron is a single-pass, disulfide-linked α/β heterodimer. The α chain is an extracellular glycoprotein, while the β chain is a transmembrane subunit with tyrosine kinase activity. The intracellular domain includes the tyrosine kinase catalytic site (azure box) flanked by distinctive juxtamembrane and carboxy-terminal sequences. Phosphorylation of two tyrosines within the kinase domain positively regulates the enzyme activity, whereas a serine residue in the juxtamembrane domain has a negative regulatory role. Two tyrosine residues in the carboxy-terminal region, when phosphorylated, form a specific docking site for multiple signal transducers and adaptors. GRB2 binds preferentially to the second tyrosine and activates the RAS pathway through association with SOS (modified by permission from Macmillian Publishers Ltd: [94]). **b** The constitutively active ΔRon isoform is generated through skipping of exon 11. This is controlled by two adjacent splicing elements, a silencer and an enhancer, located in the central part and at the 3′ end of exon 12, respectively. These two regulatory elements may form a ''control cassette'' that tunes the strength of the acceptor site of intron 11 and thus the ratio between Ron and ΔRon transcripts. Splicing factor SF2/ASF directly binds to the enhancer and governs its activity. The primary function of the silencer could be to antagonize the enhancer and prevent exon skipping

inclusion and skipping of this exon is governed by two adjacent regulatory elements, a silencer and an enhancer, both located in the constitutive exon 12 [95]. The activity of the enhancer is controlled by splicing factor SF2/ASF and determines the strength of the acceptor site of the upstream intron 11. By affecting the competition between acceptor sites in intron 10 and 11, SF2/ASF directs the choice between inclusion and skipping of exon 11 and the production of ΔRon. Similarly to what is observed with ΔRon, over-expression of SF2/ASF profoundly affects the cell morphology and triggers nuclear accumulation of β-catenin, reorganization of actin cytoskeleton, and down-regulation of E-cadherin, a tumor and invasion suppressor in human carcinomas. All these morphological and molecular changes represent hallmarks of the epithelial to mesenchymal transition (EMT), which is implicated in the metastatic spreading of human carcinomas [99]. Given the reported up-regulation of several SR proteins, including SF2/ASF, during tumor progression [38–41], it is tempting to speculate that splicing factor SF2/ASF could promote the malignant transformation by inducing a ΔRon-mediated EMT. This is consistent with a recent report showing that SF2/ASF is a true oncogene and its over-expression confers to mouse fibroblasts the ability to form sarcomas in mice [100].

Recently, we have investigated the possibility to use the cancer-specific variant as a potential target for the development of new anti-metastatic therapeutic strategies. We have exploited approaches based on bifunctional oligonucleotides or small-molecule inhibitors of SF2/ASF activity to modulate the pathological Δ*Ron* splicing event [101]. As a first approach, we used a targeted oligonucleotide enhancers of splicing (TOES) antisense RNA oligonucleotide complementary to *Ron* exon 11 and with an additional non-complementary RNA tail that was designed to mimic an ESE sequence and to interact with splicing factors. As an alternative approach to "correct" Δ*Ron* splicing, we used indole derived compounds (IDCs), a new class of splicing inhibitors that selectively inhibit the ESE-dependent splicing activity of individual SR proteins. Both treatments efficiently correct Δ*Ron* splicing and increase exon 11 inclusion. In addition, inhibitors of SF2/ASF activity also affect the invasive phenotype of the cells. These treatments could represent important strategies toward the development of effective anti-cancer therapeutic approaches.

2.4 Alternative Splicing and Signal Transduction

A number of studies in the last 10 years have shown that activation of signaling pathways by extracellular stimuli can impact on alternative splicing. In particular, a link between splicing regulation, mitogen-activated protein kinase (MAPK), and AKT signaling pathways has been described [102]. Little is known about the mechanisms by which signaling cascades control the nuclear splicing machinery. However, it is commonly accepted that proteins involved in pre-mRNA splicing, including abundant hnRNPs and SR splicing factors, are both targets and effectors of signal transduction cascades activated by extra-cellular stimulation.

Although the presence of 10 variant exons makes the analysis highly problematic, CD44 is an excellent example to illustrate how extra- and intra-cellular cues, by affecting the activity or sub-cellular distribution of specific splicing factors, can lead to the unscheduled expression in cancer cells of splicing isoforms involved in the formation of metastases. There is reciprocal influence between alternative splicing of CD44 and the RAS signaling pathway. Indeed splicing of exon v6 is regulated by RAS and, in turn, CD44v6 isoforms are involved in a positive feedback loop that sustains late RAS signaling, a key event for cell cycle progression [103]. CD44v6 isoforms appear to exert their activity by forming a complex with HGF and its receptor MET, which is then able to activate RAS signaling [104]. The production of different CD44 isoforms correlates with changes in the abundance of SR proteins [37, 38] and several splicing factors (including hnRNPA1, SRp55, SF2/ASF, Tra-2 beta, YB-1, SRm160 and Sam68) have been shown to regulate particular variant exons [103, 105–109]. In particular, Sam68 and SRm160 collaborate to control alternative splicing of exon v5 in response to extracellular signals and their activity is stimulated by the ERK kinase downstream of RAS [103, 106].

Another good example of splicing modulation by signaling pathways comes from the fibronectin gene. Contrary to what occurs in the adult where it is mainly skipped, the EDA exon is efficiently included in the mature fibronectin mRNA in embryos as well as during wound healing and in certain tumors. Exon inclusion is triggered by the activation of the Ras–PI3K–AKT pathway by growth factors. AKT directly phosphorylates the SR proteins 9G8 and SF2/ASF, which in turn bind and promote splicing of the EDA exon [102, 110]. Activation of the same pathway by insulin regulates the activity of another SR protein, SRp40, and stimulates the inclusion of an alternative exon in the protein kinase C (PKC) II pre-mRNA [111–113]. Based on these data, it is tempting to speculate that deregulation of the Ras/PI3K/AKT pathway by activating mutations in its components would have dramatic consequences for the splicing pattern of any of the pre-mRNAs regulated by 9G8, SF2/ASF, SRp40, and, perhaps, other SR proteins. An attractive hypothesis is that exons responsive to this signaling pathway belong to a set of genes that function cooperatively to modulate the physiology of the cell in accordance with the biological role of the signaling molecule. The identification of these exons, therefore, will be of the utmost interest.

Phosphorylation of 9G8 and SF2/ASF by AKT not only leads to inclusion of the EDA exon, but also enhances the translation of mRNAs containing the EDA exon [102]. Thus, activation of a single signal transduction pathway acts at two different points to stimulate the production of a specific protein. The net effect is a drastic increase both in the speed and strength of the signaling response as measured by production of the induced protein.

An interesting observation is that kinase activities able to modulate alternative splicing may affect signal transduction pathways. This is the case of the SRPK1 that, as stated above, is over-expressed in breast and colonic tumors. Targeted inhibition of SRPK1 has an anti-tumoral effect, which is mediated by a change in the alternative splicing of MAPK2 (also known as extracellular signal regulated kinase ERK2), one of the two major kinases responsible for phosphorylation of MAPK1 [43]. Together, these results suggest an important role for SRPK1 in MAPK and AKT pathways in deregulation of splicing profiles in cancer cells and point to SRPK1 inhibitors as novel anti-tumor drugs.

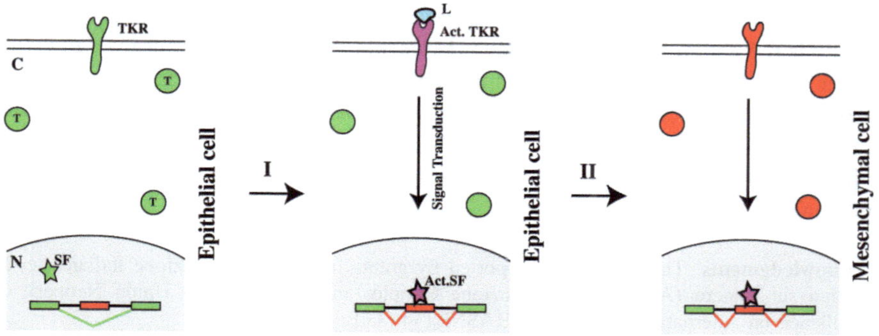

Fig. 4 A model for the role of alternative splicing in EMT. A specific splicing program is expressed in epithelial cells. *C* cytoplasm, *N* nucleus, *TRK* tyrosine kinase receptor, *SF* splicing factor, *T* protein encoded by alternative splicing variants (*green circle*). Interaction of TRKs with their ligands (*L*) activates signal transduction pathways that, through phosphorylation of splicing factors, can promote alternative splicing programs specific of mesenchymal cells. Alternative splicing would also induce the production of constitutively active isoforms of TRKs that make signal transduction pathways independent of external stimuli

3 Concluding Remarks

Cancer is an inherently complex, multi-step process of perturbation of cellular homeostasis that requires the timely accumulation of oncogenic mutations. Genetic models have suggested that 5–7 gene mutations are needed for cancer onset [114]. In recent years, alternative splicing has emerged as an important player in the development and progression of human cancer. Alternative splicing is a fundamental mechanism to modulate gene expression programs in response to different growth and environmental stimuli. There is now ample evidence that alternative splicing errors, caused by mutations in *cis*-acting elements and defects and/or imbalances in trans-acting factors, may be causatively associated to cancer progression. Moreover, a number of examples in this review strongly support the idea that the unscheduled expression of alternative splicing variants may be critical for tumor progression and the formation of metastases by promoting the EMT. As proposed in Fig. 4, the interaction between tyrosine kinase receptors (TKR) on the surface of cancer cells and specific growth factors in the tumor microenvironment would activate signal transduction cascades that target, among others, specific splicing regulators such as SR factors. A consequence of this event could be a change in alternative splicing programs leading to EMT even in the absence of gene mutations. Expression of constitutively active isoforms of TRKs (as for instance ΔRon) could be a result of this general reprogramming of alternative splicing. Activated TRKs, in turn, would make the activation of signal transduction pathways independent of external stimuli thus conferring to cancerous cells the ability to form metastases. Molecular approaches to therapy can target either the pre-mRNA or the splicing factors to change ratios between splicing isoforms and correct unscheduled splicing profiles. Hopefully, in the coming years a better understanding of the contribution of alternative splicing to carcinogenesis will be reached and novel methods will help identifying new targets for innovative anticancer therapeutic approaches.

Acknowledgments This work was supported by grants from the Associazione Italiana per la Ricerca sul Cancro (AIRC), the Fondazione Cariplo, and the European Union Network of Excellence on Alternative Splicing (EURASNET) to G.B.

References

1. Lander ES, Linton LM, Birren B et al (2001) Initial sequencing and analysis of the human genome. Nature 409:860–921
2. Black DL (2003) Mechanisms of alternative pre-messenger RNA splicing. Annu Rev Biochem 72:291–336
3. Schmucker D, Flanagan JG (2004) Generation of recognition diversity in the nervous system. Neuron 44:219–222
4. Pan Q, Shai O, Lee LJ, Frey BJ, Blencowe BJ (2008) Deep surveying of alternative splicing complexity in the human transcriptome by high-throughput sequencing. Nat Genet 40:1413–1415
5. Wang ET, Sandberg R, Luo S, Khrebtukova I, Zhang L, Mayr C, Kingsmore SF, Schroth GP, Burge CB (2008) Alternative isoform regulation in human tissue transcriptomes. Nature 456:470–476
6. Kan JL, Green MR (1999) Pre-mRNA splicing of IgM exons M1 and M2 is directed by a juxtaposed splicing enhancer and inhibitor. Genes Dev 13:462–471
7. Wang GS, Cooper TA (2007) Splicing in disease: disruption of the splicing code and the decoding machinery. Nat Rev Genet 8:749–761
8. Manley JL, Tacke R (1996) SR proteins and splicing control. Genes Dev 10:1569–1579
9. Valcarcel J, Green MR (1996) The SR protein family: pleiotropic functions in pre-mRNA splicing. Trends Biochem Sci 21:296–301
10. Fu XD (1995) The superfamily of arginine/serine-rich splicing factors. RNA 1:663–680
11. Tacke R, Manley JL (1999) Determinants of SR protein specificity. Curr Opin Cell Biol 11:358–362
12. Wu JY, Maniatis T (1993) Specific interactions between proteins implicated in splice site selection and regulated alternative splicing. Cell 75:1061–1070
13. Kohtz J, Jamison S, Will C et al (1994) Protein-protein interactions and 5′-splice-site recognition in mammalian mRNA precursors. Nature 368:119–124
14. Xiao SH, Manley JL (1997) Phosphorylation of the ASF/SF2 RS domain affects both protein–protein and protein-RNA interactions and is necessary for splicing. Genes Dev 11:334–344
15. Gui JF, Lane WS, Fu XD (1994) A serine kinase regulates intracellular localization of splicing factors in the cell cycle. Nature 369:678–682
16. Aubol BE, Chakrabarti S, Ngo J et al (2003) Processive phosphorylation of alternative splicing factor/splicing factor 2. Proc Nat Acad Sci U S A 100:12601–12606
17. Soret J, Gabut M, Dupon C et al (2003) Altered serine/arginine-rich protein phosphorylation and exonic enhancer-dependent splicing in Mammalian cells lacking topoisomerase I. Cancer Res 63:8203–8211

18. Colwill K, Feng LL, Yeakley JM et al (1996) SRPK1 and Clk/Sty protein kinases show distinct substrate specificities for serine/arginine-rich splicing factors. J Biol Chem 271:24569–24575
19. Zuo P, Maniatis T (1996) The splicing factor U2AF35 mediates critical protein–protein interactions in constitutive and enhancer-dependent splicing. Genes Dev 10:1356–1368
20. Blencowe BJ (2000) Exonic splicing enhancers: mechanism of action, diversity and role in human genetic diseases. Trends Biochem Sci 25:106–110
21. Graveley BR, Hertel KJ, Maniatis T (2001) The role of U2AF35 and U2AF65 in enhancer-dependent splicing. RNA 7:806–818
22. Ghigna C, Valacca C, Biamonti G (2008) Alternative splicing and tumor progression. Curr Genomics 9:556–570
23. Ule J, Stefani G, Mele A et al (2006) An RNA map predicting nova-dependent splicing regulation. Nature 444:580–586
24. Caceres JF, Stamm S, Helfman DM, Krainer AR (1994) Regulation of alternative splicing in vivo by overexpression of antagonistic splicing factors. Science 265:1706–1709
25. Biamonti G, Caceres JF (2009) Cellular stress and RNA splicing. Trends Biochem Sci 34:146–153
26. Denegri M, Chiodi I, Corioni M, Cobianchi F, Riva S, Biamonti G (2001) Stress-induced nuclear bodies are sites of accumulation of pre-mRNA processing factors. Mol Biol Cell 12:3502–3514
27. Caceres JF, Screaton GR, Krainer AR (1998) A specific subset of SR proteins shuttles continuously between the nucleus and the cytoplasm. Genes Dev 12:55–66
28. Wang GS, Cooper TA (2007) Splicing in disease: disruption of the splicing code and the decoding machinery. Nat Rev Genet 8:749–761
29. Ward AJ, Cooper TA (2010) The pathobiology of splicing. J Pathol 220:152–163
30. Cartegni L, Krainer AR (2003) Correction of disease-associated exon skipping by synthetic exon-specific activators. Nat Struct Biol 10:120–125
31. Lòpez-Bigas N, Audit B, Ouzounis C, Parra G, Guigò R (2005) Are splicing mutations the most frequent cause of hereditary disease? FEBS Lett 579:1900–1903
32. Liu HX, Cartegni L, Zhang MQ, Krainer AR (2001) A mechanism for exon skipping caused by nonsense or missense mutations in BRCA1 and other genes. Nat Genet 27:55–58
33. Barash Y, Calarco JA, Gao W, Pan Q, Wang X, Shai O, Blencowe BJ, Frey BJ (2010) Deciphering the splicing code. Nature 465:53–59
34. Mazoyer S, Puget N, Perrin-Vidoz L, Lynch HT, Serova-Sinilnikova OM, Lenoir GM (1998) A BRCA1 nonsense mutation causes exon skipping. Am J Hum Genet 62:713–715
35. Cartegni L, Wang J, Zhu Z, Zhang MQ, Krainer AR (2003) ESEfinder: a web resource to identify exonic splicing enhancers. Nucleic Acids Res 31:3568–3571
36. Pettigrew C, Wayte N, Lovelock PK et al (2005) Evolutionary conservation analysis increases the colocalization of predicted exonic splicing enhancers in the BRCA1 gene with missense sequence changes and in-frame deletions, but not polymorphisms. Breast Cancer Res 7:R929–R939
37. Ghigna C, Moroni M, Porta C, Riva S, Biamonti G (1998) Altered expression of heterogenous nuclear ribonucleoproteins and SR factors in human colon adenocarcinomas. Cancer Res 58:5818–5824
38. Stickeler E, Kittrell F, Medina D, Berget SM (1999) Stage-specific changes in SR splicing factors and alternative splicing in mammary tumorigenesis. Oncogene 18:3574–3582
39. Kirschbaum-Slager N, Lopes GM, Galante PA, Riggins GJ, de Souza SJ (2004) Splicing factors are differentially expressed in tumors. Genet Mol Res 3:512–520
40. Zerbe LK, Pino I, Pio R et al (2004) Relative amounts of antagonistic splicing factors, hnRNP A1 and ASF/SF2, change during neoplastic lung growth: implications for pre-mRNA processing. Mol Carcinog 41:187–196
41. Fischer DC, Noack K, Runnebaum IB et al (2004) Expression of splicing factors in human ovarian cancer. Oncol Rep 11:1085–1090

42. Kan Z, Garrett-Engele PW, Johnson JM, Castle JC (2005) Evolutionarily conserved and diverged alternative splicing events show different expression and functional profiles. Nucleic Acids Res 33:5659–5666
43. Hayes GM, Carrigan PE, Miller LJ (2007) Serine-arginine protein kinase 1 overexpression is associated with tumorigenic imbalance in mitogen-activated protein kinase pathways in breast, colonic, and pancreatic carcinomas. Cancer Res 67:2072–2080
44. Schwerk C, Schulze-Osthoff K (2005) Regulation of apoptosis by alternative pre-mRNA splicing. Mol Cell 19:1–13
45. Seol DW, Billiar TR (1999) A caspase-9 variant missing the catalytic site is an endogenous inhibitor of apoptosis. J Biol Chem 274:2072–2076
46. Akgul C, Moulding DA, Edwards SW (2004) Alternative splicing of Bcl-2-related genes: functional consequences and potential therapeutic applications. Cell Mol Life Sci 61:2189–2199
47. Paronetto MP, Achsel T, Massiello A, Chalfant CE, Sette C (2007) The RNA-binding protein Sam68 modulates the alternative splicing of Bcl-x. J Cell Biol 176:929–939
48. Dominguez C, Allain FH (2006) NMR structure of the three quasi RNA recognition motifs (qRRMs) of human hnRNP F and interaction studies with Bcl-x G-tract RNA: a novel mode of RNA recognition. Nucleic Acids Res 34:3634–3645
49. Garneau D, Revil T, Fisette JF, Chabot B (2005) Heterogeneous nuclear ribonucleoprotein F/H proteins modulate the alternative splicing of the apoptotic mediator Bcl-x. J Biol Chem 280:22641–22650
50. Li CY, Chu JY, Yu JK et al (2004) Regulation of alternative splicing of Bcl-x by IL-6, GM-CSF and TPA. Cell Res 14:473–479
51. Massiello A, Roesser JR, Chalfant CE (2006) SAP155 Binds to ceramide-responsive RNA cis-element 1 and regulates the alternative 5′ splice site selection of Bcl-x pre-mRNA. FASEB J 20:1680–1682
52. Boudrez A, Beullens M, Groenen P et al (2000) NIPP1-mediated interaction of protein phosphatase-1 with CDC5L, a regulator of pre-mRNA splicing and mitotic entry. J Biol Chem 275:25411–25417
53. Mermoud JE, Cohen PT, Lamond AI (1994) Regulation of mammalian spliceosome assembly by a protein phosphorylation mechanism. EMBO J 13:5679–5688
54. Misteli T, Spector DL (1996) Serine/threonine phosphatase 1 modulates the subnuclear distribution of pre-mRNA splicing factors. Mol Biol Cell 7:1559–1572
55. Massiello A, Chalfant CE (2006) SRp30a (ASF/SF2) regulates the alternative splicing of caspase-9 pre-mRNA and is required for ceramide-responsiveness. J Lipid Res 47:892–897
56. Naor D, Nedvetzki S, Golan I, Melnik L, Faitelson Y (2002) CD44 in cancer. Crit Rev Clin Lab Sci 39:527–579
57. Bajorath J (2000) Molecular organization, structural features, and ligand binding characteristics of CD44, a highly variable cell surface glycoprotein with multiple functions. Proteins 39:103–111
58. Heider KH, Kuthan H, Stehle G, Munzert G (2004) CD44v6: a target for antibody-based cancer therapy. Cancer Immunol Immunother 53:567–579
59. Borjesson PK, Postema EJ, Roos JC et al (2003) Phase I therapy study with (186)Re-labeled humanized monoclonal antibody BIWA 4 (bivatuzumab) in patients with head and neck squamous cell carcinoma. Clin Cancer Res 9:3961S–3972S
60. Saint-André V, Batsché E, Rachez C, Muchardt C (2011) Histone H3 lysine 9 trimethylation and HP1γ favor inclusion of alternative exons. Nat Struct Mol Biol 18:337–344
61. Vickers SM, Huang ZQ, MacMillan-Crow L, Greendorfer JS, Thompson JA (2002) Ligand activation of alternatively spliced fibroblast growth factor receptor-1 modulates pancreatic adenocarcinoma cell malignancy. J Gastrointest Surg 6:546–553
62. Luqmani YA, Mortimer C, Yiangou C et al (1995) Expression of 2 variant forms of fibroblast growth factor receptor 1 in human breast. Int J Cancer 64:274–279

63. Yamaguchi F, Saya H, Bruner JM, Morrison RS (1994) Differential expression of two fibroblast growth factor-receptor genes is associated with malignant progression in human astrocytomas. Proc Nat Acad Sci U S A 91:484–488
64. Jin W, Cote GJ (2004) Enhancer-dependent splicing of FGFR1 alpha-exon is repressed by RNA interference-mediated down-regulation of SRp55. Cancer Res 64:8901–8905
65. McCutcheon IE, Hentschel SJ, Fuller GN, Jin W, Cote GJ (2004) Expression of the splicing regulator polypyrimidine tract-binding protein in normal and neoplastic brain. Neuro Oncol 6:9–14
66. Bruno IG, Jin W, Cote GJ (2004) Correction of aberrant FGFR1 alternative RNA splicing through targeting of intronic regulatory elements. Hum Mol Genet 13:2409–2420
67. Tacconelli A, Farina AR, Cappabianca L et al (2004) TrkA alternative splicing: a regulated tumor-promoting switch in human neuroblastoma. Cancer Cell 6:347–360
68. Jang JH, Shin KH, Park YJ, Lee RJ, McKeehan WL, Park JG (2000) Novel transcripts of fibroblast growth factor receptor 3 reveal aberrant splicing and activation of cryptic splice sequences in colorectal cancer. Cancer Res 60:4049–4052
69. Lee JH, Seo YW, Park SR, Kim YJ, Kim KK (2003) Expression of a splice variant of KAI1, a tumor metastasis suppressor gene, influences tumor invasion and progression. Cancer Res 63:7247–7255
70. Wang L, Lin SH, Wu WG et al (2000) C-CAM1, a candidate tumor suppressor gene, is abnormally expressed in primary lung cancers. Clin Cancer Res 6:2988–2993
71. Lovecchio M, Maiorano E, Vacca RA et al (2003) Beta 1C Integrin expression in human endometrial proliferative diseases. Am J Pathol 163:2543–2553
72. Ryan B, O'Donovan N, Browne B et al (2005) Expression of survivin and its splice variants survivin-2B and survivin-DeltaEx3 in breast cancer. Br J Cancer 92:120–124
73. Suga K, Yamamoto T, Yamada Y, Miyatake S, Nakagawa T, Tanigawa N (2005) Correlation between transcriptional expression of survivin isoforms and clinicopathological findings in human colorectal carcinomas. Oncol Rep 13:891–897
74. Zhu X, Daffada AA, Chan CM, Dowsett M (1997) Identification of an exon 3 deletion splice variant androgen receptor mRNA in human breast cancer. Int J Cancer 72:574–580
75. Gallacchi P, Schoumacher F, Eppenberger-Castori S et al (1998) Increased expression of estrogen-receptor exon-5-deletion variant in relapse tissues of human breast cancer. Int J Cancer 79:44–48
76. Koduri S, Goldhar AS, Vonderhaar BK (2006) Activation of vascular endothelial growth factor (VEGF) by the ER-alpha variant, ERDelta3. Breast Cancer Res Treat 95:37–43
77. Wherlock M, Mellor H (2002) The Rho GTPase family: a Racs to Wrchs story. J Cell Sci 115:239–240
78. Jordan P, Brazao R, Boavida MG, Gespach C, Chastre E (1999) Cloning of a novel human Rac1b splice variant with increased expression in colorectal tumors. Oncogene 18:6835–6839
79. Egeblad M, Werb Z (2002) New functions for the matrix metalloproteinases in cancer progression. Nat Rev Cancer 2:161–174
80. Radisky DC, Levy DD, Littlepage LE et al (2005) Rac1b and reactive oxygen species mediate MMP-3-induced EMT and genomic instability. Nature 436:123–127
81. Li X, Manley JL (2005) Inactivation of the SR protein splicing factor ASF/SF2 results in genomic instability. Cell 122:365–378
82. Wagner EJ, Baraniak AP, Sessions OM, Mauger D, Moskowitz E, Garcia-Blanco MA (2005) Characterization of the intronic splicing silencers flanking FGFR2 exon IIIb. J Biol Chem 280:14017–14027
83. Baraniak AP, Chen JR, Garcia-Blanco MA (2006) Fox-2 mediates epithelial cell-specific fibroblast growth factor receptor 2 exon choice. Mol Cell Biol 26:1209–1222
84. Oltean S, Sorg BS, Albrecht T et al (2006) Alternative inclusion of fibroblast growth factor receptor 2 exon IIIc in dunning prostate tumors reveals unexpected epithelial mesenchymal plasticity. Proc Nat Acad Sci U S A 103:14116–14121

85. Warzecha CC, Sato TK, Nabet B, Hogenesch JB, Carstens RP (2009) ESRP1 and ESRP2 are epithelial cell-type-specific regulators of FGFR2 splicing. Mol Cell 33:591–601
86. Romberger DJ (1997) Fibronectin. Int J Biochem Cell Biol 29:939–943
87. Kaczmarek J, Castellani P, Nicolo G, Spina B, Allemanni G, Zardi L (1994) Distribution of oncofetal fibronectin isoforms in normal, hyperplastic and neoplastic human breast tissues. Int J Cancer 59:11–16
88. Castellani P, Viale G, Dorcaratto A et al (1994) The fibronectin isoform containing the ED-B oncofetal domain: a marker of angiogenesis. Int J Cancer 59:612–618
89. Hauptmann S, Zardi L, Siri A et al (1995) Extracellular matrix proteins in colorectal carcinomas. Expression of tenascin and fibronectin isoforms. Lab Invest 73:172–182
90. Castellani P, Borsi L, Carnemolla B et al (2002) Differentiation between high- and low-grade astrocytoma using a human recombinant antibody to the extra domain-B of fibronectin. Am J Pathol 161:1695–1700
91. Santimaria M, Moscatelli G, Viale GL et al (2003) Immunoscintigraphic detection of the ED-B domain of fibronectin, a marker of angiogenesis, in patients with cancer. Clin Cancer Res 9:571–579
92. Ebbinghaus C, Scheuermann J, Neri D, Elia G (2004) Diagnostic and therapeutic applications of recombinant antibodies: targeting the extra-domain B of fibronectin, a marker of tumor angiogenesis. Curr Pharm Des 10:1537–1549
93. Du K, Peng Y, Greenbaum LE, Haber BA, Taub R (1997) HRS/SRp40-mediated inclusion of the fibronectin EIIIB exon, a possible cause of increased EIIIB expression in proliferating liver. Mol Cell Biol 17:4096–4104
94. Trusolino L, Comoglio PM (2002) Scatter-factor and semaphorin receptors: cell signalling for invasive growth. Nat Rev Cancer 2:289–300
95. Ghigna C, Giordano S, Shen H, Benvenuto F, Castiglioni F, Comoglio PM, Green MR, Riva S, Biamonti G (2005) Cell motility is controlled by SF2/ASF through alternative splicing of the Ron protooncogene. Mol Cell 20:881–890
96. Zhou YQ, He C, Chen YQ, Wang D, Wang MH (2003) Altered expression of the RON receptor tyrosine kinase in primary human colorectal adenocarcinomas: generation of different splicing RON variants and their oncogenic potential. Oncogene 22:186–197
97. Xu XM, Zhou YQ, Wang MH (2005) Mechanisms of cytoplasmic {beta}-catenin accumulation and its involvement in tumorigenic activities mediated by oncogenic splicing variant of the receptor originated from Nantes tyrosine kinase. J Biol Chem 280:25087–25094
98. Lee JH, Gao CF, Lee CC, Kim MD, Vande Woude GF (2006) An alternatively spliced form of met receptor is tumorigenic. Exp Mol Med 38:565–573
99. Thiery JP, Sleeman JP (2006) Complex networks orchestrate epithelial-mesenchymal transitions. Nat Rev Mol Cell Biol 7:131–142
100. Karni R, de Stanchina E, Lowe SW, Sinha R, Mu D, Krainer AR (2007) The gene encoding the splicing factor SF2/ASF is a proto-oncogene. Nat Struct Mol Biol 14:185–193
101. Ghigna C, De Toledo M, Bonomi S, Valacca C, Gallo S, Apicella M, Eperon I, Tazi J, Biamonti G (2010) Pro-metastatic splicing of Ron proto-oncogene mRNA can be reversed: therapeutic potential of bifunctional oligonucleotides and indole derivatives. RNA Biol 7:495–503
102. Blaustein M, Pelisch F, Tanos T et al (2005) Concerted regulation of nuclear and cytoplasmic activities of SR proteins by AKT. Nat Struct Mol Biol 12:1037–1044
103. Cheng C, Sharp PA (2006) Regulation of CD44 alternative splicing by SRm160 and its potential role in tumor cell invasion. Mol Cell Biol 26:362–370
104. Orian-Rousseau V, Chen L, Sleeman JP, Herrlich P, Ponta H (2002) CD44 is required for two consecutive steps in HGF/c-Met signaling. Genes Dev 16:3074–3086
105. Matter N, Marx M, Weg-Remers S, Ponta H, Herrlich P, Konig H (2000) Heterogeneous ribonucleoprotein A1 is part of an exon-specific splice-silencing complex controlled by oncogenic signaling pathways. J Biol Chem 275:35353–35360

106. Matter N, Herrlich P, Konig H (2002) Signal-dependent regulation of splicing via phosphorylation of Sam68. Nature 420:691–695
107. Watermann DO, Tang Y, Zur Hausen A, Jager M, Stamm S, Stickeler E (2006) Splicing factor Tra2-beta1 is specifically induced in breast cancer and regulates alternative splicing of the CD44 gene. Cancer Res 66:4774–4780
108. Pind MT, Watson PH (2003) SR protein expression and CD44 splicing pattern in human breast tumours. Breast Cancer Res Treat 79:75–82
109. Galiana-Arnoux D, Lejeune F, Gesnel MC, Stevenin J, Breathnach R, Del Gatto-Konczak F (2003) The CD44 alternative v9 exon contains a splicing enhancer responsive to the SR proteins 9G8, ASF/SF2, and SRp20. J Biol Chem 278:32943–32953
110. Blaustein M, Pelisch F, Coso OA, Bissell MJ, Kornblihtt AR, Srebrow A (2004) Mammary epithelial-mesenchymal interaction regulates fibronectin alternative splicing via phosphatidylinositol 3-kinase. J Biol Chem 279:21029–21037
111. Patel NA, Chalfant CE, Watson JE et al (2001) Insulin regulates alternative splicing of protein kinase C beta II through a phosphatidylinositol 3-kinase-dependent pathway involving the nuclear serine/arginine-rich splicing factor, SRp40, in skeletal muscle cells. J Biol Chem 276:22648–22654
112. Patel NA, Kaneko S, Apostolatos HS et al (2005) Molecular and genetic studies imply Akt-mediated signaling promotes protein kinase CbetaII alternative splicing via phosphorylation of serine/arginine-rich splicing factor SRp40. J Biol Chem 280:14302–14309
113. Li H, Weinstein IB (2006) Protein kinase C beta enhances growth and expression of cyclin D1 in human breast cancer cells. Cancer Res 66:11399–11408
114. Tomlinson IP, Novelli MR, Bodmer WF (1996) The mutation rate and cancer. Proc Nat Acad Sci U S A 93:14800–14803

MicroRNAs in Cancer

Jianzhong Jeff Xi

Abstract

MicroRNAs (miRNAs) are a group of endogenous, small noncoding RNAs of approximately 22 nucleotides in lengths. As a new class of signaling modulators, miRNAs have attracted great attention for their unique features, including multitarget regulation, tissue specificity, and evolutionary conservation. These small endogenous RNAs are able to interact with many important genes and play critical roles in a wide range of biological processes, including cell proliferation and differentiation. Strikingly, miRNAs are frequently dysregulated in human cancers. A number of studies have shown that miRNAs are involved in cancer pathogenesis by regulating oncogenes or tumor suppressor genes. Here, we review recent studies of miRNAs in cancer development and discuss their potential applications in cancer therapeutics.

Keywords

miRNA · microRNA · Global dysregulation · Noncoding RNA · Cancer therapeutics · Diagnostic marker

Contents

J. J. Xi (✉)
Department of Biomedical Engineering, College of Engineering,
Peking University, Beijing 100871, China
e-mail: jzxi@pku.edu.cn

J. Y. Wu (ed.), *RNA and Cancer*, Cancer Treatment and Research,
DOI: 10.1007/978-3-642-31659-3_5,

1 Introduction

MicroRNAs (miRNAs) are a group of endogenous, small noncoding RNAs of $\sim$22 nucleotides. The human genome contains at least one thousand of distinct miRNAs, which potentially regulate over 30 % of the transcriptome. So far, a number of evidence shows that miRNAs make significant contribution to the formation and development of tumors, especially metastasis. In this chapter, we will start with the introduction of miRNA biogenesis, and summarize the global dysregulation of miRNAs in cancer, and then explain the roles of miRNAs in metastasis and their interaction with conventional protein modulators in several signaling pathways, and finally discuss the potential of miRNAs in therapeutical applications.

2 Biogenesis of miRNAs

The majority of primary miRNA (pri-miRNA) transcripts are produced by RNA polymerase II [9, 72]. The lengths of these pri-miRNAs vary from a few hundred to thousands of nucleotides with one or more double-stranded regions. Some pri-miRNAs have independent transcriptional units with mono- (e.g. miR-21) or polycistronic miRNA-precursor structure (e.g. the miR-17-92-1 cluster) [8, 45], whereas others locate in the intron (e.g. miR-10b) or extron (e.g. miR-198) of messenger RNAs [8, 106]. These polymerase II-directed pri-miRNAs are post-transcriptionally capped at 5′ end or polyadenylated at 3′ end, respectively. However, recent data indicate that a subset of miRNAs may instead be transcribed by RNA Polymerase III, such as C19MC, one of the largest human miRNA clusters [111]. Expression of individual miRNAs is controlled by transcription factors, such as c-Myc or p53. However, the regulatory mechanism of miRNAs at the transcriptional level remains unclear [22, 46, 96, 135].

Following transcription, the pri-miRNA is cleaved by a complex of Drosha and DGCR8 proteins (also known as Pasha), which contains two double-stranded RNA-binding domains [21, 36, 42, 68, 71]. DGCR8 directly interacts with the pri-miRNA and determines the accurate cleavage site. Then the Drosha finishes the cleavage step. An imperfect stem-loop structure of $\sim$50–70 nt in length is released, containing a hairpin stem, a terminal loop and two single-stranded

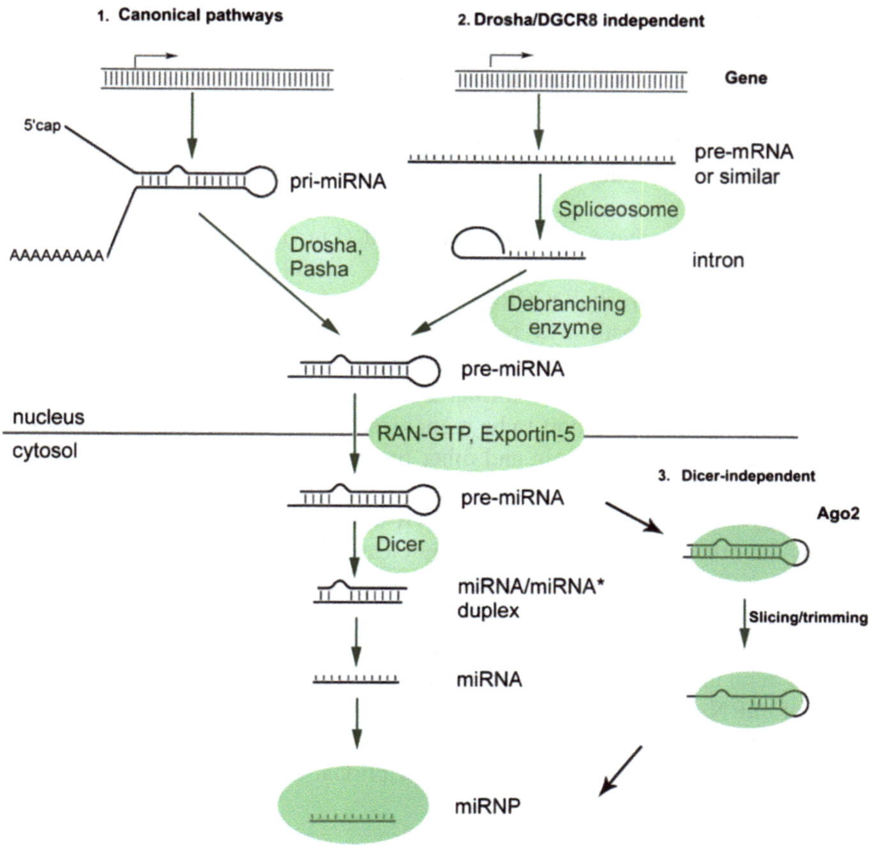

Fig. 1 An illustration of three miRNA biogenesis pathways, including (1) canonical pathway; (2) Drosha/DGCR-independent pathway; or (3) Dicer-independent pathway (adapted from http://en.wikipedia.org/wiki/MicroRNA. With permission from Creative Commons Attribution-ShareAlike 3.0 License)

flanking regions as the precursor miRNA (pre-miRNA). The double-stranded stem and the flanking regions are indispensable for the processing of pre-miRNA, but the loop region is less critical for this step [43, 141, 142].

After processing in the nucleus, the pre-miRNAs are transported to the cytoplasm by the nucleocytoplasmic shuttling protein, exportin-5, which recognizes a two-nucleotide overhang left by Drosha at the 3′ end of the pre-miRNA hairpin. Exportin-5-mediated transport to the cytoplasm is an energy-dependent process, in which GTP is bound to the Ran protein [139]. In the nucleus, in the presence of a high concentration of RanGTP, exportin-5 induces the Drosha/DGCR8 complex to release pre-miRNA and transport pre-miRNA out of the nucleus. In the cytoplasm, the low concentration of RanGTP results in the separation of pre-miRNA from exportin-5. During the subsequent step, another RNase III enzyme, Dicer, cleaves the loop portion of the hairpin structure and yielding ~22 nt small RNA duplexes, consisting of a mature miRNA strand and a partially complementary strand. Knocking out Dicer blocks the formation of mature miRNAs, indicating that this cleavage is essential for miRNA biogenesis [6, 37, 51, 62]. Dicer cleavage activity is regulated by TRBP, which binds to the amino-terminal DExD/H-box helicase domain of Dicer and induces a conformational rearrangement of Dicer [84].

In addition to the above described canonical miRNA biogenesis pathway, alternative pathways have also been proposed (Fig. 1) [12, 21, 109, 137]. For example, a pre-miRNA-like hairpin structure, which serves as Dicer substrate without cleaving by Drosha/DGCR8 complex, can be generated by many Drosha/DGCR8-independent pathways (e.g. miR-62 or mir-1071) [2, 14, 97, 109]. Another type of miRNAs does not require the cleavage of Dicer. Pri-miR-451 is processed by Drosha/DGCR8 to format a short pre-miRNA with only ~18 nt of duplex stem, which is too short to be recognized by Dicer. Instead, pre-mir-451 is directly cleaved by Ago protein and other proteins [12, 15, 138].

After the miRNA duplex is generated, one strand (named as the guide strand) is loaded into a protein complex called RNA-induced silencing complex (RISC), whereas the other strand gets degraded by cleavage or a bypass mechanism [41]. Argonaute proteins (AGOs) are the catalytic components of the RISC. AGOs have eight related family members in human, including four AGOs and four PIWI proteins. Typically, the mature miRNA-RISC binds to the 3′ untranslated region (3′UTR) of an mRNA containing a partially complementary sequence with the seed region of miRNAs (the 2nd to 8th nt of the mature miRNA). If the seed region of a miRNA can anneal with mRNAs, RISC cleaves these target mRNAs or suppresses their translation without affecting the transcriptional level of these miRNAs.

3 The Dysregulation of miRNAs in Cancer

In 2004, Croce and colleagues reported that miRNAs are not randomly distributed in the human genome [10]. For example, chromosome 4 has fewer than average miRNAs, whereas chromosomes 17 and 19 have significantly more miRNAs. Indeed, over 50 % miRNAs are located at fragile sites or chromosomal regions that are associated with cancers. After systematic analysis of over 200 miRNAs from more than 300 samples, Lu and colleagues revealed distinct expression profiles of miRNAs between normal and tumor cells or tissues [82]. Another interesting finding demonstrated in that work is that miRNA expression profiles can be used to classify poorly differentiated tumors with higher accuracy than mRNA expression files, thus indicating that miRNAs may be used as diagnostic markers.

With the development of high-throughput sequencing technology or gene chip technology, the expression patterns of miRNAs have been intensively investigated in a variety of cells or tissues. A global picture of dysregulation of miRNAs in cancers is emerging, with many miRNAs found down-regulated or overexpressed in different types of tumors. For example, miR-21 or miR-17-92 cluster is up-regulated in a range of tumors [89].

miRNAs may suppress or promote carcinogenesis, acting as either tumor suppressors or oncogenes. Those miRNAs as tumor suppressors are often downregulated in tumors and can regulate oncogenes. For example, let-7 family has been found to negatively regulate expression of RAS, an oncogene that contributes to the pathogenesis of human tumors [56]. Those miRNAs are frequently inactivated either by gene deletion or promoter modification, such as methylation.

Another group of miRNAs, referred to as oncomirs, are found to be overexpressed in cancers. For example, miR-17-92 cluster with six miRNA genes: miR-17, miR-18a, miR-19a, miR-20a, miR-19b-1, and miR-92a-1, can induce cell proliferation, inhibit apoptosis or promote tumorigenesis by cooperating with MYC in lymphomas [33, 96].

miRNAs are also involved in the epigenetic process: either as players or targets in the epigenetic regulation. The methylation of CpG islands in promoter regions leads to silencing of miRNA expression. For example, miR-127, targeting an oncogene-BCL6, is silenced in bladder tumors, but this silence could be rescued using demethylating agents [111]. On the other hand, miRNAs could also regulate enzymes that involves in methylation of CpG islands, such as DNA methyltransferases (DNMT). miR-29 could target DNMT3A and DNMT3B, thus resulting in reactivating p16 tumor suppressor gene [128].

One key question is whether dysregulation of miRNAs is cause or consequence to cancer? [17] Components of the miRNA-machinery have been implicated in tumorigenesis. For example, it was reported that expression of Dicer was downregulated in lung cancer and this downregulation correlated with shortened postoperative survival [57]. In addition, three human Argonaute genes—AGO3, AGO1, and AGO4, which are clustered on chromosome 1 (1p34–35)—are frequently deleted in Wilm's tumor of the kidney and have also been associated with other tumors [24]. In the next section, we will discuss the role or miRNAs in cancer development or metastasis.

4 miRNAs and Cancer Metastasis

Metastases account for 90 % deaths among cancer patients [40]. However, our understanding of the molecular mechanism underlying metastatic dissemination remains obscure [127]. The invasion-metastasis cascade is a dynamic and multistep process. In brief, primary tumor cells break away from neighbouring cells, invade adjacent tissue, enter the circulation systems, extravasate out of the vasculature, seed at distant sites, enter the foreign tissue parenchyma, and finally proliferate from microscopic growths into macroscopic secondary tumors [26]. A large number of studies have showed that miRNAs play a critical role in the initiation and progression of different cancers.

A number of miRNAs act to promote cancer metastasis. For example, miRNA-10b is highly expressed in metastatic breast cancer cells and regulates cell migration and invasion [86]. Overexpression of miR-10b in otherwise nonmetastatic breast tumor cells endows them with invasive and metastatic capability. Significantly, the level of miR-10b expression in primary breast carcinomas correlates with clinical progression. The expression of miR-10b is under the control of Twist, a transcription factor that orchestrates epithelial–mesenchymal transitions (EMT). miR-10b inhibits translation of HOXD10 protein, resulting in the increase of RHOC, a well-characterized prometastatic gene. In addition, miR-373 and miR-520c were identified as another metastasis promoting genes [49]. Overexpression of miR-373 or miR-520c promoted an in vitro migration and invasion of breast cancer cells. miR-373 and miR-520c inhibit CD44, a metastatic suppressor in breast, prostate or colon cancers.

On the other hand, miRNAs can act as inhibitors of metastasis at different stages. Let-7 serves as a tumor suppressor gene by inhibiting the expression of HMGA2 and RAS [56]. Let-7 expression is lower in lung tumors, whereas RAS protein is significantly higher in these tissues. miR-31, another anti-metastatic human miRNA, represses multiple steps of the invasion-metastasis cascade. Down-regulation of miR-31 enhances the migration and invasion in human breast cancer cells. This miRNA can repress a cohort of prometastatic target genes, including Fzd3, ITGA5, MMP16, RDX, and RhoA [88, 110, 113, 127].

Angiogenesis plays a critical role in the tumorigenesis and cancer progression. Vascular endothelial growth factor (VEGF) is a potent proangiogenic factor that is up-regulated in human tumors. miR-126 can directly target the 3′UTRs of Spred-1, VCAM-1, and PIK3R2 [27], negative regulators of VEGF/FGF signaling. In mammals, miR-126 is encoded by intron 7 of the EGF-like domain7 (Egfl7) gene, an endothelial cell-specific secreted peptide that inhibits migration of smooth muscle cell [120]. Thus, miR-126 shows a parallel expression pattern with Egfl7 in tissues or cell lines [28, 99]. Indeed, miR-126 regulates multiple aspects of endothelial cell biology, including cell migration, capillary network stability, and cell survival [27]. Thus, miR-126 promotes VEGF/FGF signaling and angiogenesis by repressing endogenous inhibitors in endothelial cells.

MiR-23b is highly conserved in all vertebrates. Several studies have demonstrated that miR-23b is involved in invasion and metastasis, but the molecular mechanism remains to be elucidated [107, 112]. We have recently demonstrated that miR-23b, which is down-regulated in human colon cancer samples, can potently repress cancer cell migration, invasion, growth, and angiogenesis both in vitro and in vivo [143]. miR-23b can also inhibit VEGF at both transcriptional and translational levels. This miRNA significantly inhibited tubule elongation and branching in vascular formation assay using human umbilical vein endothelial cells (HUVEC). However, miR-23 may regulate angiogenesis by indirectly suppressing VEGF. This miRNA regulates a cohort of prometastatic genes or oncogenes, including FZD7, MAP3K1, PAK2, TGFβR2, RRAS2, or uPA. Re-expression of these individual targets largely reversed effects of miR-23, whereas siRNA silencing of each target genes suppresses metastasis. These six genes participate in critical signaling pathways, including the ERK, JNK, NFκB, PI3K, TGFβ, and Wnt pathways.

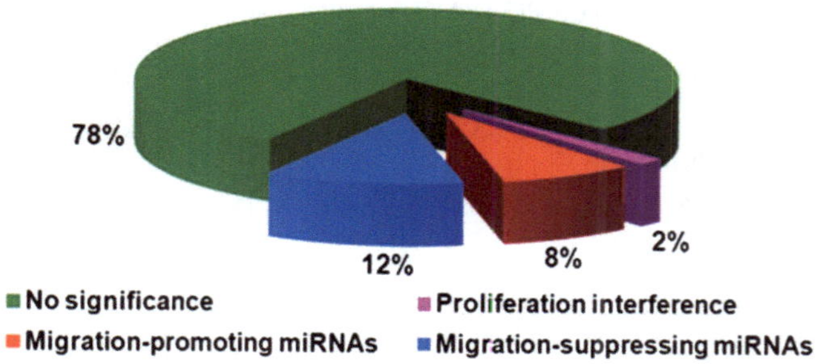

Fig. 2 A pie diagram showing the distribution of miRNAs tested in the migration and proliferation assay (Reprinted from [143]. With permission from Nature Publishing Group)

As described above, miRNAs are frequently dysregulated in human cancers [17, 82]. However, our understanding of role of miRNAs in tumor cell migration remains limited. It is not clear how many miRNAs may affect cancer cell migration, or whether the same miRNA regulates cell migration in different types of cancer cells in a similar manner.

To address these questions, we have systematically investigated regulatory capability of known human miRNAs on cancer cell migration, invasion, or apoptosis [143]. Strikingly, it was found that over one quarter of the human miRNAs tested demonstrated regulatory activities on cancer cell migration (Fig. 2). Interestingly, many of the miRNAs initially identified in a screen in HeLa cells behave in the same manner in four other epithelial cancer cell lines.

Endothelial cell migration plays an important role in the angiogenesis associated with other pathological processes such as atherosclerosis. Thus, we have continued to expand our studies to endothelial cells. It seems that the cell migration regulatory activity of miRNAs is not specific to epithelial cancer cells. It is now well established that miRNAs regulate expression and function of target genes in both physiological and pathological processes. miRNAs modulate many cellular processes including cell migration.

5 miRNAs, Key Modulators in Cell Signaling Pathways

miRNAs play important regulatory roles in a wide range of cellular processes. Individual miRNAs often have multiple target genes. Here, we focus on the roles of miRNAs as modulators in several critical cancer-related signaling pathways, including PI3K/Akt, Erk, MAPK, NF-κB, TGF-β, and mTOR.

5.1 PTEN/PI3K/AKT Signaling Pathway

The PTEN/PI3K/AKT pathway is important in regulating cell proliferation, cellular metabolism, apoptosis, and cell survival. PI3K phosphorylates PIP2 to

Table 1 miRNAs regulating PTEN/PI3 K/AKT signaling pathway

miRNAs	Targets	Effect on AKT pathway	References
miR-126	P85beta	Down	[38]
MiR-7	EGFR	Down	[60]
miR-125b		Down	[74]
miR-184	MicroRNA-205, AKT2	Down	[29, 140]
miR-331-3p	ERBB-2	Down	[23]
miR-8/miR-200	USH/FOG2	Down	[52]
miR-330	E2F1	Down	[70]
miR-320	p85 subunit	Down	[78]
miR-196a	HoxA7, HoxB8, HoxC8 and HoxD8	Up	[116]
miR-146b-5p	EGFR	Down	[58]
miR-149*	Akt1,E2F1	Down	[76]
miR-451	Akt1, CyclinD1, MMP-2, MMP-9 and Bcl-2	Down	[93]
miR-375	PDK1	Down	[124]
miR-222	PPP2R2A	Up	[133]
miR-217	KRAS	Down	[146]
miR-190	PHLPP	Up	[5]
miR-107		Down	[19]
miR-216b	KRAS	Down	[20]
miR-1		Up	[34]
miR-133, miR-223	IGF-1R	Down	[48]
miR-143	ERK5 and/or Akt	Down	[95]
miR-181d	K-ras and Bcl-2	Down	[132]

generate PIP3, an important second messenger, which in turn recruits PDK1 and AKT to the cell membrane. AKT is phosphorylated and activated by PIP3-dependent PDK1, and then regulates many downstream effectors [11]. On the other hand, PTEN dephosphorylates PIP3 to PIP2, thus attenuating the effects of the AKT pathway.

PTEN is a *bona fide* target of miR-21 [90]. Overexpression of miR-21 contributes to hepatocellular carcinoma (HCC) cells and vestibular schwannoma by suppressing PTEN [87, 90]. Interestingly, when PTEN is suppressed by miR-21, AKT induces the down-regulation of miR-199a-5p, leading to increased expression of hypoxia-inducible factor 1alpha (HIF α) and Sirtuin 1 (Sirt1) [114]. This is one example of miRNAs capable of regulating another miRNA. In addition, PTEN is not only regulated by miR-21, but also by Grhl3, which is a target of miR-21. The interaction of these molecules constitutes a multilayer regulatory network in PTEN/PI3K/AKT pathway [18]. A feed-forward regulatory circuit has been proposed in which miR-21 is a downstream effector of AKT [115].

Many other miRNAs are involved in this pathway through either targeting PTEN or other components. For example, miR-221 and -222 target PTEN as well as TIMP3, leading to the enhancement of TRAIL resistance and cellular migration [32]. miR-221 and -222 are down-regulated by miR-130a [1]. Similar to miR-21, miR-155 may activate AKT pathway via targeting PPP2CA, SOCS1 or SHIP-1 [3, 69]. The miR-17-92 cluster contains six individual miRNAs, among which miR-19 acts as a key component by targeting PTEN [98]. In addition, other miRNAs, including miR-205, 214, 26a, 29a, 29b, 23b, 301, 216a, or 217, can also target PTEN [35, 50, 59, 65, 94, 117, 131, 136] (Table 1).

5.2 MAPK/ERK Signaling Pathway

Mitogen-Activated Protein Kinase (MAPK) or Extracellular signal-Regulated Kinase (ERK) is well-studied protein kinases involved in multiple cellular processes including cell cycle regulation. MAPK/ERK Pathway consists of a series of proteins, which respond to extracellular signals by phosphorylating downstream substrates [64]. Disruption of this pathway leads to cancer and other diseases [63].

MiR-17-5p can target more than 20 genes involved in the G1/S transition in cell cycle, many of which are negative regulators of MAPK signaling cascade [16]. Overall, miR-17-5p promotes the migration of HCC cells through p38 MAPK activation. In addition, miR-17-5 can target E2F1. E2F1-dependent down-regulation of Wip1 is necessary in the activation of p38.

Let-7 family of miRNAs regulates many cellular processes, including cell growth and differentiation [108]. Let-7 reduces the expression of RAS and inhibits the MAPK/ERK pathway in papillary thyroid cancer [104]. In breast cancers, let-7 g plays an antitumor role by reducing p44/42 MAPK [102]. As a modulator of K-RAS, miR-143 decreases the proliferation and migration of prostate cancer cells [134]. Many other miRNAs, including miR-18*, miR-143, miR-181, and miR-622, also target K-RAS [31, 44, 118, 123, 132].

Spred1 is a negative regulator in MAPK/ERK pathway. miR-126 can enhance the proliferation of mast cell by inhibiting spred1 [54]. In mesenchymal stem cells, overexpression of miR-126 enhances ischemic angiogenesis by increasing the protein levels of ERK1, pErk1, AKT, or pAKT [13]. miR-133b can promote the development of cervical carcinoma by targeting MST2, CDC42, or RHOA [103]. In addition to modulating the PTEN/PI3K/AKT pathway, miR-21 regulates Spry1, Spry2, Btg2, and Pdcd4, known negative regulators in the Ras/MEK/ERK pathway. Other miRNAs are capable of regulating downstream effectors in MAPK/ERK pathway, including miR-146 and miR-221/222 [83, 100, 122].

5.3 NF-κB Signaling Pathway

NF-κB (nuclear factor kappa-light-chain-enhancer of activated B cells) is a protein complex that controls the transcription of many genes. When bound to an inhibitor-IκB, NF-κB is kept inactive in the cytoplasm. When cells are stimulated, an IκB kinase, IKK, is activated to phosphorylate IκB, resulting in the degradation of IκB and the activation of NF-κB. NF-κB then translocates into the nucleus and turns on the expression of its target genes.

The expression of miR-9 can be regulated by the activated NF-κB. On the other hand, miR-9 can affect the expression of NF-κB, forming a feedback regulation [4]. It was also found that NFKB1 was suppressed when miR-9 was overexpressed in ovarian cancer [39]. miR-146 can indirectly suppress NF-κB pathway by targeting IL-1 receptor-associated kinase or TNF receptor-associated factor 6 [7], thereby regulating IL-1 and Toll-like receptor signaling pathways.

Many other miRNAs also participate in the regulation of NF-κB pathway, including miR-98, let-7, miR-21, miR-124, miR-155, miR-15, and -16 [47, 53, 75, 77, 81, 105, 130]. On the other hand, NF-κB signaling pathway controls the expression of many genes, including miR-146, 147, or 143 [79, 121, 144].

5.4 TGF-β and mTOR Pathways

miR-21, miR-133 and 590, miR-17 cluster, miR200a, miR-106b-25 cluster, miR-210, miR-26a, or miR520/373 regulate the effectors in the TGF-β signaling pathway [61, 91, 119, 129]. The key modulators in the mTOR signaling pathway can be regulated by miR-199a-3p, miR-100, miR-221, miR-223, miR-99a, miR-218, miR-7, miR-376b, miR-520c and -373 [25, 30, 55, 66, 73, 80, 92, 101, 125].

From the limited examples described above, it is clear that miRNAs are emerging as a group of important modulators of many signaling pathways important for tumorigenesis and cancer metastasis. In a number of cases, miRNAs and their target genes can form feedback regulatory loops. It is conceivable that disruption of certain critical regulatory networks may contribute to tumor development and progression.

6 Therapeutic Potential for miRNAs

As discussed above, aberrant expression and regulation of miRNA genes have been associated with a wide range of human cancers. A number of miRNAs play critical roles in cancer development and metastasis. Such miRNAs may have great potential in serving as diagnostic biomarkers or therapeutic targets for human cancers. Indeed, several miRNAs have been identified to inhibit cancer metastasis in cellular or animal models. For example, Weinberg and colleagues demonstrated that systemic administration of miR-10b antagomirs, an inhibitor against miR-10b, inhibited breast cancer metastasis in tumor-bearing mice [85]. In another study, systemic administration of miR-26a in a mouse model of HCC using adeno-associated virus (AAV) results in inhibition of cancer cell proliferation, induction of tumor-specific apoptosis, and dramatic protection from disease progression without obvious toxicity [67]. Their unique features, including multitarget regulation and tissue specificity make miRNAs attractive target genes for developing cancer therapeutics, although much more work is needed to make this a reality.

7 Concluding Remarks

One miRNA may regulate up to hundreds of genes. Accumulating data support that miRNAs behave as buffer molecules capable of tuning the expression of target genes to appropriate levels. Expression of a certain miRNA in tumors is expected to regulate a cohort of functionally relevant genes. Although the target-specific delivery of siRNA/miRNA is still a challenging issue, detections of miRNAs in the serum suggest a new strategy to package or deliver miRNAs into specific cells or tissues [126, 145]. Another challenge is that we still lack a powerful approach to systematically identify the target genes regulated by miRNAs. A deeper understanding of the relationship between miRNAs and their targets is necessary for developing applications of these non-coding RNAs in cancer diagnostics and therapeutics.

Acknowledgments I thank Yang Hao, Junyu Yang, Ming Ma, Mingjun Jiang, Hanshuo Zhang, and Yanzhen Ye for their collecting literature and manuscription preparation. I also thank Dr. Jane Wu for manuscrition editing and discussion. This work was supported by projects of NSFC (Grant No. 81030040), MOST (Grant No. 2008ZX09401—002, 2011CB809106), NSFC (20733001, 30600142), and Coulter Foundation Seed Grant.

References

1. Acunzo M, Visone R, Romano G, Veronese A, Lovat F, Palmieri D, Bottoni A, Garofalo M, Gasparini P, Condorelli G et al (2012) miR-130a targets MET and induces TRAIL-sensitivity in NSCLC by downregulating miR-221 and 222. Oncogene 31:634–642
2. Babiarz JE, Ruby JG, Wang Y, Bartel DP, Blelloch R (2008) Mouse ES cells express endogenous shRNAs, siRNAs, and other microprocessor-independent, dicer-dependent small RNAs. Genes Dev 22:2773–2785
3. Bakirtzi K, Hatziapostolou M, Karagiannides I, Polytarchou C, Jaeger S, Iliopoulos D, Pothoulakis C (2011) Neurotensin signaling activates microRNAs-21 and -155 and Akt, promotes tumor growth in mice, and is increased in human colon tumors. Gastroenterology 141(1749–1761):e1741
4. Bazzoni F, Rossato M, Fabbri M, Gaudiosi D, Mirolo M, Mori L, Tamassia N, Mantovani A, Cassatella MA, Locati M (2009) Induction and regulatory function of miR-9 in human monocytes and neutrophils exposed to proinflammatory signals. Proc Natl Acad Sci U S A 106:5282–5287
5. Beezhold K, Liu J, Kan H, Meighan T, Castranova V, Shi X, Chen F (2011) miR-190-mediated downregulation of PHLPP contributes to arsenic-induced Akt activation and carcinogenesis. Toxicol Sci 123:411–420

6. Bernstein E, Caudy AA, Hammond SM, Hannon GJ (2001) Role for a bidentate ribonuclease in the initiation step of RNA interference. Nature 409:363–366
7. Bhaumik D, Scott GK, Schokrpur S, Patil CK, Campisi J, Benz CC (2008) Expression of microRNA-146 suppresses NF-kappaB activity with reduction of metastatic potential in breast cancer cells. Oncogene 27:5643–5647
8. Borchert GM, Lanier W, Davidson BL (2006) RNA polymerase III transcribes human microRNAs. Nat Struct Mol Biol 13:1097–1101
9. Cai X, Hagedorn CH, Cullen BR (2004) Human microRNAs are processed from capped, polyadenylated transcripts that can also function as mRNAs. RNA 10:1957–1966
10. Calin GA, Sevignani C, Dumitru CD, Hyslop T, Noch E, Yendamuri S, Shimizu M, Rattan S, Bullrich F, Negrini M et al (2004) Human microRNA genes are frequently located at fragile sites and genomic regions involved in cancers. Proc Natl Acad Sci U.S.A 101:2999–3004
11. Carnero A, Blanco-Aparicio C, Renner O, Link W, Leal JF (2008) The PTEN/PI3 K/AKT signaling pathway in cancer, therapeutic implications. Curr Cancer Drug Targets 8:187–198
12. Cheloufi S, Dos Santos CO, Chong MM, Hannon GJ (2010) A dicer-independent miRNA biogenesis pathway that requires Ago catalysis. Nature 465:584–589
13. Chen JJ, Zhou SH (2011) Mesenchymal stem cells overexpressing MiR-126 enhance ischemic angiogenesis via the AKT/ERK-related pathway. Cardiol J 18:675–681
14. Chung WJ, Agius P, Westholm JO, Chen M, Okamura K, Robine N, Leslie CS, Lai EC (2011) Computational and experimental identification of mirtrons in Drosophila melanogaster and Caenorhabditis elegans. Genome Res 21:286–300
15. Cifuentes D, Xue H, Taylor DW, Patnode H, Mishima Y, Cheloufi S, Ma E, Mane S, Hannon GJ, Lawson ND et al (2010) A novel miRNA processing pathway independent of Dicer requires Argonaute2 catalytic activity. Science 328:1694–1698
16. Cloonan N, Brown MK, Steptoe AL, Wani S, Chan WL, Forrest AR, Kolle G, Gabrielli B, Grimmond SM (2008) The miR-17-5p microRNA is a key regulator of the G1/S phase cell cycle transition. Genome Biol 9:R127
17. Croce CM (2009) Causes and consequences of microRNA dysregulation in cancer. Nat Rev Genet 10:704–714
18. Darido C, Georgy SR, Wilanowski T, Dworkin S, Auden A, Zhao Q, Rank G, Srivastava S, Finlay MJ, Papenfuss AT et al (2011) Targeting of the tumor suppressor GRHL3 by a miR-21-dependent proto-oncogenic network results in PTEN loss and tumorigenesis. Cancer Cell 20:635–648
19. Datta J, Smith A, Lang JC, Islam M, Dutt D, Teknos TN, Pan Q (2011) microRNA-107 functions as a candidate tumor-suppressor gene in head and neck squamous cell carcinoma by downregulation of protein kinase Cvarepsilon. Oncogene doi:10.1038/onc.2011.565
20. Deng M, Tang H, Zhou Y, Zhou M, Xiong W, Zheng Y, Ye Q, Zeng X, Liao Q, Guo X et al (2011) miR-216b suppresses tumor growth and invasion by targeting KRAS in nasopharyngeal carcinoma. J Cell Sci 124:2997–3005
21. Denli AM, Tops BB, Plasterk RH, Ketting RF, Hannon GJ (2004) Processing of primary microRNAs by the Microprocessor complex. Nature 432:231–235
22. Diederichs S, Haber DA (2006) Sequence variations of microRNAs in human cancer: alterations in predicted secondary structure do not affect processing. Cancer Res 66:6097–6104
23. Epis MR, Giles KM, Barker A, Kendrick TS, Leedman PJ (2009) miR-331-3p regulates ERBB-2 expression and androgen receptor signaling in prostate cancer. J Biol Chem 284:24696–24704
24. Esquela-Kerscher A, Slack FJ (2006) Oncomirs—microRNAs with a role in cancer. Nat Rev Cancer 6:259–269
25. Fang YX, Xue JL, Shen Q, Chen J, L (2012) miR-7 inhibits tumorgrowth and metastasis by targeting the PI3K/AKT pathway in hepatocellularcarcinoma. Hepatology 55(6):1852–1862
26. Fidler IJ (2003) The pathogenesis of cancer metastasis: the 'seed and soil' hypothesis revisited. Nat Rev Cancer 3:453–458

27. Fish JE, Santoro MM, Morton SU, Yu S, Yeh RF, Wythe JD, Ivey KN, Bruneau BG, Stainier DY, Srivastava D (2008) miR-126 regulates angiogenic signaling and vascular integrity. Dev Cell 15:272–284
28. Fitch MJ, Campagnolo L, Kuhnert F, Stuhlmann H (2004) Egfl7, a novel epidermal growth factor-domain gene expressed in endothelial cells. Dev Dyn 230:316–324
29. Foley NH, Bray IM, Tivnan A, Bryan K, Murphy DM, Buckley PG, Ryan J, O'Meara A, O'Sullivan M, Stallings RL (2010) MicroRNA-184 inhibits neuroblastoma cell survival through targeting the serine/threonine kinase AKT2. Mol Cancer 9:83
30. Fornari F, Milazzo M, Chieco P, Negrini M, Calin GA, Grazi GL, Pollutri D, Croce CM, Bolondi L, Gramantieri L (2010) MiR-199a-3p regulates mTOR and c-Met to influence the doxorubicin sensitivity of human hepatocarcinoma cells. Cancer Res 70:5184–5193
31. Gao JS, Zhang Y, Tang X, Tucker LD, Tarwater PM, Quesenberry PJ, Rigoutsos I, Ramratnam B (2011) The Evi1, microRNA-143, K-Ras axis in colon cancer. FEBS Lett 585:693–699
32. Garofalo M, Di Leva G, Romano G, Nuovo G, Suh SS, Ngankeu A, Taccioli C, Pichiorri F, Alder H, Secchiero P et al (2009) miR-221&222 regulate TRAIL resistance and enhance tumorigenicity through PTEN and TIMP3 downregulation. Cancer Cell 16:498–509
33. Garzon R, Heaphy CE, Havelange V, Fabbri M, Volinia S, Tsao T, Zanesi N, Kornblau SM, Marcucci G, Calin GA et al (2009) MicroRNA 29b functions in acute myeloid leukemia. Blood 114:5331–5341
34. Glass C, Singla DK (2011) MicroRNA-1 transfected embryonic stem cells enhance cardiac myocyte differentiation and inhibit apoptosis by modulating the PTEN/Akt pathway in the infarcted heart. Am J Physiol Heart Circ Physiol 301:2038–2049
35. Greene SB, Gunaratne PH, Hammond SM, Rosen JM (2010) A putative role for microRNA-205 in mammary epithelial cell progenitors. J Cell Sci 123:606–618
36. Gregory RI, Yan KP, Amuthan G, Chendrimada T, Doratotaj B, Cooch N, Shiekhattar R (2004) The Microprocessor complex mediates the genesis of microRNAs. Nature 432:235–240
37. Grishok A, Pasquinelli AE, Conte D, Li N, Parrish S, Ha I, Baillie DL, Fire A, Ruvkun G, Mello CC (2001) Genes and mechanisms related to RNA interference regulate expression of the small temporal RNAs that control C. elegans developmental timing. Cell 106:23–34
38. Guo C, Sah JF, Beard L, Willson JK, Markowitz SD, Guda K (2008) The noncoding RNA, miR-126, suppresses the growth of neoplastic cells by targeting phosphatidylinositol 3-kinase signaling and is frequently lost in colon cancers. Genes Chromosomes Cancer 47:939–946
39. Guo LM, Pu Y, Han Z, Liu T, Li YX, Liu M, Li X, Tang H (2009) MicroRNA-9 inhibits ovarian cancer cell growth through regulation of NF-kappaB1. FEBS J 276:5537–5546
40. Gupta GP, Massague J (2006) Cancer metastasis: building a framework. Cell 127:679–695
41. Hammond SM, Bernstein E, Beach D, Hannon GJ (2000) An RNA-directed nuclease mediates post-transcriptional gene silencing in Drosophila cells. Nature 404:293–296
42. Han J, Lee Y, Yeom KH, Kim YK, Jin H, Kim VN (2004) The Drosha-DGCR8 complex in primary microRNA processing. Gene Dev 18:3016–3027
43. Han J, Lee Y, Yeom KH, Nam JW, Heo I, Rhee JK, Sohn SY, Cho Y, Zhang BT, Kim VN (2006) Molecular basis for the recognition of primary microRNAs by the Drosha-DGCR8 complex. Cell 125:887–901
44. Han Z, Yang Q, Liu B, Wu J, Li Y, Yang C, Jiang Y (2012) MicroRNA-622 functions as a tumor suppressor by targeting K-Ras and enhancing the anticarcinogenic effect of resveratrol. Carcinogenesis 33:131–139
45. Hayashita Y, Osada H, Tatematsu Y, Yamada H, Yanagisawa K, Tomida S, Yatabe Y, Kawahara K, Sekido Y, Takahashi T (2005) A polycistronic microRNA cluster, miR-17-92, is overexpressed in human lung cancers and enhances cell proliferation. Cancer Res 65:9628–9632

46. He L, He X, Lim LP, de Stanchina E, Xuan Z, Liang Y, Xue W, Zender L, Magnus J, Ridzon D et al (2007) A microRNA component of the p53 tumor suppressor network. Nature 447:1130–1134
47. Hu G, Zhou R, Liu J, Gong AY, Eischeid AN, Dittman JW, Chen XM (2009) MicroRNA-98 and let-7 confer cholangiocyte expression of cytokine-inducible Src homology 2-containing protein in response to microbial challenge. J Immunol 183:1617–1624
48. Huang MB, Xu H, Xie SJ, Zhou H, Qu LH (2011) Insulin-like growth factor-1 receptor is regulated by microRNA-133 during skeletal myogenesis. PLoS One 6:e29173
49. Huang Q, Gumireddy K, Schrier M, le Sage C, Nagel R, Nair S, Egan DA, Li A, Huang G, Klein-Szanto AJ et al (2008) The microRNAs miR-373 and miR-520c promote tumor invasion and metastasis. Nat Cell Biol 10:202–210
50. Huse JT, Brennan C, Hambardzumyan D, Wee B, Pena J, Rouhanifard SH, Sohn-Lee C, le Sage C, Agami R, Tuschl T et al (2009) The PTEN-regulating microRNA miR-26a is amplified in high-grade glioma and facilitates gliomagenesis in vivo. Gene Dev 23:1327–1337
51. Hutvagner G, McLachlan J, Pasquinelli AE, Balint E, Tuschl T, Zamore PD (2001) A cellular function for the RNA-interference enzyme Dicer in the maturation of the let-7 small temporal RNA. Science 293:834–838
52. Hyun S, Lee JH, Jin H, Nam J, Namkoong B, Lee G, Chung J, Kim VN (2009) Conserved MicroRNA miR-8/miR-200 and its target USH/FOG2 control growth by regulating PI3 K. Cell 139:1096–1108
53. Iliopoulos D, Hirsch HA, Struhl K (2009) An epigenetic switch involving NF-kappaB, Lin28, Let-7 MicroRNA, and IL6 links inflammation to cell transformation. Cell 139:693–706
54. Ishizaki T, Tamiya T, Taniguchi K, Morita R, Kato R, Okamoto F, Saeki K, Nomura M, Nojima Y, Yoshimura A (2011) miR126 positively regulates mast cell proliferation and cytokine production through suppressing Spred1. Genes Cells 16:803–814
55. Jia CY, Li HH, Zhu XC, Dong YW, Fu D, Zhao QL, Wu W, Wu XZ (2011) MiR-223 suppresses cell proliferation by targeting IGF-1R. PLoS One 6:e27008
56. Johnson SM, Grosshans H, Shingara J, Byrom M, Jarvis R, Cheng A, Labourier E, Reinert KL, Brown D, Slack FJ (2005) RAS is regulated by the let-7 microRNA family. Cell 120:635–647
57. Karube Y, Tanaka H, Osada H, Tomida S, Tatematsu Y, Yanagisawa K, Yatabe Y, Takamizawa J, Miyoshi S, Mitsudomi T et al (2005) Reduced expression of Dicer associated with poor prognosis in lung cancer patients. Cancer Sci 96:111–115
58. Katakowski M, Zheng X, Jiang F, Rogers T, Szalad A, Chopp M (2010) MiR-146b-5p suppresses EGFR expression and reduces in vitro migration and invasion of glioma. Cancer Invest 28:1024–1030
59. Kato M, Putta S, Wang M, Yuan H, Lanting L, Nair I, Gunn A, Nakagawa Y, Shimano H, Todorov I et al (2009) TGF-beta activates Akt kinase through a microRNA-dependent amplifying circuit targeting PTEN. Nat Cell Biol 11:881–889
60. Kefas B, Godlewski J, Comeau L, Li Y, Abounader R, Hawkinson M, Lee J, Fine H, Chiocca EA, Lawler S et al (2008) microRNA-7 inhibits the epidermal growth factor receptor and the Akt pathway and is down-regulated in glioblastoma. Cancer Res 68:3566–3572
61. Keklikoglou I, Koerner C, Schmidt C, Zhang JD, Heckmann D, Shavinskaya A, Allgayer H, Guckel B, Fehm T, Schneeweiss A et al (2011) MicroRNA-520/373 family functions as a tumor suppressor in estrogen receptor negative breast cancer by targeting NF-kappaB and TGF-beta signaling pathways. Oncogene
62. Ketting RF, Fischer SE, Bernstein E, Sijen T, Hannon GJ, Plasterk RH (2001) Dicer functions in RNA interference and in synthesis of small RNA involved in developmental timing in C. elegans. Gene Dev 15:2654–2659
63. Khavari TA, Rinn J (2007) Ras/Erk MAPK signaling in epidermal homeostasis and neoplasia. Cell Cycle 6:2928–2931

64. Kolch W (2005) Coordinating ERK/MAPK signaling through scaffolds and inhibitors. Nat Rev Mol Cell Biol 6:827–837
65. Kong G, Zhang J, Zhang S, Shan C, Ye L, Zhang X (2011) Upregulated microRNA-29a by hepatitis B virus X protein enhances hepatoma cell migration by targeting PTEN in cell culture model. PLoS One 6:e19518
66. Korkmaz G, le Sage C, Tekirdag KA, Agami R, Gozuacik D (2012) miR-376b controls starvation and mTOR inhibition-related autophagy by targeting ATG4C and BECN1. Autophagy 8(2):165–176
67. Kota J, Chivukula RR, O'Donnell KA, Wentzel EA, Montgomery CL, Hwang HW, Chang TC, Vivekanandan P, Torbenson M, Clark KR et al (2009) Therapeutic microRNA delivery suppresses tumorigenesis in a murine liver cancer model. Cell 137:1005–1017
68. Landthaler M, Yalcin A, Tuschl T (2004) The human DiGeorge syndrome critical region gene 8 and Its D. melanogaster homolog are required for miRNA biogenesis. Curr Biol 14:2162–2167
69. Lee DW, Futami M, Carroll M, Feng Y, Wang Z, Fernandez M, Whichard Z, Chen Y, Kornblau S, Shpall EJ et al (2012) Loss of SHIP-1 protein expression in high-risk myelodysplastic syndromes is associated with miR-210 and miR-155. Oncogene doi: 10.1038/onc.2011.579
70. Lee KH, Chen YL, Yeh SD, Hsiao M, Lin JT, Goan YG, Lu PJ (2009) MicroRNA-330 acts as tumor suppressor and induces apoptosis of prostate cancer cells through E2F1-mediated suppression of Akt phosphorylation. Oncogene 28:3360–3370
71. Lee Y, Ahn C, Han J, Choi H, Kim J, Yim J, Lee J, Provost P, Radmark O, Kim S et al (2003) The nuclear RNase III Drosha initiates microRNA processing. Nature 425:415–419
72. Lee Y, Kim M, Han J, Yeom KH, Lee S, Baek SH, Kim VN (2004) MicroRNA genes are transcribed by RNA polymerase II. EMBO J 23:4051–4060
73. Li D, Liu X, Lin L, Hou J, Li N, Wang C, Wang P, Zhang Q, Zhang P, Zhou W et al (2011) MicroRNA-99a inhibits hepatocellular carcinoma growth and correlates with prognosis of patients with hepatocellular carcinoma. J Biol Chem 286:36677–36685
74. Li W, Xie L, He X, Li J, Tu K, Wei L, Wu J, Guo Y, Ma X, Zhang P et al (2008) Diagnostic and prognostic implications of microRNAs in human hepatocellular carcinoma. Int J Cancer 123:1616–1622
75. Li Y, Li W, Yang Y, Lu Y, He C, Hu G, Liu H, Chen J, He J, Yu H (2009) MicroRNA-21 targets LRRFIP1 and contributes to VM-26 resistance in glioblastoma multiforme. Brain Res 1286:13–18
76. Lin RJ, Lin YC, Yu AL (2010) miR-149* induces apoptosis by inhibiting Akt1 and E2F1 in human cancer cells. Mol Carcinog 49:719–727
77. Lindenblatt C, Schulze-Osthoff K, Totzke G (2009) IkappaBzeta expression is regulated by miR-124a. Cell Cycle 8:2019–2023
78. Ling HY, Ou HS, Feng SD, Zhang XY, Tuo QH, Chen LX, Zhu BY, Gao ZP,Tang CK, Yin WD et al (2009) Changes in microRNA profile and effects ofmiR-320 in insulin-resistant 3T3-L1 adipocytes. Clin Exp Pharmacol Physiol 36(9):e32–e39
79. Liu G, Friggeri A, Yang Y, Park YJ, Tsuruta Y, Abraham E (2009) miR-147, a microRNA that is induced upon Toll-like receptor stimulation, regulates murine macrophage inflammatory responses. Proc Natl Acad Sci U S A 106:15819–15824
80. Liu P, Wilson MJ (2012) miR-520c and miR-373 upregulate MMP9 expression by targeting mTOR and SIRT1, and activate the Ras/Raf/MEK/Erk signaling pathway and NF-kappaB factor in human fibrosarcoma cells. J Cell Physiol 227:867–876
81. Lu F, Weidmer A, Liu CG, Volinia S, Croce CM, Lieberman PM (2008) Epstein-Barr virus-induced miR-155 attenuates NF-kappaB signaling and stabilizes latent virus persistence. J Virol 82:10436–10443
82. Lu J, Getz G, Miska EA, Alvarez-Saavedra E, Lamb J, Peck D, Sweet-Cordero A, Ebert BL, Mak RH, Ferrando AA et al (2005) MicroRNA expression profiles classify human cancers. Nature 435:834–838

83. Lu Y, Roy S, Nuovo G, Ramaswamy B, Miller T, Shapiro C, Jacob ST, Majumder S (2011) Anti-microRNA-222 (anti-miR-222) and -181B suppress growth of tamoxifen-resistant xenografts in mouse by targeting TIMP3 protein and modulating mitogenic signal. J Biol Chem 286:42292–42302
84. Ma E, MacRae IJ, Kirsch JF, Doudna JA (2008) Autoinhibition of human dicer by its internal helicase domain. J Mol Biol 380:237–243
85. Ma L, Reinhardt F, Pan E, Soutschek J, Bhat B, Marcusson EG, Teruya-Feldstein J, Bell GW, Weinberg RA (2010) Therapeutic silencing of miR-10b inhibits metastasis in a mouse mammary tumor model. Nat Biotechnol 28:341–347
86. Ma L, Teruya-Feldstein J, Weinberg RA (2007) Tumor invasion and metastasis initiated by microRNA-10b in breast cancer. Nature 449:682–688
87. Ma X, Kumar M, Choudhury SN, Becker Buscaglia LE, Barker JR, Kanakamedala K, Liu MF, Li Y (2011) Loss of the miR-21 allele elevates the expression of its target genes and reduces tumorigenesis. In: Proceedings of the National Academy of Sciences of the United States of America, vol 108, pp 10144–10149
88. McClatchey AI (2003) Merlin and ERM proteins: unappreciated roles in cancer development? Nat Rev Cancer 3:877–883
89. Mendell JT (2008) miRiad roles for the miR-17-92 cluster in development and disease. Cell 133:217–222
90. Meng F, Henson R, Wehbe-Janek H, Ghoshal K, Jacob ST, Patel T (2007) MicroRNA-21 regulates expression of the PTEN tumor suppressor gene in human hepatocellular cancer. Gastroenterology 133:647–658
91. Mizuno Y, Tokuzawa Y, Ninomiya Y, Yagi K, Yatsuka-Kanesaki Y, Suda T, Fukuda T, Katagiri T, Kondoh Y, Amemiya T et al (2009) miR-210 promotes osteoblastic differentiation through inhibition of AcvR1b. FEBS Lett 583:2263–2268
92. Nagaraja AK, Creighton CJ, Yu Z, Zhu H, Gunaratne PH, Reid JG, Olokpa E, Itamochi H, Ueno NT, Hawkins SM et al (2010) A link between mir-100 and FRAP1/mTOR in clear cell ovarian cancer. Mol Endocrinol 24:447–463
93. Nan Y, Han L, Zhang A, Wang G, Jia Z, Yang Y, Yue X, Pu P, Zhong Y, Kang C (2010) MiRNA-451 plays a role as tumor suppressor in human glioma cells. Brain Res 1359:14–21
94. Nicholls PK, Harrison CA, Walton KL, McLachlan RI, O'Donnell L, Stanton PG (2011) Hormonal regulation of sertoli cell micro-RNAs at spermiation. Endocrinology 152:1670–1683
95. Noguchi S, Mori T, Hoshino Y, Maruo K, Yamada N, Kitade Y, Naoe T, Akao Y (2011) MicroRNA-143 functions as a tumor suppressor in human bladder cancer T24 cells. Cancer Lett 307:211–220
96. O'Donnell KA, Wentzel EA, Zeller KI, Dang CV, Mendell JT (2005) c-Myc-regulated microRNAs modulate E2F1 expression. Nature 435:839–843
97. Okamura K, Hagen JW, Duan H, Tyler DM, Lai EC (2007) The mirtron pathway generates microRNA-class regulatory RNAs in Drosophila. Cell 130:89–100
98. Olive V, Bennett MJ, Walker JC, Ma C, Jiang I, Cordon-Cardo C, Li QJ, Lowe SW, Hannon GJ, He L (2009) miR-19 is a key oncogenic component of mir-17-92. Gene Dev 23:2839–2849
99. Parker LH, Schmidt M, Jin SW, Gray AM, Beis D, Pham T, Frantz G, Palmieri S, Hillan K, Stainier DY et al (2004) The endothelial-cell-derived secreted factor Egfl7 regulates vascular tube formation. Nature 428:754–758
100. Perry MM, Williams AE, Tsitsiou E, Larner-Svensson HM, Lindsay MA (2009) Divergent intracellular pathways regulate interleukin-1beta-induced miR-146a and miR-146b expression and chemokine release in human alveolar epithelial cells. FEBS Lett 583:3349–3355
101. Pineau P, Volinia S, McJunkin K, Marchio A, Battiston C, Terris B, Mazzaferro V, Lowe SW, Croce CM, Dejean A (2010) miR-221 overexpression contributes to liver tumorigenesis. Proc Natl Acad Sci U S A 107:264–269

102. Qian P, Zuo Z, Wu Z, Meng X, Li G, Zhang W, Tan S, Pandey V, Yao Y, Wang P et al (2011) Pivotal role of reduced let-7 g expression in breast cancer invasion and metastasis. Cancer Res 71:6463–6474
103. Qin W, Dong P, Ma C, Mitchelson K, Deng T, Zhang L, Sun Y, Feng X, Ding Y, Lu X et al (2011) MicroRNA-133b is a key promoter of cervical carcinoma development through the activation of the ERK and AKT1 pathways. Oncogene doi:10.1038/onc.2011.561
104. Ren J, Zhu D, Liu M, Sun Y, Tian L (2010) Downregulation of miR-21 modulates Ras expression to promote apoptosis and suppress invasion of Laryngeal squamous cell carcinoma. Eur J Cancer 46:3409–3416
105. Roccaro AM, Sacco A, Thompson B, Leleu X, Azab AK, Azab F, Runnels J, Jia X, Ngo HT, Melhem MR et al (2009) MicroRNAs 15a and 16 regulate tumor proliferation in multiple myeloma. Blood 113:6669–6680
106. Rodriguez A, Griffiths-Jones S, Ashurst JL, Bradley A (2004) Identification of mammalian microRNA host genes and transcription units. Genome Res 14:1902–1910
107. Rogler CE, Levoci L, Ader T, Massimi A, Tchaikovskaya T, Norel R, Rogler LE (2009) MicroRNA-23b cluster microRNAs regulate transforming growth factor-beta/bone morphogenetic protein signaling and liver stem cell differentiation by targeting Smads. Hepatology 50:575–584
108. Roush S, Slack FJ (2008) The let-7 family of microRNAs. Trends Cell Biol 18:505–516
109. Ruby JG, Jan CH, Bartel DP (2007) Intronic microRNA precursors that bypass Drosha processing. Nature 448:83–86
110. Sahai E, Marshall CJ (2002) RHO-GTPases and cancer. Nat Rev Cancer 2:133–142
111. Saito Y, Liang G, Egger G, Friedman JM, Chuang JC, Coetzee GA, Jones PA (2006) Specific activation of microRNA-127 with downregulation of the proto-oncogene BCL6 by chromatin-modifying drugs in human cancer cells. Cancer Cell 9:435–443
112. Salvi A, Sabelli C, Moncini S, Venturin M, Arici B, Riva P, Portolani N, Giulini SM, De Petro G, Barlati S (2009) MicroRNA-23b mediates urokinase and c-met downmodulation and a decreased migration of human hepatocellular carcinoma cells. FEBS J 276:2966–2982
113. Sanchez-Carbayo M, Socci ND, Lozano J, Saint F, Cordon-Cardo C (2006) Defining molecular profiles of poor outcome in patients with invasive bladder cancer using oligonucleotide microarrays. J Clin Oncol 24:778–789
114. Sayed D, Abdellatif M (2010) AKT-ing via microRNA. Cell Cycle 9:3213–3217
115. Sayed D, He M, Hong C, Gao S, Rane S, Yang Z, Abdellatif M (2010) MicroRNA-21 is a downstream effector of AKT that mediates its antiapoptotic effects via suppression of Fas ligand. J Biol Chem 285:20281–20290
116. Schimanski CC, Frerichs K, Rahman F, Berger M, Lang H, Galle PR, Moehler M, Gockel I (2009) High miR-196a levels promote the oncogenic phenotype of colorectal cancer cells. World J Gastroenterol 15:2089–2096
117. Shi W, Gerster K, Alajez NM, Tsang J, Waldron L, Pintilie M, Hui AB, Sykes J, P'ng C, Miller N et al (2011) MicroRNA-301 mediates proliferation and invasion in human breast cancer. Cancer Res 71:2926–2937
118. Shin KH, Bae SD, Hong HS, Kim RH, Kang MK, Park NH (2011) miR-181a shows tumor suppressive effect against oral squamous cell carcinoma cells by downregulating K-ras. Biochem Biophys Res Commun 404:896–902
119. Smith AL, Iwanaga R, Drasin DJ, Micalizzi DS, Vartuli RL, Tan AC, and Ford HL (2012). The miR-106b-25 cluster targets Smad7, activates TGF-beta signaling, and induces EMT and tumor initiating cell characteristics downstream of Six1 in human breast cancer. Oncogene doi:10.1038/onc.2012.11
120. Soncin F, Mattot V, Lionneton F, Spruyt N, Lepretre F, Begue A, Stehelin D (2003) VE-statin, an endothelial repressor of smooth muscle cell migration. EMBO J 22:5700–5711
121. Taganov KD, Boldin MP, Chang KJ, Baltimore D (2006) NF-kappaB-dependent induction of microRNA miR-146, an inhibitor targeted to signaling proteins of innate immune responses. Proc Natl Acad Sci U S A 103:12481–12486

122. Ting Y, Medina DJ, Strair RK, Schaar DG (2010) Differentiation-associated miR-22 represses Max expression and inhibits cell cycle progression. Biochem Biophys Res Commun 394:606–611
123. Tsang WP, Kwok TT (2009) The miR-18a* microRNA functions as a potential tumor suppressor by targeting on K-Ras. Carcinogenesis 30:953–959
124. Tsukamoto Y, Nakada C, Noguchi T, Tanigawa M, Nguyen LT, Uchida T, Hijiya N, Matsuura K, Fujioka T, Seto M et al (2010) MicroRNA-375 is downregulated in gastric carcinomas and regulates cell survival by targeting PDK1 and 14–3-3zeta. Cancer Res 70:2339–2349
125. Uesugi A, Kozaki K, Tsuruta T, Furuta M, Morita K, Imoto I, Omura K, Inazawa J (2011) The tumor suppressive microRNA miR-218 targets the mTOR component Rictor and inhibits AKT phosphorylation in oral cancer. Cancer Res 71:5765–5778
126. Valadi H, Ekstrom K, Bossios A, Sjostrand M, Lee JJ, Lotvall JO (2007) Exosome-mediated transfer of mRNAs and microRNAs is a novel mechanism of genetic exchange between cells. Nat Cell Biol 9:654–659
127. Valastyan S, Reinhardt F, Benaich N, Calogrias D, Szasz AM, Wang ZC, Brock JE, Richardson AL, Weinberg RA (2009) A pleiotropically acting microRNA, miR-31, inhibits breast cancer metastasis. Cell 137:1032–1046
128. Voortman J, Goto A, Mendiboure J, Sohn JJ, Schetter AJ, Saito M, Dunant A, Pham TC, Petrini I, Lee A et al (2010) MicroRNA expression and clinical outcomes in patients treated with adjuvant chemotherapy after complete resection of non-small cell lung carcinoma. Cancer Res 70:8288–8298
129. Wang B, Koh P, Winbanks C, Coughlan MT, McClelland A, Watson A, Jandeleit-Dahm K, Burns WC, Thomas MC, Cooper ME et al (2011) miR-200a Prevents renal fibrogenesis through repression of TGF-beta2 expression. Diabetes 60:280–287
130. Wang B, Majumder S, Nuovo G, Kutay H, Volinia S, Patel T, Schmittgen TD, Croce C, Ghoshal K, Jacob ST (2009) Role of microRNA-155 at early stages of hepatocarcinogenesis induced by choline-deficient and amino acid-defined diet in C57BL/6 mice. Hepatology 50:1152–1161
131. Wang C, Bian Z, Wei D, Zhang JG (2011) miR-29b regulates migration of human breast cancer cells. Mol Cell Biochem 352:197–207
132. Wang XF, Shi ZM, Wang XR, Cao L, Wang YY, Zhang JX, Yin Y, Luo H, Kang CS, Liu N et al (2011c) MiR-181d acts as a tumor suppressor in glioma by targeting K-ras and Bcl-2. J Cancer Res Clin Oncol 138(4):573–584
133. Wong QW, Ching AK, Chan AW, Choy KW, To KF, Lai PB, Wong N (2010) MiR-222 overexpression confers cell migratory advantages in hepatocellular carcinoma through enhancing AKT signaling. Clin Cancer Res 16:867–875
134. Xu B, Niu X, Zhang X, Tao J, Wu D, Wang Z, Li P, Zhang W, Wu H, Feng N et al (2011) miR-143 decreases prostate cancer cells proliferation and migration and enhances their sensitivity to docetaxel through suppression of KRAS. Mol Cell Biochem 350:207–213
135. Yanaihara N, Caplen N, Bowman E, Seike M, Kumamoto K, Yi M, Stephens RM, Okamoto A, Yokota J, Tanaka T et al (2006) Unique microRNA molecular profiles in lung cancer diagnosis and prognosis. Cancer Cell 9:189–198
136. Yang H, Kong W, He L, Zhao JJ, O'Donnell JD, Wang J, Wenham RM, Coppola D, Kruk PA, Nicosia SV et al (2008) MicroRNA expression profiling in human ovarian cancer: miR-214 induces cell survival and cisplatin resistance by targeting PTEN. Cancer Res 68:425–433
137. Yang JS, Lai EC (2011) Alternative miRNA biogenesis pathways and the interpretation of core miRNA pathway mutants. Mol Cell 43:892–903
138. Yang JS, Maurin T, Robine N, Rasmussen KD, Jeffrey KL, Chandwani R, Papapetrou EP, Sadelain M, O'Carroll D, Lai EC (2010) Conserved vertebrate mir-451 provides a platform for Dicer-independent, Ago2-mediated microRNA biogenesis. Proc Natl Acad Sci U S A 107:15163–15168

139. Yi R, Qin Y, Macara IG, Cullen BR (2003) Exportin-5 mediates the nuclear export of pre-microRNAs and short hairpin RNAs. Gene Dev 17:3011–3016
140. Yu J, Ryan DG, Getsios S, Oliveira-Fernandes M, Fatima A, Lavker RM (2008) MicroRNA-184 antagonizes microRNA-205 to maintain SHIP2 levels in epithelia. Proc Natl Acad Sci U S A 105:19300–19305
141. Zeng Y, Cullen BR (2003) Sequence requirements for micro RNA processing and function in human cells. RNA 9:112–123
142. Zeng Y, Cullen BR (2005) Efficient processing of primary microRNA hairpins by Drosha requires flanking nonstructured RNA sequences. J Biol Chem 280:27595–27603
143. Zhang H, Hao Y, Yang J, Zhou Y, Li J, Yin S, Sun C, Ma M, Huang Y, Xi J (2011) Genome-wide Functional Screening of miR-23b as a Pleiotropic Modulator Suppressing Cancer Metastasis. Nat Commun 2. doi:10.1038/ncomms1555
144. Zhang X, Liu S, Hu T, He Y, Sun S (2009) Up-regulated microRNA-143 transcribed by nuclear factor kappa B enhances hepatocarcinoma metastasis by repressing fibronectin expression. Hepatology 50:490–499
145. Zhang Y, Liu D, Chen X, Li J, Li L, Bian Z, Sun F, Lu J, Yin Y, Cai X et al (2010) Secreted monocytic miR-150 enhances targeted endothelial cell migration. Mol Cell 39:133–144
146. Zhao WG, Yu SN, Lu ZH, Ma YH, Gu YM, Chen J (2010) The miR-217 microRNA functions as a potential tumor suppressor in pancreatic ductal adenocarcinoma by targeting KRAS. Carcinogenesis 31:1726–1733

The Perinucleolar Compartment: RNA Metabolism and Cancer

John T. Norton and Sui Huang

Abstract

The perinucleolar compartment (PNC) is a nuclear substructure associated with, but structurally distinct from, the nucleolus. The PNC contains several RNA processing proteins and several RNA pol III transcripts, which form novel complexes. As determined by cell culture experiments and human tumor samples, the PNC forms exclusively in cancer cells and the percentage of cancer cells in a population that have one or more PNCs directly correlates with the malignancy of that population of cells. Therefore, the PNC is being developed as a prognostic marker for several malignancies. PNC elimination in cancer cells has proven to be a useful as screening method to discover probe compounds used to elucidate PNC biology and to discover compounds with the potential to be developed as minimally toxic anti-cancer drugs.

Keywords

Nuclear architecture · PNC · RNPs · Chromatin · Cancer

Contents

S. Huang (✉)
Department of Cell and Molecular Biology, Northwestern University Feinberg School of Medicine, 303 E. Chicago Ave, Ward Building 11-240, Chicago, IL 60614, USA
e-mail: s-huang2@northwestern.edu

J. T. Norton
Department of Cell and Molecular Biology, Northwestern University, Chicago, IL, USA

J. Y. Wu (ed.), *RNA and Cancer*, Cancer Treatment and Research,
DOI: 10.1007/978-3-642-31659-3_6, © Springer-Verlag Berlin Heidelberg 2013

1 Introduction

1.1 Structure of the PNC

The perinucleolar compartment (PNC) is a nonmembrane bound nuclear substructure associated with, but structurally distinct from, the nucleolus. The PNC is irregularly shaped with dimensions ranging from 0.25 to 4 microns. Electron microscopy studies have revealed the structure of the PNC consists of several 80–180 nm electron dense strands that form a reticulated meshwork on the surface of the nucleolus [1, 2]]. The PNC persists through interphase with limited movement, disassembles in pro-metaphase, and reassembles in late telophase along with the biogenesis of nucleoli [1]. The PNC is generally heritable from mother to daughter cells, which can be observed in newly divided daughter cells, which often display PNCs that are mirror images (Fig. 1). PNC is a dynamic structure through which some of the components shuttle in and out rapidly [[2], our unpublished data].

1.2 Molecular Components of the PNC

Although the molecular composition of the structure is not fully elucidated, the PNC is known to be enriched with several RNAs and RNA binding proteins. The PNC was initially described during the characterization of the polypyrimidine tract-binding protein (PTB) [3], which is a multi-functional RNA binding protein involved in pre-mRNA splicing, stability, and translational regulation. Although PTB shuttles between the nucleus and the cytoplasm, the protein is enriched primarily in the nucleoplasm and is highly concentrated in the PNC when the structure is present (Fig. 1). Since the discovery of PTB localization to the PNC, several other RNA binding proteins have also been found to be concentrated in the PNC. They include CUG-BP [4], KSRP [5], Raver1 [6], Raver2 [7], Rod1 [our unpublished data], and nucleolin [our unpublished data]. The PTB-associated splicing factor (PSF) [8] and the apobec editosome [9] may also localize to the

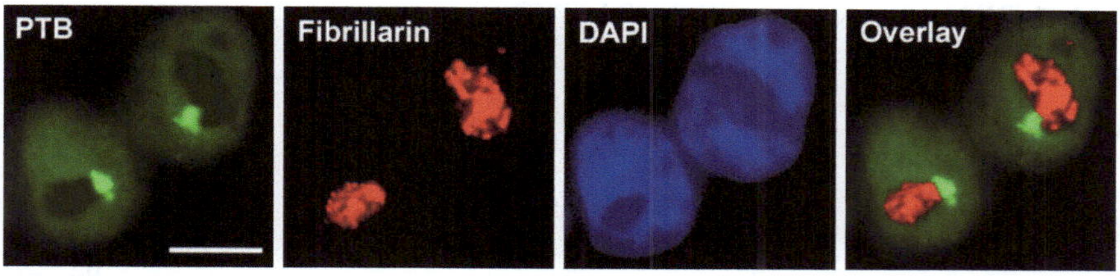

Fig. 1 The numbers and the position of the PNC in relation to the nucleolus are heritable to daughter cells during cell division as shown by immunostaining. Labeling of PTB in two newly divided daughter cells marks the PNCs (bright spots at the nucleolar periphery) and nucleoplasm. Fibrillarin marks the nucleoli and DAPI marks the nucleoplasm. Overlay of the PTB and fibrillarin signals shows the association of the PNC with the nucleolus. Scale bar = 10 μm

PNC. All these proteins are implicated primarily in the processing of pol II RNAs, with the exception of nucleolin. However, not all pre-mRNA processing factors are enriched in the PNC nor are pol II transcription factors [our unpublished data]. Since PNC is physically associated with the nucleolus and can be co-purified with nucleoli [our unpublished data], we examined the localization of several nucleolar proteins to determine if they are in the PNC. Surprisingly, many nucleolar proteins are not enriched in the PNC. These proteins include UBF, pol I subunits, SL1 components, RRN3, fibrillarin, and B23 [our unpublished data], all of which are either involved in pol I transcription or pre-rRNA processing.

In addition to proteins, a set of small non-coding pol III RNAs have also been found enriched in the PNC. They include MRP RNA [10], RNAse P RNA [10], hY RNAs (hY1, 2, and 5) [10], Alu RNA [11], and SRP (7SL) RNA [11]. MRP and RNAse P RNAs are highly conserved components of two different site specific endoribonucleases that are involved in pre-rRNA processing [12]. hY is an abundant RNA species that associates with the Ro protein, whose function remains unclear. SRP RNA is a transcript component of the signal recognition particle which functions in trafficking nascent proteins containing the endoplasmic reticulum (ER) signal and the associated ribosome to the ER [13]. Alu is a relatively newly evolved RNA that is derived from 7SL RNA and also associates with the signal recognition particle [14]. However, in situ hybridization to other pol III RNAs including U6 [[10], our unpublished data], tRNA [our unpublished data], 7SK, and hY4 [10] RNAs did not show localization of these RNAs in the PNC.

Therefore, the PNC is concentrated with RNA binding proteins that have been primarily implicated in the metabolism of pol II RNAs and is also enriched with pol III synthesized small RNAs (Table 1). Our recent observations demonstrate novel interactions among the PNC-associated RNA and the proteins [15]. The enrichment of the RNA and proteins in the PNC does not appear to be simply due to overexpression of these components in PNC containing cells, since overexpression of the protein components (PTB or CUG-BP) alone or in concert with PNC-associated RNAs (such as MRP RNA and RNase P RNA) does not induce

Table 1 RNA and protein components of the PNC

RNAs	Proteins
MRP	PTB
	CUG-BP
Alu	Raver1
	Raver2
Rnase P	Rod1
	KSRP
hY (1, 2, and 5)	nucleolin
	PSF
SRP (7SL)	apobec

Some of these components have previously been linked to cancer and metastasis. Alu RNAs have been shown to be over expressed in cancers but no functional link has been established [15]. PTB is often up regulated in cancer cells [[16], our unpublished data], may support malignant transformation [our unpublished data], and possibly promote metastasis in some cell types [[17], our unpublished data]. Nucleolin can also be unregulated in cancer cells [18] and is involved in the production of MMP-9 [19], which promotes metastatic behavior. However, how these components interact in the PNC and the function of the PNC in malignancy remains unclear

the formation of the PNCs in primary or immortalized cells [our unpublished data]. The complete molecular composition of the PNC has not been fully resolved and the interactions among the known PNC-associated components are just beginning to be explored. This chapter will discuss the possible functions of the PNC in RNA metabolism based on published and our unpublished data, the association of the PNC with the malignant phenotype, and the potential utilization of the PNC as a prognostic and drug discovery cancer marker.

2 The PNC and RNA Metabolism

2.1 The PNC is Likely Involved in RNA Processing

Although the precise function of the PNC is unknown, several lines of evidence have suggested that it might be involved in RNA metabolism. First, RNase treatment disassembles the PNC in unfixed permeabilized cells while DNase has no effect [1]. Second, pulse labeling with Br-U shows enrichment of these nucleotides in the PNC after only 5 min, indicating that the PNC is enriched with newly transcribed RNAs [2]. The third piece of evidence is the fact that all known protein components of the PNC are RNA binding proteins involved in RNA processing. Finally, the RNA-binding capacity of PTB is required for its localization to the PNC and PTB is essential for maintaining the integrity of the PNC [1]. All these findings support a role for PNC in RNA metabolism.

2.2 PNC is Enriched with Pol III Transcripts, but not Pol I or Pol II RNAs

To determine the origin of newly synthesized PNC-associated RNAs, we have performed experiments that selectively inhibit pol I, II, or III transcriptional activity. The initial experiments using a low dose of actinomycin D (0.4 μg/mL), which selectively inhibits pol I transcription [20] caused elimination the PNC [2]. However, further experiments with cycloheximide, which also selectively inhibits pol I transcription (5 h at 100 ug/ml) [21], did not induce PNC disassembly nor did it affect the labeled nucleotide enrichment in the PNC. Thus, the affect of actinomycin D on the PNC is likely due to an "off target" affect of the drug, perhaps such as DNA intercalation, rather than pol I transcription inhibition. This is further supported by the finding that neither 28S and 18S RNAs nor pre-rRNA processing factors, such as fibrillarin, are detected in the PNC through in situ hybridization and immunolabeling [[1, 10], our unpublished data]. Therefore, the source of these newly synthesized PNC-associated RNAs is unlikely rRNA. It is also unlikely that the primary source of PNC-localized RNA is from pol II as the PNC is not sensitive to pol II transcription inhibition by α-amanatin [2], nor is BrU incorporation into the PNC [our unpublished data]. In addition, in situ hybridization to several pre-mRNAs did not show any enrichment in the PNC [5], our unpublished data]; however, this does not exclude the possibility that some pol II transcripts might localize to the PNC.

The structural integrity of the PNC is dependent upon continuous pol III transcription. Injection of tagetin, a specific pol III inhibitor, into HeLa cells results in a disassembly of the PNC within 2 h [11]. This finding suggests that the majority of PNC-associated RNAs are of pol III origins and these RNAs are essential components of the PNC. Furthermore, over expression of one PNC-associated RNA, MRP RNA, from a pol II promoter followed by injection of tagetin partially blocks the tagetin-induced PNC disassembly [11], demonstrating that it is the RNA rather than activity of the polymerase that is important for the integrity of the PNC. In addition, inhibition of pol III transcription disassembles the PNC within a short period of time but does not disrupt the localization of MRP RNA to its functional RNP within the nucleolus [11]. These findings, along with the observation that none of the genes of known PNC-associated RNAs localize to the PNC [[10], our unpublished data], demonstrates that the PNC rapidly recruits a subset of newly synthesized pol III transcripts.

2.3 Novel RNP Associates with the PNC

Reciprocal precipitation experiments were used to analyze the in vivo interactions to determine whether the pol III RNAs in the PNC interact with the RNA binding proteins enriched in the PNC. MRP RNA pulled-down by a specific oligo or immunoprecipitation of PTB or CUGBP by specific antibodies show a reciprocal co-precipitation between the RNA and the RNA binding proteins [15].

Glycerol gradient analyses show that this complex is large and sediments at a different fraction from known MRP RNA containing complexes, the MRP RNP ribozyme, and hTERT. Tethering PNC components to a LacO locus recruits other PNC components, further confirming the in vivo interactions. High-resolution localization analyses demonstrate that MRP RNA, CUGBP, and PTB colocalize at the PNC as a reticulated network [15]. These findings indicate that the pol III RNA containing complexes in the PNC represent non-canonical interactions that may have novel roles in their metabolism and in the PNC.

2.4 Potential Functions of the PNC

What might be the functional significance of the enrichment of newly synthesized RNA and RNA binding proteins in the PNC? Several possibilities can be envisioned. Since PNC is not the site of transcription for the known PNC-associated RNAs, one obvious possibility is that the PNC may serve as an assembly site for the RNPs themselves. However, localization studies of the subunits of MRP RNase, RNase P, and Ro RNP, whose RNA components are associated with the PNC, show that neither the subunits nor functional RNPs localized to the PNC [[10], our unpublished data], indicating that the PNC is not likely involved in the canonical RNP assembly. These findings together with the fact that the PNC is highly enriched with newly synthesized RNA suggest that the RNAs are concentrated in the PNC prior to being assembled into mature or functional RNPs that are subsequently distributed to the nucleolus or other cellular destinations. Since live cell analyses showed that PTB shuttles in and out of PNCs rapidly [1], the association of these RNAs with the PNC is likely to be dynamic rather than long-term storage or simple aggregation. All these findings lead to a working model that the PNC is primarily involved in the metabolism of a subset of newly synthesized pol III RNA transcripts in transformed cells.

There are several possibilities for the specific role for PNC in the metabolism of these RNAs: (1) the PNC could be the site of RNA processing; (2) the RNAs could be sequestered in the PNC prior to being assembled into functional complexes, which may serve as a regulatory mechanism; (3) the PNC may act as the site of assembly for RNA export complexes for the cytoplasmic translocation of some of the PNC-associated RNAs; or (4) the PNC could also be the site for degradation of excess RNAs.

The PNC might be involved in the processing of the pol III PNC-associated transcripts; however, the post-transcriptional processing of pol III RNAs is poorly understood, with the exception of tRNAs. La, an RNA binding protein, is the only protein shown to mediate processing of newly made pol III transcripts [22]. To determine whether PNC is involved in La-mediated processes, the localization of La was evaluated through immunofluorescence and expression of tagged La with GFP and T7 individually. La was not enriched in the PNC when compared to the concentration of pol III RNAs in the structure [our unpublished data]. This finding suggests that the PNC is unlikely to be part of La-mediated pol III RNA processing, but there is increasing evidence to support that the PNC contains novel RNA–protein complexes [our unpublished data] that may be possibly involved in pol III RNA processing. Localization, RNA pull-down, and immunoprecipitation experiments reveal that the pol III RNAs and proteins primarily implicated in pol II transcription, including PTB and CUG-BP are co-enriched in the PNC and interact with each other in vivo. In addition, dynamic studies in live cells show that these RNA binding proteins have much slower dynamics in the PNC as compared to their counterparts in the nucleoplasm [our unpublished data], which suggests altered function for these proteins when in the PNC. Further, understanding of the novel RNP complexes associated with the PNC could help elucidate the function of PNC and novel mechanisms of post-transcriptional metabolism of a subset of pol III transcripts.

The PNC may also serve as a regulatory depot that sequesters a subset of pol III RNAs and regulates their functional availability. During transformation, there is an up-regulation of pol III transcription [23]. As a large number of pol III transcripts are functional RNAs (for example, the RNA components of RNase MRP, RNase P, snRNPs, and tRNA) the level of these RNAs could significantly impact a broad spectrum of cellular activities. The up-regulation of these RNAs during transformation may indeed reflect the increase demand for these RNAs throughout the process. It is possible that the PNC participates in regulating the post-transcriptional availability of these RNAs in transformed cells.

In addition, it is also possible that the PNC acts as the assembly site of RNA export complexes for the cytoplasmic translocation of some of the PNC-associated RNAs. The RNase MRP complex is known to be involved in mitochondrial DNA replication [24] and Ro RNPs are predominantly localized to the cytoplasm [25] although their function remains to be clarified. Treatment of cells with leptomycin B or ratjadone, which block the XPO1 mediated nuclear export of rRNA, some mRNAs, and several RNPs, effectively disassembles the PNC [our unpublished data]. Since inhibition of pol II transcription dose not eliminate PNCs [2], the disassembly of PNCs by leptomycin B and ratjadone is unlikely due to the loss of protein synthesis from the block of mRNA export. Therefore, the requirement of XPO1 activity for PNC suggests that the PNC could play a role XPO1 mediated export.

Finally, the PNC could also be the site for degradation of excess RNAs. The over expression of pol III transcription may trigger the RNA degradation machinery to eliminate the excess amount the RNA. Evidence supporting a possible role of PNC in this function are the following: two components of the PNC, CUG-BP, [26] and KSRP [27], are known to promote the degradation of RNAs in addition to their roles in RNA processing. Second, preliminary proteomic analyses suggest the presence of several other classes of RNA degradation proteins in the PNC [our unpublished data]. To distinguish what role the PNC actually plays in RNA metabolism, parallel studies using different techniques are underway to identify the molecular complexes that are associated with the PNC and to characterize their functional interactions.

3 The PNC and Malignant Transformation

3.1 PNC Selectively Forms in Metastatic Solid Tumor Cells

3.1.1 In Vitro Studies

During the initial characterization of the PNC, it was observed that PNC prevalence (% non-mitotic and non-apoptotic cells with one or more PNC) was invariably low (< 5 %) in normal cell lines while heterogeneous, but much higher (15–95 %) in transformed and cancerous cell lines [1]. Examination of many more (> 50) primary cells, normal cell lines, and cancer cell lines has demonstrated the same trend. The PNC can form not only in carcinomas, but also in sarcomas and blastomas; however, the PNC prevalence is invariably low in hematological malignancies. The PNC is not prevalent in primary cells or normal cell lines derived from stromal, endothelial, haematopoetic, or embryonic stem cell origins [35]. These findings suggest that PNCs selectively form in cells from solid tumors.

3.1.2 In Vivo Studies

The increased PNC prevalence in transformed and cancerous cells prompted examination of the PNC in vivo. Breast cancer has been used as a model system since the disease progression and molecular basis of the disease have been extensively characterized. Histological samples of normal breast tissue, primary tumors, affected lymph nodes, and distant metastasis were immunolabeled with SH54, an antibody to PTB, via microwave antigen retrieval protocol. For each sample, > 500 cells in the most active area (with the highest histological grading) were scored for PNC prevalence. The results showed that PNC prevalence is 0 % in normal breast tissue, but increases in the primary tumor along with the progression of the disease from benign, to ductal carcinoma in situ, to affected lymph nodes, and finally reaches near 100 % in distant metastasis. The PNC prevalence also increases in a step wise fashion from the primary tumor, to the cancerous lymph node lesions, to the distant metastasis. In addition, high PNC prevalence in primary tumors positively correlates with disease relapse and inversely correlates with disease free and overall survival in a retrospective 17 year follow-up study. A multivariate examination of the data from this study showed that PNC prevalence provides additional prognostic information for stage I, node negative patients [28]. More recently, we found similar correlations between PNC prevalence and the disease progression in colon and ovarian cancers [36]. Together with the findings that PNC forms in solid tumor cell lines derived from a wide range of tissue types, PNC prevalence has the potential to be a useful pan-cancer prognostic marker, making it the first marker of its kind.

3.2 The PNC and Metastatic Behavior

Results from the breast cancer study [28] showed that PNC prevalence increased with the progression of the disease, ultimately reaching near 100 % in distant metastasis, suggesting that PNC containing cells have a metastatic advantage over those lacking PNCs. High PNC prevalence correlates with increased risk of relapse and decreased overall survival in breast cancer patients, further supporting that the PNC marks the malignant (metastatic) breast cancer cells.

To empirically determine if PNC marks metastatic cells, the PC-3 series of cell lines, which have varying levels of metastatic capacities as selected for in mouse models, were examined for PNC prevalence. The PC-3 cell line was created from a human prostate carcinoma [29]. The PC-3 M cell line is a metastatic variant of PC-3 created by injecting PC-3 cells into a nude mouse, allowing the cells to metastasize, and then resecting the metastatic cells for culturing [30]. The PNC prevalence in PC-3 cells is 4 % and significantly increases to 85 % in the metastatic variant PC-3M [35]. The PC-3 M cell line was further enriched for metastatic cells by injecting them into the prostate of a nude mouse, allowing lymph node metastasis, resecting the metastases and reinjecting the metastatic cells into the prostate of another nude mouse. This process was iterated four times to obtain the highly metastatic variant PC-3M LN4 [31], which has a PNC prevalence of 98 % and abnormally large PNCs [our unpublished data]. Conversely, PC-3 M cells were used to create a cell line enriched with nonmetastatic cells by resecting the primary prostate tumors, reinjecting into the prostate of another nude mouse, and iterating this process four times [31]. This cell line, PC-3 M Pro4, has a PNC prevalence of 71 %, most of which are atypically small and nearly undetectable [35]. When the PNC prevalence is adjusted to the percentage of cells with PNCs greater than 2.2 μm, it correlates very closely with the metastatic behavior of these cells. These observations in cells of the same origin, but of varying metastatic capacities, further confirm that the presence of typical PNCs reflects the metastatic capability of cancer cells. To evaluate the association of PNC prevalence with metastatic behavior in an alternative system, PNC prevalence was examined in cell lines over expressing the breast cancer related metastatic suppressor protein (BRMS). BRMS is a chromatin remodeling protein that suppresses the ability of cells to proliferate at distant sites [32]. Stable over expression in two breast cancer cell lines, MB-MDA-231 and MB-MDA-435, caused a great decrease in metastasis formation compared to the parental cells when injected into a nude mouse [32]. The PNC prevalence in the BRMS overexpressing cell lines is significantly lower than in the parental cells [35] further confirming the association of the PNC with metastatic cells.

3.3 PNC is not a Marker of Differentiation or Growth Rate

Although metastasis is a trait specific to cancer cells, some characteristics of cancer cells can be shared by normal cells, including rapid proliferation, high glycolytic rate, and undifferentiation. To determine whether the PNC prevalence also correlates with traits that are shared by normal cells, the PNC prevalence was examined in several in vitro experimental systems. The proliferation of MCF-10A (normal breast epithelium) cells is over 5 times more rapid than the proliferation of MCF-7 (breast carcinoma) cells. However, the PNC prevalence of the MCF-10A cells is about 7 times lower than the MCF-7 cells [35], which dissociates PNC prevalence from proliferation. To further examine the relationship of PNC prevalence and proliferation, HeLa cells were treated under normal serum or serum starved conditions. The serum starved cells proliferated much slower than the cells grown under normal conditions, but PNC prevalence remains the same under both conditions. Thus, the PNC does not indicate rapid proliferation. In addition, peripheral blood mononuclear cells (PBMCs) were treated with the antigen phytohemagglutinin (PHA), which stimulates metabolism and proliferation of these cells. PBMCs have 0 % PNC, as they are primary cells, and their PNC prevalence remains at 0 % even after 72 h treatment with PHA demonstrating that normal cells cannot form PNC simply by increasing proliferation rate [our [35]], which further dissociates the PNC from proliferation. To address whether the PNC is associated with a high rate of glycolysis, HeLa cells were grown in a medium lacking glucose and pyruvate for 24 h, which significantly inhibits growth when compared to cells grown in normal glucose conditions. PNC prevalence remains the same in cells grown under both conditions, demonstrating that PNC does not correlate with a high rate of glycolysis [our unpublished data] and further demonstrating that the PNC does not associate with proliferation rate. Cancer cells are generally less differentiated than normal somatic cells and an undifferentiated state is also characteristic of normal progenitor cells. To determine whether PNC formation reflects an undifferentiated state, the PNC prevalence was examined in human embryonic stem cells and the results show a 0 % PNC prevalence. In addition, a blastoma cell line (NIE-115) and teratoma cell line (F9) that can each be differentiated by specific chemical treatment [[33, 34] respectively] showed no change in PNC prevalence after induced differentiation, demonstrating that PNC is not a marker of an undifferentiated state [our unpublished data]. These observations together show that PNC formation does not associate with cellular proliferation rate, glycolytic rate, or the differentiation state, all of which are characteristics shared by normal and cancer cells. Therefore, PNC prevalence selectively associates with the metastatic capability of cancer cells.

3.4 Why does the PNC Form in Transformed Cells?

The unique association of the PNC with metastatic capable cancer cells from solid tumors suggests that it forms due to cellular conditions specific to these cells. Two possible mechanisms for PNC formation, which are not mutually exclusive, can be speculated. (1) PNC formation could partially be due to increased need for metabolism or regulation of PNC-associated components in cancer cells. Pol III transcription is significantly increased during transformation [23], which may lead to an excess of RNP RNAs, allowing increased interaction with the protein components of the PNC, leading to the nucleation of the PNC. While the interactions between the protein and RNA components of the PNC have not yet been fully characterized, initial studies suggest that several of the protein and RNA components are in the same complex in vivo as determined by

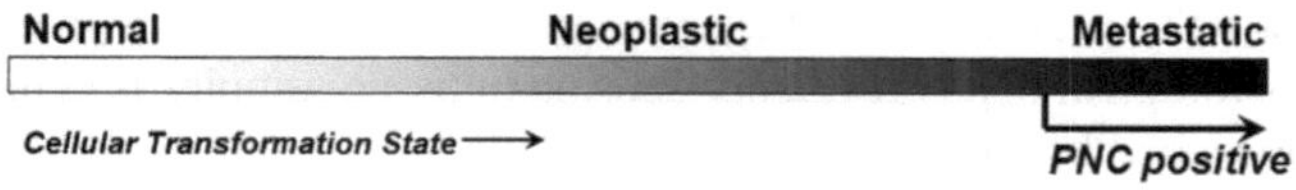

Fig. 2 The PNC forms at a late stage in the multi-step process of malignant transformation and is indicative of metastatic cells

immunoprecipitation and RNA pull-down experiments [[10], our unpublished data]. (2) Another possibility is that yet to be identified factors in the PNC are altered at the level of expression or function specifically in solid tumor cells, which nucleate the RNAs and RNA binding proteins in the PNC. Formation of the PNC is likely a late event during malignant transformation (Fig. 2), possibly as a result of the heterogeneous multi-step process of malignant transformation. These steps can include: increased pol III transcription, altered molecular complex expression levels or functions, and possibly alterations in expression or function of unidentified PNC-nucleation factors. While PNC is most likely a result of an advanced cellular transformation state, the PNC may also functionally promote or maintain malignant phenotype through regulating the molecular complexes associated with the PNC. Studies are currently underway to identify these molecular complexes, their functions in the PNC, and how they impact malignant phenotype.

4 Potential Utilization of the PNC

4.1 Prognostic Marker for Solid Tumors

Our findings in breast, ovary, and colon cancers, as well as cancer cell lines from multiple tissue origins suggest that PNC is an ideal candidate to be a pan-cancer marker for solid tumors. The PNC is a multi-component complex structure whose presence may reflect the malignant behavior of cancer cells more comprehensively than molecular markers, since malignancy is induced by complex and heterogeneous mechanisms among, and even with in, tumors. In addition, PNC is selectively associated with metastasis without obvious links to proliferation, glycolysis, or differentiation state. Such specific association with malignant behavior makes the PNC a unique tumor marker that may more selectively represent the malignant characteristics of cancer cells than other markers. Therefore, PNC prevalence can be an ideal tumor marker that increases the accuracy of disease prognosis. There is still a great need for selective and specific tumor markers to help make appropriate treatment decisions for many cancer patients. For example, stage I, node negative breast cancer patients often undergo adjuvant chemotherapy, which causes severe side effects and long-term health problems. Yet, the majority of the patients will not have relapses even without the chemotherapy. The lack of accurate prognostic markers that distinguish high risk from low risk patients causes a large proportion of the patients to be over-treated. PNC prevalence provides additional prognostic information for this group of patients than the existing markers [28], demonstrating the potential for PNC prevalence to be developed into a useful prognostic marker. Currently, histological PNC prevalence scoring in tissue samples is being refined to make it a reproducible and reliable marker.

4.2 Anti-Cancer Drug Discovery Marker

As the PNC marks metastatic cells in vitro and in vivo, PNC elimination could serve as a surrogate marker that indicates changes in cancer cell behavior toward a more benign phenotype (Fig. 2). This hypothesis rationalizes the use of PNC elimination as a drug discovery marker with the goal of discovering broadly efficacious and selective anti-cancer compounds. Since the PNC is unique to cancer cells and marks metastatic cells, it is reasonable to expect discoveries of compounds that inhibit metastatic behavior of cancer cells while minimally affecting normal cells. The findings from our lab that clinically used cytotoxic cancer drugs and experimental cancer drugs are enriched with PNC reducing compounds while random small molecule libraries are not [34], preliminarily validating that PNC prevalence reduction is a sound screening strategy that should be pursued further [34]. Compounds that eliminate the PNC not only have potential to be developed into novel drugs [37], but can also be used as chemical biology tools to help understand the biology driving PNC formation, maintenance, and its function in malignant cells. Further elucidation of PNC function will lead to a better understanding of novel biology underlying all solid tumor cells and potentially provide novel targeted pan-cancer treatment strategies.

Acknowledgments We would like to thank the partial funding from the Robert H. Lurie Comprehensive Cancer Center, and grant to SH from NIH, R01 GM078555.

References

1. Huang S, Deerinck TJ, Ellisman MH, Spector DL (1997) The dynamic organization of the perinucleolar compartment in the cell nucleus. J Cell Biol 137(5):965–974
2. Huang S, Deerinck TJ, Ellisman MH, Spector DL (1998) The perinucleolar compartment and transcription. J Cell Biol 143(1):35–47
3. Ghetti A, Piñol-Roma S, Michael WM, Morandi C, Dreyfuss G (1992) hnRNP I, the polypyrimidine tract-binding protein: distinct nuclear localization and association with hnRNAs. Nucleic Acids Res 20(14):3671–3678
4. Timchenko LT, Miller JW, Timchenko NA, DeVore DR, Datar KV, Lin L et al (1996) Identification of a (CUG)n triplet repeat RNA-binding protein and its expression in myotonic dystrophy. Nucleic Acids Res 24:4407–4414
5. Hall MP, Huang S, Black DL (2004) Differentiation-induced colocalization of the KH-type splicing regulatory protein with polypyrimidine tract binding protein and the c-src pre-mRNA. Mol Biol Cell 15(2):774–786
6. Hüttelmaier S, Illenberger S, Grosheva I, Rüdiger M, Singer RH, Jockusch BM (2001) Raver1, a dual compartment protein, is a ligand for PTB/hnRNPI and microfilament attachment proteins. J Cell Biol 155(5):775–786

7. Kleinhenz M, Fabienke S, Swiniarski N, Wittenmayer J, Kirsch B, Jockusch H et al (2005) Raver2, a new member of the hnRNP family. FEBS Lett 579(20):4254–4258
8. Shav-Tal Y, Lee BC, Bar-Haim S, Schori H, Zipori D (2001) Reorganization of nuclear factors during myeloid differentiation. J Cell Biochem 81:379–392
9. Lau PP, Chan L (2003) Involvement of a chaperone regulator, Bcl2-associated athanogene-4, in apolipoprotein B mRNA editing. J Biol Chem 278(52):52988–52996
10. Matera AG, Frey MR, Margelot K, Wolin SL (1995) A perinucleolar compartment contains several RNA polymerase III transcripts as well as the polypyrimidine tract-binding protein, hnRNP I. J Cell Biol 129(5):1181–1193
11. Wang C, Politz JC, Pederson T, Huang S (2003) RNA polymerase III transcripts and the PTB protein are essential for the integrity of the perinucleolar compartment. Mol Biol Cell 14:2425–2435
12. Pollock C, Daily K, Nguyen VT, Wang C, Lewandowska M, Bensaude O, Huang S (2011) Characterization of MRP RNA-protein interactions within the perinucleolar compartment. Mol Biol Cell 22(6):858–867
13. Koch HG, Moser M, Müller M (2003) Signal recognition particle-dependent protein targeting, universal to all kingdoms of life. Rev Physiol Biochem Pharmacol 146:55–94
14. Häsler J, Strub K (2006) Alu elements as regulators of gene expression. Nucleic Acids Res 34(19):5491–5497
15. Fähling M, Steege A, Perlewitz A, Nafz B, Mrowka R, Persson PB, Thiele BJ (2005) Role of nucleolin in posttranscriptional control of MMP-9 expression. Biochim Biophys Acta 1731(1):32–40
16. Perry RP (1963) Selective effects of actinomycin D on the intracellular distribution of RNA synthesis in tissue culture cells. Exp Cell Res 29:400–406
17. Higashi K, Matsuhisa T, Kitao A, Sakamoto Y (1968) Selective suppression of nucleolar RNA metabolism in the absence of protein synthesis. Biochim Biophys Acta 166:388–393
18. Wolin SL, Cedervall T (2002) The La protein. Annu Rev Biochem 71:375–403
19. White RJ (2004) RNA polymerase III transcription and cancer. Oncogene 23:3208–3216
20. Lee DY, Clayton DA (1998) Initiation of mitochondrial DNA replication by transcription and R-loop processing. Biol Chem 273:30614–30621
21. Pruijn GJ, Simons FH, van Venrooij WJ (1997) Intracellular localization and nucleocytoplasmic transport of Ro RNP components. Eur J Cell Biol 74:123–132
22. Paillard L, Legagneux V, Beverley OH (2003) A functional deadenylation assay identifies human CUG-BP as a deadenylation factor. Biol Cell 95:107–113
23. Norton JT, Wang C, Gjidoda A, Henry RW, Huang S (2009) Perinucleolar compartment is directly associated with DNA. J Biol Chem 284:4090–4101
24. Gherzi R, Lee KY, Briata P, Wegmüller D, Moroni C, Karin M, Chen CY (2004) A KH domain RNA binding protein, KSRP, promotes ARE-directed mRNA turnover by recruiting the degradation machinery. Mol Cell 14:571–583
25. Norton JT, Pollock CB, Wang C, Schink JC, Kim JJ, Huang S (2008) Perinucleolar compartment prevalence is a phenotypic pan-cancer marker of malignancy. Cancer 113:861–869
26. Kamath RV, Thor AD, Wang C, Edgerton SM, Slusarczyk A, Leary DJ et al (2005) Perinucleolar compartment prevalence has an independent prognostic value for breast cancer. Cancer Res 65(1):246–253
27. Kaighn ME, Lechner JF, Narayan KS, Jones LW (1978) Prostate carcinoma: tissue culture cell lines. Natl Cancer Inst Monogr 49:17–21
28. Kozlowski JM, Fidler IJ, Campbell D, Xu ZL, Kaighn ME, Hart IR (1984) Metastatic behavior of human tumor cell lines grown in the nude mouse. Cancer Res 44:3522–3529
29. Pettaway CA, Pathak S, Greene G, Ramirez E, Wilson MR, Killion JJ et al (1996) Selection of highly metastatic variants of different human prostatic carcinomas using orthotopic implantation in nude mice. Clin Cancer Res 2:1627–1636
30. Oh JE, Karlmark KR, Shin JH, Pollak A, Freilinger A, Hengstschlager M et al (2005) Differentiation of neuroblastoma cell line N1E − 115 involves several signaling cascades. Neurochem Res 30(3):333–348

31. Strickland S, Smith KK, Marotti KR (1980) Hormonal induction of differentiation in teratocarcinoma stem cells: generation of parietal endoderm by retinoic acid and dibutyryl cAMP. Cell 21(2):347–355
32. Slusarczyk A, Kamath R, Wang C, Anchel D, Pollock C, Lewandowska MA, Fitzpatrick T, Bazett-Jones DP, Huang S (2010) Structure and Function of the Perinucleolar Compartment in Cancer Cells. Cold Spring Harb Symp Quant Biol 75:599–605 Epub 2011
33. McCutcheon IE, Hentschel SJ, Fuller GN, Jin W, Cote GJ (2004) Expression of the splicing regulator polypyrimidine tract-binding protein in normal and neoplastic brain. Neuro Oncol 6(1):9–14
34. He X, Pool M, Darcy KM, Lim SB, Auersperg N, Coon JS, Beck WT (2007) Knockdown of polypyrimidine tract-binding protein suppresses ovarian tumor cell growth and invasiveness in vitro. Oncogene 26(34):4961–4968
35. Storck S, Shukla M, Dimitrov S, Bouvet P (2007) Functions of the histone chaperone nucleolin in diseases. Subcell Biochem 41:125–144
36. Samant RS, Seraj MJ, Saunders MM, Sakamaki TS, Shevde LA, Harms JF et al (2000) Analysis of mechanisms underlying BRMS1 suppression of metastasis. Clin Exp Metastasis 18(8):683–693
37. Liu Y, Norton JT, Witshi MA, Xu Q, Lou G, hen Wang C, Appella DH, Chen Z, Huang S (2011) Methoxyethlyamino-numonafide is an efficacious and minimally toxic amonafide derivative in murine models of human cancer. Neoplasia 13(5):453–460

Regulation of ARE-mRNA Stability by Cellular Signaling: Implications for Human Cancer

Christian Kroun Damgaard and Jens Lykke-Andersen

Abstract

During recent years, it has become clear that regulation of mRNA stability is an important event in the control of gene expression. The stability of a large class of mammalian mRNAs is regulated by AU-rich elements (AREs) located in the mRNA 3′ UTRs. mRNAs with AREs are inherently labile but as a response to different cellular cues they can become either stabilized, allowing expression of a given gene, or further destabilized to silence their expression. These tightly regulated mRNAs include many that encode growth factors, proto-oncogenes, cytokines, and cell cycle regulators. Failure to properly regulate their stability can therefore lead to uncontrolled expression of factors associated with cell proliferation and has been implicated in several human cancers. A number of transfactors that recognize AREs and regulate the translation and degradation of ARE-mRNAs have been identified. These transfactors are regulated by signal transduction pathways, which are often misregulated in cancers. This chapter focuses on the function of ARE-binding proteins with an emphasis on their regulation by signaling pathways and the implications for human cancer.

C. K. Damgaard
Department of Molecular Biology and Genetics, University of Aarhus, DK-8000, Aarhus C, Denmark

J. Lykke-Andersen (✉)
Division of Biological Sciences, University of California, San Diego, CA 92093, USA
e-mail: jlykkeandersen@ucsd.edu

J. Y. Wu (ed.), *RNA and Cancer*, Cancer Treatment and Research,
DOI: 10.1007/978-3-642-31659-3_7,

Keywords
mRNA stability · AU-rich element · MAP kinase pathway · TTP · BRF-1 · BRF-2 · KSRP · AUF1 · HuR · Cancer

Contents

1 Introduction

Gene expression in higher eukaryotes is a tightly regulated process, which ensures proper and timely expression of proteins, for example during development, throughout the cell cycle and as a response to cellular stimuli. Regulation of gene expression does not only occur during the transcriptional or post-transcriptional events that take place in the nucleus, but also in the cytoplasm at the level of mRNA translation and turnover. Many mammalian mRNAs that are highly regulated at the level of translation and turnover contain AU-rich elements (AREs) in their 3′ untranslated regions (3′ UTRs). AREs function as heterogeneous binding platforms for a number of cellular proteins, which in turn decide the fate of the given mRNA [1]. For example, a subset of AU-binding proteins (AUBPs) function to stabilize ARE-containing mRNAs, whereas others induce their rapid degradation [2]. ARE-mRNAs are normally unstable with half-lives in mammalian cells ranging from ≈15 min to a few hours, whereas stable mRNAs, generally show half-lives in the 12–24 h range. Since many ARE-containing mRNAs encode growth factors, proto-oncogenes, cytokines, and cell cycle regulators, misregulation of their decay has been associated with a number of human cancers [3–7]. Over the past few years, a large body of evidence has demonstrated an intimate link between cellular signaling and the activity of AUBPs, which ultimately affects ARE-mRNA decay rates. Here we discuss the function of AUBPs, their regulation by signaling pathways, and their misregulation in cancer.

2 AU-Rich Elements

Numerous reports have over the last 25 years provided evidence for the involvement of AREs in rapid turnover (recently reviewed in [2, 5, 7, 8]). AREs were first noted in cytokine mRNAs [9]. Several studies have since demonstrated that AREs from a variety of mRNAs confer instability to otherwise stable transcripts when fused to their 3′ UTRs (e.g. [10–19]). AREs usually span 50–150 nucleotides and are situated in the 3′ UTRs of many inherently unstable mRNAs. Although AREs remain poorly defined, a recent bioinformatics survey estimates that more than 8 % of the transcriptome contains AREs [20]. AREs have been grouped into three classes based on characteristic sequence and mRNA decay features [1]: Class I AREs that contain dispersed AUUUA pentamer-sequences coupled with one or more U-rich stretches, class II AREs that contain consecutive AUUUA sequences, and class III AREs that lack the AUUUA pentamer altogether, but require U-rich and possibly additional unknown sequences to exert their destabilizing function. However, the relevance of this classification remains unclear. For example, certain AUBPs promote decay of mRNAs containing any of the three classes of AREs [21]. Moreover, an AUUUA-sequence within a 3′ UTR is not sufficient to render its cognate transcript unstable [1]. In line with this, regions outside the core AUUUA sequences may greatly influence the rate of mRNA decay via diverse mechanisms [18, 22, 23]. Perhaps contributing to this complexity, RNA secondary structure has in a number of cases been implicated as an important determinant for ARE function [4, 24–28]. Moreover, although sharing common sequence features, different AREs found in various transcripts cannot necessarily substitute for each other in various mRNA and cellular contexts [29, 30]. AREs are most likely defined by the specific subset of AUBPs with which they associate, and their apparent complexity may, at least in part, be explained by differences in expression levels, sub-cellular localizations, and activities of AUBPs under various cellular conditions.

3 ARE-Binding Proteins

The regulation of mRNA by AREs is mediated through AUBPs, which in turn interface with the general translation and mRNA decay machineries (reviewed in [2, 7, 8]. While a number of AUBPs have been identified, the mechanisms by which they regulate ARE-mRNA decay and translation are poorly understood. However, some AUBPs have been shown to interact with mRNA decapping, deadenylation, and exonucleolytic activities to stimulate ARE-mRNA decay [31–35]. Other AUBPs stabilize or modulate translation of ARE-mRNAs [13, 36–47]. Thus, the stability and translatability of specific ARE-mRNAs appears to be modulated by multiple AUBPs. In addition, certain general mRNA decay factors have been reported to directly bind ARE-mRNAs to enhance their turnover [48, 49].

Although ARE-mRNAs are intrinsically short lived, their translation and decay rates can be tightly regulated in response to cellular stimuli. The mechanism by which individual ARE-mRNAs are regulated upon specific cellular cues remains poorly understood, but evidence for signal-dependent modulation of the levels, localizations or activities of specific AUBPs has been reported [34, 35, 43, 44, 50–67] and reviewed in [68]. The expression levels and activities of stabilizing or destabilizing AUBPs are regulated according to cell type, differentiation state, and a multitude of cellular stimuli, which along with the aforementioned diversity of AREs provides a combinatorial network that ultimately may determine the fate of specific ARE-containing mRNAs under given conditions. Adding to the complexity of this regulatory network of AREs/AUBPs is the observation that many ARE-mRNAs also encompass microRNA (miRNA) binding sites, which also regulate target mRNA stability, and translation efficiency (reviewed in [69]). Recent evidence suggests that the regulatory roles of miRNAs and AUBPs may be interconnected and seem, at least in some cases, to influence the efficiency of one another [70–74].

Importantly, many ARE-mRNAs encode proteins, which, when deregulated, can contribute to transformation and tumorigenesis. In order to further the understanding of the molecular mechanisms underlying these forms of cancers, it will be important to delineate how AUBPs function in combination with each other in different cellular settings. The next section provides a brief overview of the functions of individual AUBPs.

3.1 TTP, BRF-1, and BRF-2

A well-established family of AUBPs includes the paralogs tristetraprolin (TTP; also called ZFP36 or TIS11A), butyrate responsive factor-1 (BRF-1; also called ZFP36L1, hsERF1 or TIS11B), and BRF-2 (also called ZFP36L2, hsERF2 or TIS11D). The rodent TTP-family also includes a member ZFP36L3, which appears to be exclusively expressed in placental tissue [75]. Historically, the prototypic member of this protein family, TTP, was identified as the product of an immediate early response gene to stimuli such as insulin and other growth factors [76–80] and reviewed in [5, 7, 81]. Several lines of evidence suggest that TTP and BRF-proteins stimulate ARE-mRNA decay. For example, overexpression of TTP, BRF-1, or BRF-2 in cell lines enhances the degradation of a number of tested ARE-containing mRNAs [33, 82–86], whereas expression of dominant negative forms of TTP, RNA interference (RNAi)-mediated depletion, or knock-out of TTP and BRF-proteins results in stabilization of subsets of ARE-mRNAs [33, 87–90]. TTP and BRF-proteins bind AREs through two tandem CCCH-type zinc-finger domains. Flanking the zinc-finger domains are N- and C-terminal activation domains that both serve to activate mRNA decay [33]. These may, at least in part, act by serving as scaffolds for recruitment of decay factors including those involved in decapping, deadenylation, and exonucleolytic decay [33, 91], and recent evidence suggests that this function can be regulated by phosphorylation

[34, 35]. Moreover, TTP and BRF-1 are able to nucleate large complexes of decay factors on ARE-containing mRNAs to form cytoplasmic mRNP granules termed processing bodies (PBs) [92].

Further functional implications have come from the phenotype of TTP and BRF-1/BRF-2 knockout mice. Whereas BRF-1 and BRF–2 are essential for development [93–95], TTP knockout mice are seemingly normal, but suffer from severe inflammation (e.g., arthritis, dermatitis and cachexia) [96]. This phenotype correlates with abnormally high levels of ARE-mRNAs encoding GM-CSF and TNFα [97, 98]. In line with this, TTP, as well as BRF-1 and BRF–2 have been reported to bind TNFα- and GM-CSF-encoding ARE-mRNAs in vitro and to promote their deadenylation and degradation in tissue culture cells [33, 83, 97–99]. TTP has also been implicated in regulating the decay of its own mRNA [100], as well as mRNAs encoding, BRF-1 and BRF-2 [20, 101], interleukin 2 (IL-2) [102], interleukin 10 (IL-10) [101], inducible nitric oxide synthase (iNOS) [103], cyclooxygenase 2 (COX-2) [104], and vascular endothelial growth factor (VEGF) [105]. Moreover, a global analysis screening for stabilized transcripts in mouse embryonic fibroblasts lacking TTP (TTP-/- MEFs), identified more than 250 mRNAs of which several were identified as bona fide TTP-targets [90]. Another microarray-based analysis identified more than 100 mRNAs specifically associated with TTP in macrophages [101]. Consistent with prevalent sequence elements within many of these target mRNAs, in vitro RNA-binding studies have revealed that TTP favors iterative AUUUA sequences and that UUAUUUAUU can function as a minimum high-affinity binding sequence [106–110]. Interestingly, knockdown of TTP in macrophages does not stabilize all of its associated ARE-mRNAs, perhaps reflecting functional redundancy between TTP-family members [101].

3.2 KSRP

hnRNP K homology-type splicing regulatory protein (KSRP) was first identified as a component of a pre-mRNA splicing regulatory complex in neurons [111]. In agreement with a function in pre-mRNA splicing, KSRP is predominantly nuclear in both neuronal and epithelial cells [112]. However, more recently KSRP has been implicated also as an activator of ARE-mRNA decay [31, 32, 113, 114], as well as a regulator of miRNA biogenesis [115]. Global analyses to identify mRNAs associated with KSRP and stabilized upon siRNA-mediated knockdown of KSRP revealed a group of approximately 100 mRNAs, of which a large subset encode inflammatory regulators [116].

KSRP contains four hnRNP K homology (KH) domains, surrounded by N- and C-terminal domains. Functionally, the central KH-spanning region (KH domains 1–4) is sufficient to promote ARE-mRNA decay [21, 32], whereas KH domains 3 and 4 can act independently as ARE-binding moieties [117]. Consistent with a role in stimulating ARE-mRNA decay, KSRP associates with a wide range of mRNA decay factors, including factors involved in decapping, deadenylation, and exonucleolytic decay, via both the central four KH domains and the C-terminal domain [21, 31, 32]. In addition, recent evidence suggests that KSRP promotes endoribonucleolytic cleavage to initiate parathyroid hormone (PTH) mRNA decay, and that this is mediated by KSRP-dependent recruitment of the endoribonuclease PMR1 [118]. Interestingly, KSRP activity is regulated by an interaction with Pin1 (a prolyl isomerase), which leads to dephosphorylation and activation of KSRP [119]. It remains to be investigated whether KSRP functions to destabilize ARE-mRNAs in the nucleus, where it is primarily localized, or via relocalization to the cytoplasmic compartment.

3.3 AUF1/hnRNP D

ARE/poly (U)-binding/degradation factor 1 (AUF1; also known as hnRNP D) was first identified as a cytoplasmic fraction of K562 cells able to activate ARE-mRNA decay [120]. Subsequent cloning revealed that four AUF1 isoforms exist, p37, p40, p42, and p45, which are produced by translation of a single alternatively spliced pre-mRNA [121]. All four isoforms contain two classical RNA recognition motifs (RRMs), which are both necessary for high-affinity ARE-binding but apparently not sufficient, since flanking sequences also seem important [122]. In vitro binding studies suggest that p37 displays the highest binding affinity for various ARE-mRNAs, followed by p42, p45, and p40 [12, 121, 122]. Unlike the well-documented mRNA-destabilizing effects of the TTP/BRF-protein family and KSRP, AUF1 isoforms seem to exert either destabilizing or stabilizing effects on ARE-mRNAs, in an isoform- and cell type-specific manner [19, 26, 123–128]. Consistent with a destabilizing function, AUF1 knockout mice show symptoms of severe endotoxic shock, including vascular hemorrhage and intravascular coagulation, which correlates with overproduction of TNFα and IL-1β, both of which are encoded by ARE-mRNAs [129]. Early studies suggested that the degree to which different AUF1 isoforms are able to stabilize or destabilize ARE-mRNAs correlates with their RNA-binding affinity (p37 > p42 > p45 > p40) [53, 123, 125, 130]. However, a recent study, which identified a signature AU-rich RNA-binding motif for AUF1, suggests that a robust AUF1-mRNA interaction does not necessarily promote mRNA destabilization [131]. This is in agreement with evidence suggesting that AUF1, in addition to a role in mRNA decay, also regulates the translation efficiency of target mRNAs [38, 132]. Consistent with an important function in regulating translation, AUF1 has been shown to co-purify with eukaryotic translation initiation factor 4G (eIF4G) and the cytoplasmic poly(A) binding protein PABPC1 [14], but it remains to be determined whether AUF1 modulates mRNA degradation or translation through these interactions [133].

Although all four isoforms are mainly nuclear in most tested cell lines, the subcellular localization of the individual isoforms differs according to the investigated cell type and the nature of cellular stimuli [14, 53, 123, 130, 134]. Several studies have provided evidence that AUF1 activity is regulated by signaling, and that AUF1 activity often correlates with its cellular localization. For example, AUF1 becomes sequestered in the nuclear and perinuclear compartments of the cell upon heat shock, which correlates with ARE-mRNA stabilization [14, 135]. Furthermore, the p37 isoform of AUF1 was observed to become sequestered in the cytoplasm of chinese hamster ovary (CHO) cells upon binding to a specific phosphoserine-binding 14-3-3 protein, 14-3-3σ, which in turn correlates with activation of ARE-mRNA decay [53]. Moreover, LPS-stimulated induction of melanoma cell IL-10, which is encoded by an ARE-mRNA, is associated with low cytoplasmic AUF1 levels [136], and is dependent on the AUF1 p40 isoform [126]. Phosphorylation of the p40 isoform has been reported in macrophages and in vitro through protein kinase A (PKA) and glycogen synthase kinase 3 (GSK3), which in turn modulates its ARE-RNA-binding and mRNA decay-activating capacity [137, 138]. The cellular level of AUF1, and the stability and translation efficiency of select ARE-mRNAs, is also regulated by MAPK/MK2-dependent Hsp27 phosphorylation, which in turn promotes proteasomal degradation of AUF1 [139, 140].

3.4 HuR

Another class of AUBPs that regulates ARE-mRNA decay is the Hu-family of RNA-binding proteins [141–143]. Expression of two of the Hu proteins, HuB and HuC, is restricted to neurons, whereas HuD is expressed in neurons, testes, and ovaries [144–148]. Expression of these Hu proteins can be observed in both nuclear and cytoplasmic compartments in cells of neuronal origin, and have been implicated in neurite outgrowth [147, 149]. In contrast, HuR (also referred to as HuA) is ubiquitously expressed and predominantly localized to the nucleus [143, 150, 151]. Each of the Hu proteins contains three classical RRMs important for high-affinity binding to ARE-sequences [143, 152–156]. Several lines of evidence suggest that HuR stabilizes target ARE-mRNAs [13, 15, 39, 40, 43, 44, 55, 157–172]. For example, various ARE-mRNAs have been observed to be destabilized upon antisense- or RNAi-mediated depletion of HuR and/or stabilized upon HuR overexpression. The mechanism by which HuR stabilizes target mRNAs is unclear. However, there is evidence that HuR, at least on some mRNAs, may displace destabilizing AUBPs or translational repressors from target mRNAs [168]. Interestingly, early evidence suggested that HuR may stabilize some ARE-mRNAs at a step after deadenylation [15].

HuR has been shown not only to stabilize its target ARE-mRNAs, but also to regulate their translation. For example, HuR has been reported to stimulate the translation of p53, ProTα, MKP1, and HIF-1α mRNA in UV-irradiated cells [40, 173], to stabilize and increase translation of the mitogen-activated protein (MAP) kinase phosphatase 1 (MKP-1) mRNA in H_2O_2 treated cells [168] and to repress translation of c-Myc mRNA in competition with AUF1 [38]. HuR also regulates mRNA translation in a more indirect fashion by stabilizing eIF4E mRNA in competition with AUF1 through mutually exclusive binding to an AU-rich element in the 3' UTR [174].

Although HuR localizes mainly to the nucleus, it is thought to exert its mRNA-stabilizing role in the cytoplasm [175, 176]. Hence, it contains an HuR nucleo-cytoplasmic shuttling sequence (HNS), situated in the hinge region between the second and the third RRM, that enables the protein to shuttle between the nuclear and cytoplasmic compartments [177]. Importin-α and transportin-1 and -2 import receptors have all been proposed to mediate nuclear import of HuR [59, 178, 179]. The shuttling function of HuR seems important for nuclear export of at least some ARE-mRNAs [180, 181]. Accordingly, re-localization of HuR to the cytoplasmic compartment has been suggested as an important mechanism by which HuR controls ARE-mRNA decay [15, 59, 141, 175, 176, 182]. Supporting this notion is the finding that increased cytoplasmic localization of HuR, induced by either exposure to UV-light, heat shock, nutrient starvation, or expression of a dominant negative mutant AMP-activated protein kinase (AMPK), correlates with increased ARE-mRNA stability [15, 43, 44, 59, 182–185]. The factors that control the cytoplasmic localization of HuR remain obscure, but two HuR interaction partners pp32 and APRIL, have been proposed to modulate HuR shuttling [141, 180]. HuR activity, and in some cases also its subcellular localization, is regulated by several cellular signaling pathways, including the mitogen-activated protein kinase (MAPK) [55, 60], AMPK [43, 59], protein kinase C (PKC) pathways [52, 56], as well as by the cell cycle checkpoint kinase 1/2 (Chk1/2) pathway [50]; recently reviewed in [175, 176]. Moreover, HuR may also be regulated via methylation by coactivator-associated arginine methyltransferase 1 (CARM1), which correlates with increased stability of TNFα mRNA [186].

3.5 TIA-1 and TIAR

T cell-restricted intracellular antigen-1 (TIA-1) and TIA-1-related protein (TIAR; also called TIAL1) were first characterized as regulators of apoptosis, since they both induce DNA-fragmentation when added to permeabilized thymocytes [187, 188]. A function in regulating pre-mRNA splicing has also been attributed to these proteins [189–191]. TIA-1 and TIAR both contain three N-terminal RRMs and a C-terminal prion-like glutamine-rich motif [187, 188], consistent with its ability to promote the formation of mRNP granules called stress granules (SGs) [192]. Initially, TIA-proteins were shown to bind uridine-rich sequences and AREs of TNFα, GM-CSF, and COX-2 mRNAs [42, 193–195]. More recently, an immunoprecipitation/microarray approach identified more than 180 potential TIA-1 target mRNAs under heat shock conditions, many of which contain AREs [39]. Several lines of evidence suggest that TIA-1 and TIAR repress translation during various stress conditions without activating mRNA decay [36–39, 41, 42, 194]. For example, TIA-$1^{-/-}$ mouse embryonic fibroblasts (MEFs), display an increased concentration of TNFα and COX-2 proteins, but no change in their mRNA levels [42, 194]. Recent evidence challenges this notion by suggesting that the translational silencing exerted by TIA-1 may, at least in some cases, render certain mRNAs prone to increased turnover by exposing these to the general decay machinery [196]. Arguing for an important function in regulating translation, numerous reports have provided evidence that TIA-1 and TIAR are key components of SGs, where translationally repressed mRNAs accumulate during stress (reviewed by [197–199]). Under such conditions, bulk translation initiation is inhibited, in many cases by phosphorylation of eIF2α, which in turn efficiently inhibits formation of the ternary eIF2-GTP-tRNA^{iMet} complex [200–205]. As a result, mRNAs stalled at a step in translation initiation are sequestered by TIA-1 and TIAR-proteins into SGs [206]. The glutamine-rich domain of TIA-1 plays an important role in this aggregation, since cells expressing a mutant lacking this domain are refractory to SG assembly [192]. Global proteomics analyses have identified five phosphorylation sites within each of TIA-1 and TIAR, but the involved kinase(s) and the functional consequences have not been identified [207, 208].

3.6 Other ARE-Binding Proteins

Other proteins that have been reported to bind AREs, include CUG-BP, RHAU, GAPDH, NF90/NFAR1, hnRNP-A1, -A2, -A3, -C1, Nucleolin, TINO, and PAIP2 [209] and references therein. Some of these factors have been proposed to play a role in mRNA turnover but none of them have been studied in detail and only a few will be mentioned here.

A recently described DExH-box helicase, named RHAU (for RNA helicase associated with AU-rich element), was found to bind and destabilize a reporter mRNA containing the core ARE from an mRNA encoding urokinase plasminogen activator (uPA) [210]. Even though recombinant RHAU activates ARE-reporter decay in vitro, it does not display significant binding affinity for its mRNA target, suggesting that the protein may be recruited to the RNA via interaction partners [210]. However, recent evidence has shown that RHAU can interact with mRNA through its N-terminal domain, which is also necessary for recruitment of the protein to SGs [211]. Consistent with a model in which RHAU recruits the general mRNA decay machinery, RHAU co-purifies with components of the 3′ to 5′ exonucleolytic exosome complex [210].

CUG-BP-1 was first identified by its ability to bind CUG-sequences in the 3′ UTR of the DMPK mRNA [212, 213]. However, subsequent studies also revealed high affinity for both UG-rich and ARE sequences [40, 214, 215]. CUG-BP-1, and its paralog CUG-BP-2, has been found to regulate alternative pre-mRNA splicing [216, 217] and translation of various transcripts [218–220]. In one study, upregulation of CUG-BP-2 induced by irradiation of epithelial cells, correlated with ARE-dependent stabilization and translational inhibition of COX-2 mRNA [218]. Another study proposed a role for CUG-BP-1 in regulating deadenylation of ARE-mRNAs, through an interaction with the deadenylase PARN [22]. Since CUG-BP is the human homolog of the *Xenopus* protein EDEN-BP, which regulates translation of maternally deposited mRNAs in oocytes during development by controlling poly(A)-tail length, (reviewed in [221]), an interesting goal for future studies will be to test whether the ability of CUG-BP to repress translation is a consequence of its ability to activate mRNA deadenylation. More recent global analyses have identified multiple mRNAs that contain GU-rich elements and are targeted for mRNA degradation by CUG-BP1.

4 Signal Transduction Pathways Regulating ARE-mRNA Decay

During recent years it has become increasingly clear that the stability of many ARE-mRNAs is regulated by various signaling cascades, which are controlled by changes in extra- and intra-cellular environments. Cellular signaling pathways that impact ARE-mRNA decay include the MAPK [55, 57, 113, 222, 223], phosphatidylinositol 3-kinase (PI3-K)/Akt/protein kinase B (PKB)[224, 225], AMPK [182, 226], PKC [227–229], and Wnt/β-catenin pathways [230]. The next section deals with some of these signal transduction pathways and what is known about their impact on ARE-mRNA decay.

4.1 MAPK Pathways

The MAPK pathways and their role in regulating ARE-mRNA decay is by far the most studied. Activation of MAPK pathways involves receptor-mediated stimulation of a phosphorylation cascade involving MAP kinase kinase kinases (MAP3Ks), which activate MAP2Ks that in turn activate one or more MAPKs. In mammals, MAPKs have been divided into six distinct groups: (1) p38 (2) ERK1/2, (3) ERK3/4, (4) ERK5, (5) ERK7/8, and (6) JNK 1/2/3 (reviewed in [231]). Whereas the JNK and p38 pathways mainly are activated by pro-inflammatory stress signals, the ERK pathways are stimulated by growth factors and other mitogens [232].

4.1.1 p38

A number of studies have implicated the p38 MAPK pathway in the regulation of decay and translation of ARE-mRNAs [34, 35, 60, 65, 100, 113, 116, 233–246]; reviewed in [247]. Four different isoforms of p38 have been identified (α, β, γ and δ) of which the α, and β isoforms are ubiquitously expressed. p38 MAPKs are activated by several agents including cytokines, lipopolysaccharide (LPS), various hormones, or stress such as UV-irradiation, energy deprivation, osmotic stress, and heat shock (reviewed in [231, 248]). Early studies showed that inhibition of p38 in various cell types using pyridinyl imidazole agents leads to destabilization of several ARE-mRNAs [223, 238–240]. More recently, a study using transcriptional shut-off followed by microarray assays to calculate ARE-mRNA half-lives in the presence or absence of p38 inhibitors, identified 45 ARE-mRNAs that become markedly destabilized upon inhibition of p38 [242]. By contrast, when the p38 pathway is activated by overexpresssion of constitutive active mutants of the p38 MAP2Ks, MEK3, and MEK6, several tested ARE-mRNAs become stabilized e.g. [113, 243–246, 249, 250]. Moreover, studies using spleen cells and embryonic fibroblasts from mice knocked out for MAPKAP kinase 2 (MK2), which functions downstream of p38 [251], implicate MK2 in the regulation of both translation and decay of TNFα- and IL-6 mRNAs, both of which contain AREs [237, 243, 245]. Thus, it appears that the p38 MAPK pathway plays a generally stabilizing role in ARE-mRNA decay.

How does the p38 MAPK pathway cause ARE-mRNA stabilization? The AUBP, TTP has been identified as a phosphorylation target for both p38 and MK2 [60, 250, 252–254]. Phosphorylation of TTP occurs at multiple serine-residues with Ser52 and Ser178 reported as major MK2 sites [250, 253, 255]. Phosphorylation of these two residues enables binding of phophoserine-binding 14-3-3 proteins, which appear to impair the ARE-mRNA-destabilizing function of TTP [250, 253, 256]. The molecular mechanism underlying TTP inactivation by phosphorylation and association with 14-3-3 remains poorly understood. Evidence indicates that the sub-cellular localization of TTP may be modulated by phosphorylation and that 14-3-3 may act to protect TTP from active dephosphorylation by protein phosphatase 2A (PP2A) [57, 250, 256, 257]. The effect of phosphorylation of TTP on its ARE-binding activity remains controversial, e.g. [34, 35, 57, 236, 245, 252, 254], but recent evidence suggest that the ability of TTP to recruit members of the deadenylation machinery to ARE-mRNA becomes impaired upon phosphorylation by MK2 [34, 35].

p38 has also been shown to regulate the activity of KSRP [113]. Forced differentiation of myoblast cells, by expression of a constitutively active MKK6 protein (a MAP3 K acting upstream of p38), correlates with specific stabilization of ARE-containing myogenic mRNAs encoding myogenin and $p21^{CIP1/WAF}$ [113]. UV-crosslinking and in vitro mRNA decay assays identified KSRP as the AUBP conferring instability to the myogenic transcripts in uninduced cells. The mechanism underlying the differentiation-induced stabilization of myogenic transcripts involves direct phosphorylation of KSRP by the p38 MAPK during induced differentiation, which in turn inhibits the ARE-binding and decay activating ability of KSRP, although it is still able to interact with the general decay machinery [113].

HuR has been shown to function in concert with p38 and MK2 to stabilize a number of ARE-mRNAs. Early evidence suggests that expression of a constitutively active MK2 protein or treatment of cells with stimuli known to activate the p38 signaling pathway (e.g. TNFα or oxidative stress) increases the cytoplasmic accumulation of HuR by an unknown mechanism [51, 58]. More recently, in gamma irradiated cells, p38 was shown to directly phosphorylate HuR at Thr118 increasing the cytoplasmic localization of HuR and its interaction with the ARE-mRNA encoding cyclin-dependent kinase inhibitor $p21^{CIP1/WAF}$ [166]. This allows for rapid upregulation of $p21^{CIP1/WAF}$, which in turn leads to G(1)/S cell cycle arrest [166]. Thus, translocation of nuclear HuR to the cytoplasm through p38-mediated phosphorylation is likely a general phenomenon leading to increased HuR mRNA target stability and enhanced translation. HuR also regulates the activity of MAPK pathways by increasing stability and translation of the ARE-mRNA encoding MAP kinase phosphatase 1 (MKP-1) during stress, which plays an important role in dephosphorylation of ERK, JNK, and p38 [168].

4.1.2 JNK

The JNK pathway is related to the p38-signaling pathway in that both are stimulated by stress signals such as UV-light exposure, heat shock, oxidative, and osmotic stress along with pro-inflammatory cytokines IL-1 and TNFα (reviewed in [231]). Accordingly, in some cells the major MAP2Ks acting upstream of JNK, MEK4, and MEK7, also activate the p38 pathway. The JNK pathway has been demonstrated to regulate the decay of several ARE-mRNAs, including those encoding IL-3 [258], IL-2 [222, 259], VEGF [260], and iNOS [261]. However, it remains unclear in these cases if AUBPs are directly regulated by JNK pathway phosphorylation. IL-2 contains an ARE-sequence in its 3′ UTR, which is required for the intrinsic IL-2 mRNA instability [222, 259]. However, JNK-mediated stabilization of IL-2 mRNA upon T cell activation also requires a CU-rich element in the IL-2 mRNA 5′ UTR, which specifically interacts with two proteins: nucleolin and Y-box binding protein 1 (YB-1) [259]. The specific mechanism by which JNK regulates the factors that associates with the IL-2 mRNA remains unknown.

4.1.3 ERK

ERK signaling is mainly governed by mitogens and growth factors and is deregulated in approximately one-third of all human cancers (reviewed in [232]). ERK has in a number of studies been implicated in the regulation of ARE-mRNA decay [61, 96, 105, 262–267]. For example, activation of ERK signaling results in stabilization of GM-CSF ARE-mRNA in eosinophils [262, 263]. This stabilization correlates with increased phosphorylation of AUF1 and a concomitant reduction in the association of AUF1 with GM-CSF mRNA [265]. Furthermore, conformational changes in AUF1 exerted through isomerization of specific prolyl residues, which is catalyzed by peptidyl-prolyl isomerase 1 (Pin1), has been suggested to regulate the ability of AUF1 to interact with the decay machinery leading to stabilization of GM-CSF mRNA upon activation of ERKs [265]. Whether ERKs directly phosphorylate AUF1 isoforms remains to be tested.

TTP becomes phophorylated upon activation of ERK signaling in mouse fibroblasts via stimulation by various growth factors [268]. Although the effect of this event on TTP-mediated ARE-mRNA decay remains to be established, the phosphorylation may be mediated by ERK2 since it can phosphorylate recombinant TTP at serine 220 in vitro [268]. These findings are consistent with a recent study suggesting that ERK signaling in a macrophage cell line acts synergistically with p38 MAPK to promote TTP phosphorylation, which in turn regulates the subcellular localization and stability of TTP [257]. In line with this, a recent study demonstrated that an ERK-dependent stabilization of VEGF mRNA requires deactivation of TTP, possibly due to its phosphorylation [105].

Another study suggested that ERK signaling in a lung carcinoma cell line promotes stabilization of $p21^{CIP1/WAF}$ ARE-mRNA, which correlates with increased cytoplasmic localization of HuR [61]. While ERK activation stimulated the association of HuR with the $p21^{CIP1/WAF}$ mRNA, the cytoplasmic re-localization of HuR seems independent of ERK function [61]. Aside from the phosphorylation of TTP in vitro, potential AUBP targets of ERKs remain to be identified.

4.2 PI3K/Akt-PKB

Akt, also known as protein kinase B (PKB), has been implicated in tumorigenesis in numerous cases (reviewed in [269]). The three Akt family members, Akt1/PKBα, Akt2/PKBβ, and Akt3/PKBγ are activated by stimuli such as insulin and other growth factors (reviewed in [270–272]). Specifically, Akt is activated by binding of specific phosphoinositides (PtdIns) produced by phophatidylinositol 3-kinase (PI3K), which induces a conformational change in Akt allowing for phosphorylation of residues in its activation loop [273]. The involvement of Akt in regulating ARE-mRNA decay has been demonstrated in recent studies [225, 274–276]. One study found that serine 92 in BRF-1 is a target for phosphorylation by Akt in vitro and that stimulation of Akt signaling in rat fibroblasts leads to BRF-1 phosphorylation at the same residue, which in turn inhibits the ARE-mRNA-destabilizing activity of BRF-1 [225]. Similar to TTP and AUF1, phosphorylation of BRF-1 leads to binding by 14-3-3 proteins, which reportedly does not affect the ability of BRF-1 to interact with target ARE-mRNAs [225].

The activity of KSRP is also regulated by Akt signaling [274, 275]. Specifically, upon treatment of cells with insulin or overexpression of an activated form of Akt1, β-catenin ARE-mRNA becomes stabilized through phosphorylation of KSRP [274]. Phosphorylation of Ser193 in KSRP results in 14-3-3 binding and impairs the ability of KSRP to recruit the exosome, whereas an interaction with the deadenylase PARN remains intact [274]. In an attempt to identify mRNA targets that are upregulated upon activation of Akt through a KSRP-specific mechanism, a recent report combined KSRP affinity purification of mRNAs with a microarray assay to screen for binding of ARE-mRNAs [275]. Comparing the KSRP-interacting mRNAs with the mRNAs found upregulated upon activation of Akt1, allowed the identification of seven highly stabilized mRNAs including those encoding hnRNP A1, -A/B, -F, and PP2A [275]. Interestingly, PP2A has been implicated in the dephosphorylation of TTP to promote its mRNA decay activating ability [57]. It is therefore tempting to speculate that KSRP-mediated stabilization of PP2A mRNA upon stimulation of Akt signaling, represents an auto-regulatory loop in which upregulation of PP2A activates dephosphorylation of AUBPs in general, to reactivate ARE-mRNA decay.

5 Perspective: Implications for Cancer

Failure to regulate ARE-mRNA turnover has been linked to malignant transformation in a number of cases (reviewed in [3, 5, 7, 277]. Many proto-oncogenes and tumor suppressor genes encode ARE-mRNAs and mis-regulation of their decay can lead to tumorigenesis by creating an imbalance between growth promoting and growth inhibiting factors. Deregulation of MAPK and Akt signaling has been observed in association with a number of malignancies (reviewed in [232, 278]). For example, the ERK pathway is reportedly deregulated in more than 30 % of all human cancers [232]. Since these signaling pathways alter the activity of AUBPs, that either promote or inhibit decay of ARE-mRNAs directly implicated in tumorigenesis, AUBP levels and/or activities may be nodal points at which the potential for transformation and tumorigenesis is decided. For example, the observation that transgenic mice that overexpress the p37 isoform of AUF1 develop sarcomas provides a correlation between deregulation of AUBPs and cancer [279].

Examples of ARE-mRNAs that are deregulated in cancers include those encoding regulators of cell proliferation (e.g. the proto-oncogenes c-fos, c-jun or c-myc, and the growth factor GM-CSF), regulators of the cell cycle (e.g. cyclins A, -B, -D, -E, p53, or $p21^{CIP1/WAF}$), regulators of angiogenesis and extracellular matrix degradation (e.g. VEGF, uPA, uPAR, and MMP13), and regulators of apoptosis (e.g. Bcl-2, Mcl-1, COX-2, SIRT-1, p53, or $p21^{CIP1/WAF}$) [3, 5, 277, 280]. Many of these ARE-mRNAs are regulated by HuR, TTP, and BRF-proteins, each of which have been found to be deregulated in a number of cancers [277, 281–284].

An emerging notion is that mRNA-destabilizing AUBPs (e.g., the TTP family) are important for maintaining low levels of growth promoting factors, in order to prevent oncogenesis. For example, TTP protein expression was recently reported to be virtually lost in a number of human cancer cell lines and tumor tissues (e.g., colon, breast, cervix, lung, and prostate), when compared to normal tissue [282–284] and low TTP expression is associated with bad prognosis in breast cancer [282]. In line with this, global gene expression profiling has revealed a significant increase in the steady-state levels of ARE-mRNAs encoding cancer-promoting factors when comparing normal and tumor tissue [285]. Could TTP-family proteins function as bona fide tumor suppressors? A recent study tested this question by intratumoral injections of recombinant BRF-1 protein fused to a cell-penetrating peptide [286]. This treatment significantly reduced tumor growth, which correlated with diminished levels of several angiogenic cytokines, including VEGF, IL-1α, and IL-6 [286]. Taken together, these results suggest that there is a correlation between the general level of ARE-mRNAs and their potential in promoting oncogenesis. However, this view is likely too simplistic, due to the fact that not all ARE-mRNAs encode oncogenic proteins. For example, the prototypic tumor suppressor, p53, is encoded by an ARE-mRNA and is downregulated or otherwise impaired in an estimated 50 % of all cancers [287]. The posttranscriptional regulation of p53 is highly complex and involves numerous mechanisms aside from ARE-mRNA decay and translational regulation (reviewed in [288]). Another example of an ARE-mRNA that is reportedly downregulated in cancer, includes the $p21^{CIP1/WAF}$mRNA, which function as a tumor suppressor by promoting G(1)/S cell cycle arrest [289]. Interestingly, both p53 and $p21^{CIP1/WAF}$ are regulated by HuR-mediated stabilization and enhancement of translation [40, 166, 172].

Taken together, it is conceivable that many of the oncogenic mutations reported in components of MAPK and Akt pathways represent a major mechanism by which the level or activity of AUBPs are modulated, which eventually may lead to tumorigenesis. Although deregulation of a number of factors encoded by ARE-mRNAs are implicated in transformation and cancer, many aspects of these processes remain unresolved. Future studies will undoubtedly add numerous factors encoded by ARE-mRNAs to the already long list of proteins implicated in cancer and further our understanding of how these are regulated. This process will be of importance in the development of novel regimens to treat various cancers.

References

1. Chen CY, Shyu AB (1995) AU-rich elements: characterization and importance in mRNA degradation. Trends Biochem Sci 20:465–470
2. Garneau NL, Wilusz J, Wilusz CJ (2007) The highways and byways of mRNA decay. Nat Rev Mol Cell Biol 8:113–126
3. Audic Y, Hartley RS (2004) Post-transcriptional regulation in cancer. Biol Cell 96:479–498
4. Bevilacqua A, Ceriani MC, Capaccioli S, Nicolin A (2003) Post-transcriptional regulation of gene expression by degradation of messenger RNAs. J Cell Physiol 195:356–372
5. Eberhardt W, Doller A, el Akool S, Pfeilschifter J (2007) Modulation of mRNA stability as a novel therapeutic approach. Pharmacol Ther 114:56–73
6. Lopez de Silanes I, Quesada MP, Esteller M (2007) Aberrant regulation of messenger RNA 3'-untranslated region in human cancer. Cell Oncol 29:1–17
7. Sanduja S, Blanco FF, Dixon DA (2010) The roles of TTP and BRF proteins in regulated mRNA decay. WIREs RNA 2:42–57
8. Reznik B, Lykke-Andersen J (2010) Regulated and quality-control mRNA turnover pathways in eukaryotes. Biochem Soc Trans 38:1506–1510
9. Caput D, Beutler B, Hartog K, Thayer R, Brown-Shimer S, Cerami A (1986) Identification of a common nucleotide sequence in the 3'-untranslated region of mRNA molecules specifying inflammatory mediators. Proc Natl Acad Sci U S A 83:1670–1674
10. Chen CY, Chen TM, Shyu AB (1994) Interplay of two functionally and structurally distinct domains of the c-fos AU-rich element specifies its mRNA-destabilizing function. Mol Cell Biol 14:416–426
11. Chen CY, Xu N, Shyu AB (1995) mRNA decay mediated by two distinct AU-rich elements from c-fos and granulocyte-macrophage colony-stimulating factor transcripts: different deadenylation kinetics and uncoupling from translation. Mol Cell Biol 15:5777–5788
12. DeMaria CT, Brewer G (1996) AUF1 binding affinity to A + U-rich elements correlates with rapid mRNA degradation. J Biol Chem 271:12179–12184
13. Fan XC, Steitz JA (1998) Overexpression of HuR, a nuclear-cytoplasmic shuttling protein, increases the in vivo stability of ARE-containing mRNAs. EMBO J 17:3448–3460
14. Laroia G, Cuesta R, Brewer G, Schneider RJ (1999) Control of mRNA decay by heat shock-ubiquitin-proteasome pathway. Science 284:499–502
15. Peng SS, Chen CY, Xu N, Shyu AB (1998) RNA stabilization by the AU-rich element binding protein, HuR, an ELAV protein. EMBO J 17:3461–3470
16. Shaw G, Kamen R (1986) A conserved AU sequence from the 3' untranslated region of GM-CSF mRNA mediates selective mRNA degradation. Cell 46:659–667
17. Treisman R (1985) Transient accumulation of c-fos RNA following serum stimulation requires a conserved 5' element and c-fos 3' sequences. Cell 42:889–902
18. Xu N, Chen CY, Shyu AB (1997) Modulation of the fate of cytoplasmic mRNA by AU-rich elements: key sequence features controlling mRNA deadenylation and decay. Mol Cell Biol 17:4611–4621
19. Xu N, Chen CY, Shyu AB (2001) Versatile role for hnRNP D isoforms in the differential regulation of cytoplasmic mRNA turnover. Mol Cell Biol 21:6960–6971
20. Bakheet T, Williams BR, Khabar KS (2006) ARED 3.0: the large and diverse AU-rich transcriptome. Nucleic Acids Res 34:D111–D114
21. Gherzi R, Lee KY, Briata P et al (2004) A KH domain RNA binding protein, KSRP, promotes ARE-directed mRNA turnover by recruiting the degradation machinery. Mol Cell 14:571–583
22. Moraes KC, Wilusz CJ, Wilusz J (2006) CUG-BP binds to RNA substrates and recruits PARN deadenylase. RNA 12:1084–1091

23. Stoecklin G, Lu M, Rattenbacher B, Moroni C (2003) A constitutive decay element promotes tumor necrosis factor alpha mRNA degradation via an AU-rich element-independent pathway. Mol Cell Biol 23:3506–3515
24. Brown CY, Lagnado CA, Goodall GJ (1996) A cytokine mRNA-destabilizing element that is structurally and functionally distinct from A + U-rich elements. Proc Natl Acad Sci U S A 93:13721–13725
25. Claffey KP, Shih SC, Mullen A et al (1998) Identification of a human VPF/VEGF 3' untranslated region mediating hypoxia-induced mRNA stability. Mol Biol Cell 9:469–481
26. Paschoud S, Dogar AM, Kuntz C, Grisoni-Neupert B, Richman L, Kuhn LC (2006) Destabilization of interleukin-6 mRNA requires a putative RNA stem-loop structure, an AU-rich element, and the RNA-binding protein AUF1. Mol Cell Biol 26:8228–8241
27. Putland RA, Sassinis TA, Harvey JS et al (2002) RNA destabilization by the granulocyte colony-stimulating factor stem-loop destabilizing element involves a single stem-loop that promotes deadenylation. Mol Cell Biol 22:1664–1673
28. Wilson GM, Sutphen K, Moutafis M, Sinha S, Brewer G (2001) Structural remodeling of an A + U-rich RNA element by cation or AUF1 binding. J Biol Chem 276:38400–38409
29. Nair AP, Hahn S, Banholzer R, Hirsch HH, Moroni C (1994) Cyclosporin A inhibits growth of autocrine tumour cell lines by destabilizing interleukin-3 mRNA. Nature 369:239–242
30. Schuler GD, Cole MD (1988) GM-CSF and oncogene mRNA stabilities are independently regulated in trans in a mouse monocytic tumor. Cell 55:1115–1122
31. Chen CY, Gherzi R, Ong SE et al (2001) AU binding proteins recruit the exosome to degrade ARE-containing mRNAs. Cell 107:451–464
32. Chou CF, Mulky A, Maitra S et al (2006) Tethering KSRP, a decay-promoting AU-rich element-binding protein, to mRNAs elicits mRNA decay. Mol Cell Biol 26:3695–3706
33. Lykke-Andersen J, Wagner E (2005) Recruitment and activation of mRNA decay enzymes by two ARE-mediated decay activation domains in the proteins TTP and BRF-1. Genes Dev 19:351–361
34. Marchese FP, Aubareda A, Tudor C, Saklatvala J, Clark AR, Dean JL (2010) MAPKAP kinase 2 blocks tristetraprolin-directed mRNA decay by inhibiting CAF1 deadenylase recruitment. J Biol Chem 285:27590–27600
35. Clement SL, Scheckel C, Stoecklin G, Lykke-Andersen J (2011) Phosphorylation of tristetraprolin by MK2 impairs AU-rich element mRNA decay by preventing deadenylase recruitment. Mol Cell Biol 31:256–266
36. Kawai T, Lal A, Yang X, Galban S, Mazan-Mamczarz K, Gorospe M (2006) Translational control of cytochrome c by RNA-binding proteins TIA-1 and HuR. Mol Cell Biol 26:3295–3307
37. Lal A, Abdelmohsen K, Pullmann R et al (2006) Posttranscriptional derepression of GADD45alpha by genotoxic stress. Mol Cell 22:117–128
38. Liao B, Hu Y, Brewer G (2007) Competitive binding of AUF1 and TIAR to MYC mRNA controls its translation. Nat Struct Mol Biol 14:511–518
39. Lopez de Silanes I, Fan J, Galban CJ, Spencer RG, Becker KG, Gorospe M (2004) Global analysis of HuR-regulated gene expression in colon cancer systems of reducing complexity. Gene Expr 12:49–59
40. Mazan-Mamczarz K, Galban S (2003) Lopez de Silanes I, et al. RNA-binding protein HuR enhances p53 translation in response to ultraviolet light irradiation. Proc Natl Acad Sci U S A 100:8354–8359
41. Mazan-Mamczarz K, Lal A, Martindale JL, Kawai T, Gorospe M (2006) Translational repression by RNA-binding protein TIAR. Mol Cell Biol 26:2716–2727
42. Piecyk M, Wax S, Beck AR et al (2000) TIA-1 is a translational silencer that selectively regulates the expression of TNF-alpha. EMBO J 19:4154–4163
43. Wang W, Caldwell MC, Lin S, Furneaux H, Gorospe M (2000) HuR regulates cyclin A and cyclin B1 mRNA stability during cell proliferation. EMBO J 19:2340–2350
44. Wang W, Furneaux H, Cheng H et al (2000) HuR regulates p21 mRNA stabilization by UV light. Mol Cell Biol 20:760–769

45. Kuwano Y, Pullmann R Jr, Marasa BS et al (2010) NF90 selectively represses the translation of target mRNAs bearing an AU-rich signature motif. Nucleic Acids Res 38:225–238
46. Bergalet J, Fawal M, Lopez C et al (2011) HuR-Mediated Control of C/EBP{beta} mRNA Stability and Translation in ALK-Positive Anaplastic Large Cell Lymphomas. Mol Cancer Res 9:485–496
47. Ishimaru D, Ramalingam S, Sengupta TK et al (2009) Regulation of Bcl-2 expression by HuR in HL60 leukemia cells and A431 carcinoma cells. Mol Cancer Res 7:1354–1366
48. Anderson JR, Mukherjee D, Muthukumaraswamy K, Moraes KC, Wilusz CJ, Wilusz J (2006) Sequence-specific RNA binding mediated by the RNase PH domain of components of the exosome. RNA 12:1810–1816
49. Mukherjee D, Gao M, O'Connor JP et al (2002) The mammalian exosome mediates the efficient degradation of mRNAs that contain AU-rich elements. EMBO J 21:165–174
50. Abdelmohsen K, Pullmann R Jr, Lal A et al (2007) Phosphorylation of HuR by Chk2 regulates SIRT1 expression. Mol Cell 25:543–557
51. Atasoy U, Curry SL (2003) Lopez de Silanes I, et al. Regulation of eotaxin gene expression by TNF-alpha and IL-4 through mRNA stabilization: involvement of the RNA-binding protein HuR. J Immunol 171:4369–4378
52. Doller A, Huwiler A, Muller R, Radeke HH, Pfeilschifter J, Eberhardt W (2007) Protein Kinase C alpha-dependent phosphorylation of the mRNA-stabilizing factor HuR: implications for posttranscriptional regulation of cyclooxygenase-2. Mol Biol Cell 18:2137–2148
53. He C, Schneider R (2006) 14–3-3sigma is a p37 AUF1-binding protein that facilitates AUF1 transport and AU-rich mRNA decay. EMBO J 25:3823–3831
54. Lal A, Mazan-Mamczarz K, Kawai T, Yang X, Martindale JL, Gorospe M (2004) Concurrent versus individual binding of HuR and AUF1 to common labile target mRNAs. EMBO J 23:3092–3102
55. Ming XF, Stoecklin G, Lu M, Looser R, Moroni C (2001) Parallel and independent regulation of interleukin-3 mRNA turnover by phosphatidylinositol 3-kinase and p38 mitogen-activated protein kinase. Mol Cell Biol 21:5778–5789
56. Pascale A, Amadio M, Scapagnini G et al (2005) Neuronal ELAV proteins enhance mRNA stability by a PKCalpha-dependent pathway. Proc Natl Acad Sci U S A 102:12065–12070
57. Sun L, Stoecklin G, Van Way S et al (2007) Tristetraprolin (TTP)-14-3-3 complex formation protects TTP from dephosphorylation by protein phosphatase 2a and stabilizes tumor necrosis factor-alpha mRNA. J Biol Chem 282:3766–3777
58. Tran H, Maurer F, Nagamine Y (2003) Stabilization of urokinase and urokinase receptor mRNAs by HuR is linked to its cytoplasmic accumulation induced by activated mitogen-activated protein kinase-activated protein kinase 2. Mol Cell Biol 23:7177–7188
59. Wang W, Yang X, Kawai T et al (2004) AMP-activated protein kinase-regulated phosphorylation and acetylation of importin alpha1: involvement in the nuclear import of RNA-binding protein HuR. J Biol Chem 279:48376–48388
60. Winzen R, Kracht M, Ritter B et al (1999) The p38 MAP kinase pathway signals for cytokine-induced mRNA stabilization via MAP kinase-activated protein kinase 2 and an AU-rich region-targeted mechanism. EMBO J 18:4969–4980
61. Yang X, Wang W, Fan J et al (2004) Prostaglandin A2-mediated stabilization of p21 mRNA through an ERK-dependent pathway requiring the RNA-binding protein HuR. J Biol Chem 279:49298–49306
62. Qian X, Ning H, Zhang J, et al (2011) Posttranscriptional Regulation of IL-23 Expression by IFN-{gamma} through Tristetraprolin. J Immunol 186:6454–6464
63. Lee WH, Lee HH, Vo MT et al (2011) Casein kinase 2 regulates the mRNA-destabilizing activity of tristetraprolin. J Biol Chem 286:21577–21587
64. Schaljo B, Kratochvill F, Gratz N et al (2009) Tristetraprolin is required for full anti-inflammatory response of murine macrophages to IL-10. J Immunol 183:1197–1206
65. Tudor C, Marchese FP, Hitti E et al (2009) The p38 MAPK pathway inhibits tristetraprolin-directed decay of interleukin-10 and pro-inflammatory mediator mRNAs in murine macrophages. FEBS Lett 583:1933–1938

66. Suswam E, Li Y, Zhang X et al (2008) Tristetraprolin down-regulates interleukin-8 and vascular endothelial growth factor in malignant glioma cells. Cancer Res 68:674–682
67. Datta S, Biswas R, Novotny M et al (2008) Tristetraprolin regulates CXCL1 (KC) mRNA stability. J Immunol 180:2545–2552
68. Ronkina N, Menon MB, Schwermann J et al (2010) MAPKAP kinases MK2 and MK3 in inflammation: complex regulation of TNF biosynthesis via expression and phosphorylation of tristetraprolin. Biochem Pharmacol 80:1915–1920
69. Fabian MR, Sonenberg N, Filipowicz W (2010) Regulation of mRNA translation and stability by microRNAs. Annu Rev Biochem 79:351–379
70. Jing Q, Huang S, Guth S et al (2005) Involvement of microRNA in AU-rich element-mediated mRNA instability. Cell 120:623–634
71. Kim HH, Kuwano Y, Srikantan S, Lee EK, Martindale JL, Gorospe M (2009) HuR recruits let-7/RISC to repress c-Myc expression. Genes Dev 23:1743–1748
72. Jacobsen A, Wen J, Marks DS, Krogh A (2010) Signatures of RNA binding proteins globally coupled to effective microRNA target sites. Genome Res 20:1010–1019
73. Glorian V, Maillot G, Poles S, Iacovoni JS, Favre G, Vagner S (2011) HuR-dependent loading of miRNA RISC to the mRNA encoding the Ras-related small GTPase RhoB controls its translation during UV-induced apoptosis. Cell Death Differ 18:1692–1701
74. Leibovich L, Mandel-Gutfreund Y, Yakhini Z (2010) A structural-based statistical approach suggests a cooperative activity of PUM1 and miR-410 in human 3'-untranslated regions. Silence 1:17
75. Blackshear PJ, Phillips RS, Ghosh S, Ramos SB, Richfield EK, Lai WS (2005) Zfp36l3, a rodent X chromosome gene encoding a placenta-specific member of the Tristetraprolin family of CCCH tandem zinc finger proteins. Biol Reprod 73:297–307
76. Blackshear PJ (2002) Tristetraprolin and other CCCH tandem zinc-finger proteins in the regulation of mRNA turnover. Biochem Soc Trans 30:945–952
77. DuBois RN, McLane MW, Ryder K, Lau LF, Nathans D (1990) A growth factor-inducible nuclear protein with a novel cysteine/histidine repetitive sequence. J Biol Chem 265:19185–19191
78. Lai WS, Stumpo DJ, Blackshear PJ (1990) Rapid insulin-stimulated accumulation of an mRNA encoding a proline-rich protein. J Biol Chem 265:16556–16563
79. Ma Q, Herschman HR (1991) A corrected sequence for the predicted protein from the mitogen-inducible TIS11 primary response gene. Oncogene 6:1277–1278
80. Varnum BC, Lim RW, Kujubu DA et al (1989) Granulocyte-macrophage colony-stimulating factor and tetradecanoyl phorbol acetate induce a distinct, restricted subset of primary-response TIS genes in both proliferating and terminally differentiated myeloid cells. Mol Cell Biol 9:3580–3583
81. Baou M, Jewell A, Murphy JJ (2009) TIS11 family proteins and their roles in posttranscriptional gene regulation. J Biomed Biotechnol 2009:634520
82. Lai WS, Blackshear PJ (2001) Interactions of CCCH zinc finger proteins with mRNA: tristetraprolin-mediated AU-rich element-dependent mRNA degradation can occur in the absence of a poly(A) tail. J Biol Chem 276:23144–23154
83. Lai WS, Carballo E, Thorn JM, Kennington EA, Blackshear PJ (2000) Interactions of CCCH zinc finger proteins with mRNA. Binding of tristetraprolin-related zinc finger proteins to Au-rich elements and destabilization of mRNA. J Biol Chem 275: 17827–17837
84. Stoecklin G, Colombi M, Raineri I et al (2002) Functional cloning of BRF1, a regulator of ARE-dependent mRNA turnover. EMBO J 21:4709–4718
85. Lee HH, Vo MT, Kim HJ et al (2010) Stability of the LATS2 tumor suppressor gene is regulated by tristetraprolin. J Biol Chem 285:17329–17337
86. Lee HH, Son YJ, Lee WH et al (2010) Tristetraprolin regulates expression of VEGF and tumorigenesis in human colon cancer. Int J Cancer 126:1817–1827
87. Lai WS, Kennington EA, Blackshear PJ (2002) Interactions of CCCH zinc finger proteins with mRNA: non-binding tristetraprolin mutants exert an inhibitory effect on degradation of AU-rich element-containing mRNAs. J Biol Chem 277:9606–9613

88. Marderosian M, Sharma A, Funk AP et al (2006) Tristetraprolin regulates Cyclin D1 and c-Myc mRNA stability in response to rapamycin in an Akt-dependent manner via p38 MAPK signaling. Oncogene 25:6277–6290
89. Al-Souhibani N, Al-Ahmadi W, Hesketh JE, Blackshear PJ, Khabar KS (2010) The RNA-binding zinc-finger protein tristetraprolin regulates AU-rich mRNAs involved in breast cancer-related processes. Oncogene 29:4205–4215
90. Lai WS, Parker JS, Grissom SF, Stumpo DJ, Blackshear PJ (2006) Novel mRNA targets for tristetraprolin (TTP) identified by global analysis of stabilized transcripts in TTP-deficient fibroblasts. Mol Cell Biol 26:9196–9208
91. Sandler H, Kreth J, Timmers HT, Stoecklin G (2011) Not1 mediates recruitment of the deadenylase Caf1 to mRNAs targeted for degradation by tristetraprolin. Nucleic Acids Res 39:4373–4386
92. Franks TM, Lykke-Andersen J (2007) TTP and BRF proteins nucleate processing body formation to silence mRNAs with AU-rich elements. Genes Dev 21:719–735
93. Stumpo DJ, Byrd NA, Phillips RS et al (2004) Chorioallantoic fusion defects and embryonic lethality resulting from disruption of Zfp36L1, a gene encoding a CCCH tandem zinc finger protein of the Tristetraprolin family. Mol Cell Biol 24:6445–6455
94. Ramos SB, Stumpo DJ, Kennington EA et al (2004) The CCCH tandem zinc-finger protein Zfp36l2 is crucial for female fertility and early embryonic development. Development 131:4883–4893
95. Bell SE, Sanchez MJ, Spasic-Boskovic O et al (2006) The RNA binding protein Zfp36l1 is required for normal vascularisation and post-transcriptionally regulates VEGF expression. Dev Dyn 235:3144–3155
96. Taylor GA, Carballo E, Lee DM et al (1996) A pathogenetic role for TNF alpha in the syndrome of cachexia, arthritis, and autoimmunity resulting from tristetraprolin (TTP) deficiency. Immunity 4:445–454
97. Carballo E, Lai WS, Blackshear PJ (1998) Feedback inhibition of macrophage tumor necrosis factor-alpha production by tristetraprolin. Science 281:1001–1005
98. Carballo E, Lai WS, Blackshear PJ (2000) Evidence that tristetraprolin is a physiological regulator of granulocyte-macrophage colony-stimulating factor messenger RNA deadenylation and stability. Blood 95:1891–1899
99. Lai WS, Carballo E, Strum JR, Kennington EA, Phillips RS, Blackshear PJ (1999) Evidence that tristetraprolin binds to AU-rich elements and promotes the deadenylation and destabilization of tumor necrosis factor alpha mRNA. Mol Cell Biol 19:4311–4323
100. Tchen CR, Brook M, Saklatvala J, Clark AR (2004) The stability of tristetraprolin mRNA is regulated by mitogen-activated protein kinase p38 and by tristetraprolin itself. J Biol Chem 279:32393–32400
101. Stoecklin G, Tenenbaum SA, Mayo T et al (2008) Genome-wide analysis identifies interleukin-10 mRNA as target of tristetraprolin. J Biol Chem 283:11689–11699
102. Raghavan A, Robison RL, McNabb J, Miller CR, Williams DA, Bohjanen PR (2001) HuA and tristetraprolin are induced following T cell activation and display distinct but overlapping RNA binding specificities. J Biol Chem 276:47958–47965
103. Fechir M, Linker K, Pautz A et al (2005) Tristetraprolin regulates the expression of the human inducible nitric-oxide synthase gene. Mol Pharmacol 67:2148–2161
104. Phillips K, Kedersha N, Shen L, Blackshear PJ, Anderson P (2004) Arthritis suppressor genes TIA-1 and TTP dampen the expression of tumor necrosis factor alpha, cyclooxygenase 2, and inflammatory arthritis. Proc Natl Acad Sci U S A 101:2011–2016
105. Essafi-Benkhadir K, Onesto C, Stebe E, Moroni C, Pages G (2007) Tristetraprolin inhibits Ras-dependent tumor vascularization by inducing vascular endothelial growth factor mRNA degradation. Mol Biol Cell 18:4648–4658
106. Blackshear PJ, Lai WS, Kennington EA, et al (2003) Characteristics of the interaction of a synthetic human tristetraprolin tandem zinc finger peptide with AU-rich element-containing RNA substrate. Interactions of CCCH zinc finger proteins with mRNA: non-binding tristetraprolin mutants exert an inhibitory effect on degradation of AU-rich element-containing mRNAs. J Biol Chem 278:19947–19955. Epub 2003 Mar 14

107. Brewer BY, Malicka J, Blackshear PJ, Wilson GM (2004) RNA sequence elements required for high affinity binding by the zinc finger domain of tristetraprolin: conformational changes coupled to the bipartite nature of Au-rich MRNA-destabilizing motifs. J Biol Chem 279:27870–27877
108. Lai WS, Carrick DM, Blackshear PJ (2005) Influence of nonameric AU-rich tristetraprolin-binding sites on mRNA deadenylation and turnover. J Biol Chem 280:34365–34377
109. Worthington MT, Pelo JW, Sachedina MA, Applegate JL, Arseneau KO, Pizarro TT (2002) RNA binding properties of the AU-rich element-binding recombinant Nup475/TIS11/tristetraprolin protein. J Biol Chem 277:48558–48564
110. Lai WS, Kennington EA, Blackshear PJ (2002) Interactions of CCCH zinc finger proteins with mRNA: non-binding tristetraprolin mutants exert an inhibitory effect on degradation of AU-rich element-containing mRNAs. J Biol Chem 277:9606–9613
111. Min H, Turck CW, Nikolic JM, Black DL (1997) A new regulatory protein, KSRP, mediates exon inclusion through an intronic splicing enhancer. Genes Dev 11:1023–1036
112. Hall MP, Huang S, Black DL (2004) Differentiation-induced colocalization of the KH-type splicing regulatory protein with polypyrimidine tract binding protein and the c-src pre-mRNA. Mol Biol Cell 15:774–786
113. Briata P, Forcales SV, Ponassi M et al (2005) p38-dependent phosphorylation of the mRNA decay-promoting factor KSRP controls the stability of select myogenic transcripts. Mol Cell 20:891–903
114. Gherzi R, Lee KY, Briata P et al (2004) A KH domain RNA binding protein, KSRP, promotes ARE-directed mRNA turnover by recruiting the degradation machinery. Mol Cell 14:571–583
115. Trabucchi M, Briata P, Garcia-Mayoral M et al (2009) The RNA-binding protein KSRP promotes the biogenesis of a subset of microRNAs. Nature 459:1010–1014
116. Winzen R, Thakur BK, Dittrich-Breiholz O et al (2007) Functional analysis of KSRP interaction with the AU-rich element of interleukin-8 and identification of inflammatory mRNA targets. Mol Cell Biol 27:8388–8400
117. Garcia-Mayoral MF, Hollingworth D, Masino L et al (2007) The structure of the C-terminal KH domains of KSRP reveals a noncanonical motif important for mRNA degradation. Structure 15:485–498
118. Nechama M, Peng Y, Bell O et al (2009) KSRP-PMR1-exosome association determines parathyroid hormone mRNA levels and stability in transfected cells. BMC Cell Biol 10:70
119. Nechama M, Uchida T, Mor Yosef-Levi I, Silver J, Naveh-Many T (2009) The peptidyl-prolyl isomerase Pin1 determines parathyroid hormone mRNA levels and stability in rat models of secondary hyperparathyroidism. J Clin Invest 119:3102–3114
120. Brewer G, An A (1991) + U-rich element RNA-binding factor regulates c-myc mRNA stability in vitro. Mol Cell Biol 11:2460–2466
121. Wagner BJ, DeMaria CT, Sun Y, Wilson GM, Brewer G (1998) Structure and genomic organization of the human AUF1 gene: alternative pre-mRNA splicing generates four protein isoforms. Genomics 48:195–202
122. DeMaria CT, Sun Y, Wagner BJ, Long L, Brewer GA (1997) Structural determination in AUF1 required for high affinity binding to A + U-rich elements. Nucleic Acids Symp Ser (36):12–14
123. Loflin P, Chen CY, Shyu AB (1999) Unraveling a cytoplasmic role for hnRNP D in the in vivo mRNA destabilization directed by the AU-rich element. Genes Dev 13:1884–1897
124. Raineri I, Wegmueller D, Gross B, Certa U, Moroni C (2004) Roles of AUF1 isoforms, HuR and BRF1 in ARE-dependent mRNA turnover studied by RNA interference. Nucleic Acids Res 32:1279–1288
125. Sarkar B, Xi Q, He C, Schneider RJ (2003) Selective degradation of AU-rich mRNAs promoted by the p37 AUF1 protein isoform. Mol Cell Biol 23:6685–6693
126. Sarkar S, Sinsimer KS, Foster RL, Brewer G, Pestka S (2008) AUF1 isoform-specific regulation of anti-inflammatory IL10 expression in monocytes. J Interferon Cytokine Res 28:679–691

127. Chen TM, Hsu CH, Tsai SJ, Sun HS (2010) AUF1 p42 isoform selectively controls both steady-state and PGE2-induced FGF9 mRNA decay. Nucleic Acids Res 38:8061–8071
128. Ishimaru D, Zuraw L, Ramalingam S et al (2010) Mechanism of regulation of bcl-2 mRNA by nucleolin and A + U-rich element-binding factor 1 (AUF1). J Biol Chem 285: 27182–27191
129. Lu JY, Sadri N, Schneider RJ (2006) Endotoxic shock in AUF1 knockout mice mediated by failure to degrade proinflammatory cytokine mRNAs. Genes Dev 20:3174–3184
130. Xu N, Chen CY, Shyu AB (2001) Versatile role for hnRNP D isoforms in the differential regulation of cytoplasmic mRNA turnover. Mol Cell Biol 21:6960–6971
131. Mazan-Mamczarz K, Kuwano Y, Zhan M et al (2009) Identification of a signature motif in target mRNAs of RNA-binding protein AUF1. Nucleic Acids Res 37:204–214
132. Sarkar S, Han J, Sinsimer KS et al (2011) RNA-binding protein AUF1 regulates lipopolysaccharide-induced IL10 expression by activating IkappaB kinase complex in monocytes. Mol Cell Biol 31:602–615
133. Lu JY, Bergman N, Sadri N, Schneider RJ (2006) Assembly of AUF1 with eIF4G-poly(A) binding protein complex suggests a translation function in AU-rich mRNA decay. RNA 12:883–893
134. Sarkar B, Lu JY, Schneider RJ (2003) Nuclear import and export functions in the different isoforms of the AUF1/heterogeneous nuclear ribonucleoprotein protein family. J Biol Chem 278:20700–20707
135. Laroia G, Schneider RJ (2002) Alternate exon insertion controls selective ubiquitination and degradation of different AUF1 protein isoforms. Nucleic Acids Res 30:3052–3058
136. Brewer G, Saccani S, Sarkar S, Lewis A, Pestka S (2003) Increased interleukin-10 mRNA stability in melanoma cells is associated with decreased levels of A + U-rich element binding factor AUF1. J Interferon Cytokine Res 23:553–564
137. Wilson GM, Lu J, Sutphen K et al (2003) Phosphorylation of p40AUF1 regulates binding to A + U-rich mRNA-destabilizing elements and protein-induced changes in ribonucleoprotein structure. J Biol Chem 278:33039–33048
138. Wilson GM, Lu J, Sutphen K, Sun Y, Huynh Y, Brewer G (2003) Regulation of A + U-rich element-directed mRNA turnover involving reversible phosphorylation of AUF1. J Biol Chem 278:33029–33038
139. Sinsimer KS, Gratacos FM, Knapinska AM et al (2008) Chaperone Hsp27, a novel subunit of AUF1 protein complexes, functions in AU-rich element-mediated mRNA decay. Mol Cell Biol 28:5223–5237
140. Knapinska AM, Gratacos FM, Krause CD et al (2011) Chaperone Hsp27 modulates AUF1 proteolysis and AU-rich element-mediated mRNA degradation. Mol Cell Biol 31:1419–1431
141. Brennan CM, Gallouzi IE, Steitz JA (2000) Protein ligands to HuR modulate its interaction with target mRNAs in vivo. J Cell Biol 151:1–14
142. Good PJ (1995) A conserved family of elav-like genes in vertebrates. Proc Natl Acad Sci U S A 92:4557–4561
143. Ma WJ, Cheng S, Campbell C, Wright A, Furneaux H (1996) Cloning and characterization of HuR, a ubiquitously expressed Elav-like protein. J Biol Chem 271:8144–8151
144. Szabo A, Dalmau J, Manley G et al (1991) HuD, a paraneoplastic encephalomyelitis antigen, contains RNA-binding domains and is homologous to Elav and Sex-lethal. Cell 67:325–333
145. Abe R, Uyeno Y, Yamamoto K, Sakamoto H (1994) Tissue-specific expression of the gene encoding a mouse RNA binding protein homologous to human HuD antigen. DNA Res 1:175–180
146. Sakai K, Gofuku M, Kitagawa Y et al (1994) A hippocampal protein associated with paraneoplastic neurologic syndrome and small cell lung carcinoma. Biochem Biophys Res Commun 199:1200–1208
147. Okano HJ, Darnell RB (1997) A hierarchy of Hu RNA binding proteins in developing and adult neurons. J Neurosci 17:3024–3037
148. Wakamatsu Y, Weston JA (1997) Sequential expression and role of Hu RNA-binding proteins during neurogenesis. Development 124:3449–3460

149. Kasashima K, Terashima K, Yamamoto K, Sakashita E, Sakamoto H (1999) Cytoplasmic localization is required for the mammalian ELAV-like protein HuD to induce neuronal differentiation. Genes Cells 4:667–683
150. Antic D, Keene JD (1997) Embryonic lethal abnormal visual RNA-binding proteins involved in growth, differentiation, and posttranscriptional gene expression. Am J Hum Genet 61:273–278
151. King PH, Levine TD, Fremeau RT Jr, Keene JD (1994) Mammalian homologs of Drosophila ELAV localized to a neuronal subset can bind in vitro to the 3' UTR of mRNA encoding the Id transcriptional repressor. J Neurosci 14:1943–1952
152. Park S, Myszka DG, Yu M, Littler SJ, Laird-Offringa IA (2000) HuD RNA recognition motifs play distinct roles in the formation of a stable complex with AU-rich RNA. Mol Cell Biol 20:4765–4772
153. Fialcowitz-White EJ, Brewer BY, Ballin JD, Willis CD, Toth EA, Wilson GM (2007) Specific protein domains mediate cooperative assembly of HuR oligomers on AU-rich mRNA-destabilizing sequences. J Biol Chem 282:20948–20959
154. Fan XC, Myer VE, Steitz JA (1997) AU-rich elements target small nuclear RNAs as well as mRNAs for rapid degradation. Genes Dev 11:2557–2568
155. Myer VE, Fan XC, Steitz JA (1997) Identification of HuR as a protein implicated in AUUUA-mediated mRNA decay. EMBO J 16:2130–2139
156. Kim HS, Wilce MC, Yoga YM et al (2011) Different modes of interaction by TIAR and HuR with target RNA and DNA. Nucleic Acids Res 39:1117–1130
157. el Akool S, Kleinert H, Hamada FM et al (2003) Nitric oxide increases the decay of matrix metalloproteinase 9 mRNA by inhibiting the expression of mRNA-stabilizing factor HuR. Mol Cell Biol 23:4901–4916
158. Dean JL, Wait R, Mahtani KR, Sully G, Clark AR, Saklatvala J (2001) The 3' untranslated region of tumor necrosis factor alpha mRNA is a target of the mRNA-stabilizing factor HuR. Mol Cell Biol 21:721–730
159. van der Giessen K, Di-Marco S, Clair E, Gallouzi IE (2003) RNAi-mediated HuR depletion leads to the inhibition of muscle cell differentiation. J Biol Chem 278:47119–47128
160. Sully G, Dean JL, Wait R et al (2004) Structural and functional dissection of a conserved destabilizing element of cyclo-oxygenase-2 mRNA: evidence against the involvement of AUF-1 [AU-rich element/poly(U)-binding/degradation factor-1], AUF-2, tristetraprolin, HuR (Hu antigen R) or FBP1 (far-upstream-sequence-element-binding protein 1). Biochem J 377:629–639
161. Garcia-Dominguez DJ, Morello D, Cisneros E, Kontoyiannis DL, Frade JM (2011) Stabilization of Dll1 mRNA by Elavl1/HuR in neuroepithelial cells undergoing mitosis. Mol Biol Cell 22:1227–1239
162. Ramgolam VS, DeGregorio SD, Rao GK et al (2010) T cell LFA-1 engagement induces HuR-dependent cytokine mRNA stabilization through a Vav-1, Rac1/2, p38MAPK and MKK3 signaling cascade. PLoS One 5:e14450
163. Nowotarski SL, Shantz LM (2010) Cytoplasmic accumulation of the RNA-binding protein HuR stabilizes the ornithine decarboxylase transcript in a murine nonmelanoma skin cancer model. J Biol Chem 285:31885–31894
164. Drury GL, Di Marco S, Dormoy-Raclet V, Desbarats J, Gallouzi IE (2010) FasL expression in activated T lymphocytes involves HuR-mediated stabilization. J Biol Chem 285:31130–31138
165. Zhang X, Zou T, Rao JN et al (2009) Stabilization of XIAP mRNA through the RNA binding protein HuR regulated by cellular polyamines. Nucleic Acids Res 37: 7623–7637
166. Lafarga V, Cuadrado A, Lopez de Silanes I, Bengoechea R, Fernandez-Capetillo O, Nebreda AR (2009) p38 Mitogen-activated protein kinase- and HuR-dependent stabilization of p21(Cip1) mRNA mediates the G(1)/S checkpoint. Mol Cell Biol 29:4341–4351
167. Lopez de Silanes I, Gorospe M, Taniguchi H, et al (2009) The RNA-binding protein HuR regulates DNA methylation through stabilization of DNMT3b mRNA. Nucleic Acids Res 37:2658–2671

168. Kuwano Y, Kim HH, Abdelmohsen K et al (2008) MKP-1 mRNA stabilization and translational control by RNA-binding proteins HuR and NF90. Mol Cell Biol 28:4562–4575
169. Rzymski T, Paantjens A, Bod J, Harris AL (2008) Multiple pathways are involved in the anoxia response of SKIP3 including HuR-regulated RNA stability, NF-kappaB and ATF4. Oncogene 27:4532–4543
170. Doller A, el Akool S, Huwiler A et al (2008) Posttranslational modification of the AU-rich element binding protein HuR by protein kinase Cdelta elicits angiotensin II-induced stabilization and nuclear export of cyclooxygenase 2 mRNA. Mol Cell Biol 28:2608–2625
171. Dormoy-Raclet V, Menard I, Clair E et al (2007) The RNA-binding protein HuR promotes cell migration and cell invasion by stabilizing the beta-actin mRNA in a U-rich-element-dependent manner. Mol Cell Biol 27:5365–5380
172. Zou T, Mazan-Mamczarz K, Rao JN et al (2006) Polyamine depletion increases cytoplasmic levels of RNA-binding protein HuR leading to stabilization of nucleophosmin and p53 mRNAs. J Biol Chem 281:19387–19394
173. Kim HH, Abdelmohsen K, Lal A et al (2008) Nuclear HuR accumulation through phosphorylation by Cdk1. Genes Dev 22:1804–1815
174. Topisirovic I, Siddiqui N, Orolicki S et al (2009) Stability of eukaryotic translation initiation factor 4E mRNA is regulated by HuR, and this activity is dysregulated in cancer. Mol Cell Biol 29:1152–1162
175. Doller A, Pfeilschifter J, Eberhardt W (2008) Signalling pathways regulating nucleo-cytoplasmic shuttling of the mRNA-binding protein HuR. Cell Signal 20:2165–2173
176. Kim HH, Abdelmohsen K, Gorospe M (2010) Regulation of HuR by DNA damage response kinases. J Nucleic Acids 25 july pii:981487
177. Fan XC, Steitz JA (1998) HNS, a nuclear-cytoplasmic shuttling sequence in HuR. Proc Natl Acad Sci U S A 95:15293–15298
178. Guttinger S, Muhlhausser P, Koller-Eichhorn R, Brennecke J, Kutay U (2004) Transportin2 functions as importin and mediates nuclear import of HuR. Proc Natl Acad Sci U S A 101:2918–2923
179. Rebane A, Aab A, Steitz JA (2004) Transportins 1 and 2 are redundant nuclear import factors for hnRNP A1 and HuR. RNA 10:590–599
180. Gallouzi IE, Brennan CM, Steitz JA (2001) Protein ligands mediate the CRM1-dependent export of HuR in response to heat shock. RNA 7:1348–1361
181. Gallouzi IE, Steitz JA (2001) Delineation of mRNA export pathways by the use of cell-permeable peptides. Science 294:1895–1901
182. Wang W, Fan J, Yang X et al (2002) AMP-activated kinase regulates cytoplasmic HuR. Mol Cell Biol 22:3425–3436
183. Xu YZ, Di Marco S, Gallouzi I, Rola-Pleszczynski M, Radzioch D (2005) RNA-binding protein HuR is required for stabilization of SLC11A1 mRNA and SLC11A1 protein expression. Mol Cell Biol 25:8139–8149
184. Yaman I, Fernandez J, Sarkar B et al (2002) Nutritional control of mRNA stability is mediated by a conserved AU-rich element that binds the cytoplasmic shuttling protein HuR. J Biol Chem 277:41539–41546
185. Atasoy U, Watson J, Patel D, Keene JD (1998) ELAV protein HuA (HuR) can redistribute between nucleus and cytoplasm and is upregulated during serum stimulation and T cell activation. J Cell Sci 111(Pt 21):3145–3156
186. Li H, Park S, Kilburn B et al (2002) Lipopolysaccharide-induced methylation of HuR, an mRNA-stabilizing protein, by CARM1. Coactivator-associated arginine methyltransferase. J Biol Chem 277:44623–44630
187. Kawakami A, Tian Q, Duan X, Streuli M, Schlossman SF, Anderson P (1992) Identification and functional characterization of a TIA-1-related nucleolysin. Proc Natl Acad Sci U S A 89:8681–8685
188. Tian Q, Streuli M, Saito H, Schlossman SF, Anderson P (1991) A polyadenylate binding protein localized to the granules of cytolytic lymphocytes induces DNA fragmentation in target cells. Cell 67:629–639

189. Del Gatto-Konczak F, Bourgeois CF, Le Guiner C et al (2000) The RNA-binding protein TIA-1 is a novel mammalian splicing regulator acting through intron sequences adjacent to a 5' splice site. Mol Cell Biol 20:6287–6299
190. Forch P, Puig O, Kedersha N et al (2000) The apoptosis-promoting factor TIA-1 is a regulator of alternative pre-mRNA splicing. Mol Cell 6:1089–1098
191. Le Guiner C, Lejeune F, Galiana D et al (2001) TIA-1 and TIAR activate splicing of alternative exons with weak 5' splice sites followed by a U-rich stretch on their own pre-mRNAs. J Biol Chem 276:40638–40646
192. Gilks N, Kedersha N, Ayodele M et al (2004) Stress granule assembly is mediated by prion-like aggregation of TIA-1. Mol Biol Cell 15:5383–5398
193. Dember LM, Kim ND, Liu KQ, Anderson P (1996) Individual RNA recognition motifs of TIA-1 and TIAR have different RNA binding specificities. J Biol Chem 271:2783–2788
194. Dixon DA, Balch GC, Kedersha N et al (2003) Regulation of cyclooxygenase-2 expression by the translational silencer TIA-1. J Exp Med 198:475–481
195. Gueydan C, Droogmans L, Chalon P, Huez G, Caput D, Kruys V (1999) Identification of TIAR as a protein binding to the translational regulatory AU-rich element of tumor necrosis factor alpha mRNA. J Biol Chem 274:2322–2326
196. Yamasaki S, Stoecklin G, Kedersha N, Simarro M, Anderson P (2007) T-cell intracellular antigen-1 (TIA-1)-induced translational silencing promotes the decay of selected mRNAs. J Biol Chem 282:30070–30077
197. Balagopal V, Parker R (2009) Polysomes, P bodies and stress granules: states and fates of eukaryotic mRNAs. Curr Opin Cell Biol 21:403–408
198. Buchan JR, Parker R (2009) Eukaryotic stress granules: the ins and outs of translation. Mol Cell 36:932–941
199. Anderson P, Kedersha N (2009) Stress granules. Curr Biol 19:R397–R398
200. Harding HP, Novoa I, Zhang Y et al (2000) Regulated translation initiation controls stress-induced gene expression in mammalian cells. Mol Cell 6:1099–1108
201. Harding HP, Zhang Y, Bertolotti A, Zeng H, Ron D (2000) Perk is essential for translational regulation and cell survival during the unfolded protein response. Mol Cell 5:897–904
202. Jefferson LS, Kimball SR (2003) Amino acids as regulators of gene expression at the level of mRNA translation. J Nutr 133:2046S–2051S
203. Kaufman RJ (1999) Stress signaling from the lumen of the endoplasmic reticulum: coordination of gene transcriptional and translational controls. Genes Dev 13:1211–1233
204. Kimball SR (2001) Regulation of translation initiation by amino acids in eukaryotic cells. Prog Mol Subcell Biol 26:155–184
205. Srivastava SP, Kumar KU, Kaufman RJ (1998) Phosphorylation of eukaryotic translation initiation factor 2 mediates apoptosis in response to activation of the double-stranded RNA-dependent protein kinase. J Biol Chem 273:2416–2423
206. Kedersha NL, Gupta M, Li W, Miller I, Anderson P (1999) RNA-binding proteins TIA-1 and TIAR link the phosphorylation of eIF-2 alpha to the assembly of mammalian stress granules. J Cell Biol 147:1431–1442
207. Brill LM, Motamedchaboki K, Wu S, Wolf DA (2009) Comprehensive proteomic analysis of Schizosaccharomyces pombe by two-dimensional HPLC-tandem mass spectrometry. Methods 48:311–319
208. Tao WA, Wollscheid B, O'Brien R et al (2005) Quantitative phosphoproteome analysis using a dendrimer conjugation chemistry and tandem mass spectrometry. Nat Methods 2:591–598
209. Barreau C, Paillard L, Osborne HB (2005) AU-rich elements and associated factors: are there unifying principles? Nucleic Acids Res 33:7138–7150
210. Tran H, Schilling M, Wirbelauer C, Hess D, Nagamine Y (2004) Facilitation of mRNA deadenylation and decay by the exosome-bound, DExH protein RHAU. Mol Cell 13:101–111
211. Chalupnikova K, Lattmann S, Selak N, Iwamoto F, Fujiki Y, Nagamine Y (2008) Recruitment of the RNA helicase RHAU to stress granules via a unique RNA-binding domain. J Biol Chem 283:35186–35198

212. Timchenko LT, Miller JW, Timchenko NA et al (1996) Identification of a (CUG)n triplet repeat RNA-binding protein and its expression in myotonic dystrophy. Nucleic Acids Res 24:4407–4414
213. Barreau C, Paillard L, Mereau A, Osborne HB (2006) Mammalian CELF/Bruno-like RNA-binding proteins: molecular characteristics and biological functions. Biochimie 88:515–525
214. Charlet BN, Logan P, Singh G, Cooper TA (2002) Dynamic antagonism between ETR-3 and PTB regulates cell type-specific alternative splicing. Mol Cell 9:649–658
215. Savkur RS, Philips AV, Cooper TA (2001) Aberrant regulation of insulin receptor alternative splicing is associated with insulin resistance in myotonic dystrophy. Nat Genet 29:40–47
216. Ho TH, Bundman D, Armstrong DL, Cooper TA (2005) Transgenic mice expressing CUG-BP1 reproduce splicing mis-regulation observed in myotonic dystrophy. Hum Mol Genet 14:1539–1547
217. Ladd AN, Taffet G, Hartley C, Kearney DL, Cooper TA (2005) Cardiac tissue-specific repression of CELF activity disrupts alternative splicing and causes cardiomyopathy. Mol Cell Biol 25:6267–6278
218. Mukhopadhyay D, Houchen CW, Kennedy S, Dieckgraefe BK, Anant S (2003) Coupled mRNA stabilization and translational silencing of cyclooxygenase-2 by a novel RNA binding protein, CUGBP2. Mol Cell 11:113–126
219. Timchenko NA, Cai ZJ, Welm AL, Reddy S, Ashizawa T, Timchenko LT (2001) RNA CUG repeats sequester CUGBP1 and alter protein levels and activity of CUGBP1. J Biol Chem 276:7820–7826
220. Timchenko NA, Wang GL, Timchenko LT (2005) RNA CUG-binding protein 1 increases translation of 20-kDa isoform of CCAAT/enhancer-binding protein beta by interacting with the alpha and beta subunits of eukaryotic initiation translation factor 2. J Biol Chem 280:20549–20557
221. Osborne HB, Gautier-Courteille C, Graindorge A et al (2005) Post-transcriptional regulation in Xenopus embryos: role and targets of EDEN-BP. Biochem Soc Trans 33:1541–1543
222. Chen CY, Del Gatto-Konczak F, Wu Z, Karin M (1998) Stabilization of interleukin-2 mRNA by the c-Jun NH2-terminal kinase pathway. Science 280:1945–1949
223. Dean JL, Sully G, Clark AR, Saklatvala J (2004) The involvement of AU-rich element-binding proteins in p38 mitogen-activated protein kinase pathway-mediated mRNA stabilisation. Cell Signal 16:1113–1121
224. Gherzi R, Trabucchi M, Ponassi M et al (2006) The RNA-binding protein KSRP promotes decay of beta-catenin mRNA and is inactivated by PI3 K-AKT signaling. PLoS Biol 5:e5
225. Schmidlin M, Lu M, Leuenberger SA et al (2004) The ARE-dependent mRNA-destabilizing activity of BRF1 is regulated by protein kinase B. EMBO J 23:4760–4769
226. Wang W, Yang X, Lopez de Silanes I, Carling D, Gorospe M (2003) Increased AMP:ATP ratio and AMP-activated protein kinase activity during cellular senescence linked to reduced HuR function. J Biol Chem 278:27016–27023
227. Carpenter L, Cordery D, Biden TJ (2001) Protein kinase Cdelta activation by interleukin-1beta stabilizes inducible nitric-oxide synthase mRNA in pancreatic beta-cells. J Biol Chem 276:5368–5374
228. Gringhuis SI, Garcia-Vallejo JJ, van Het Hof B, van Dijk W (2005) Convergent actions of I kappa B kinase beta and protein kinase C delta modulate mRNA stability through phosphorylation of 14–3-3 beta complexed with tristetraprolin. Mol Cell Biol 25:6454–6463
229. Perrone-Bizzozero NI, Cansino VV, Kohn DT (1993) Posttranscriptional regulation of GAP-43 gene expression in PC12 cells through protein kinase C-dependent stabilization of the mRNA. J Cell Biol 120:1263–1270
230. Briata P, Ilengo C, Corte G et al (2003) The Wnt/beta-catenin Pitx2 pathway controls the turnover of Pitx2 and other unstable mRNAs. Mol Cell 12:1201–1211
231. Raman M, Chen W, Cobb MH (2007) Differential regulation and properties of MAPKs. Oncogene 26:3100–3112
232. Dhillon AS, Hagan S, Rath O, Kolch W (2007) MAP kinase signalling pathways in cancer. Oncogene 26:3279–3290

233. Brook M, Sully G, Clark AR, Saklatvala J (2000) Regulation of tumour necrosis factor alpha mRNA stability by the mitogen-activated protein kinase p38 signalling cascade. FEBS Lett 483:57–61
234. Clark AR, Dean JL, Saklatvala J (2003) Post-transcriptional regulation of gene expression by mitogen-activated protein kinase p38. FEBS Lett 546:37–44
235. Dean JL, Brook M, Clark AR, Saklatvala J (1999) p38 mitogen-activated protein kinase regulates cyclooxygenase-2 mRNA stability and transcription in lipopolysaccharide-treated human monocytes. J Biol Chem 274:264–269
236. Hitti E, Iakovleva T, Brook M et al (2006) Mitogen-activated protein kinase-activated protein kinase 2 regulates tumor necrosis factor mRNA stability and translation mainly by altering tristetraprolin expression, stability, and binding to adenine/uridine-rich element. Mol Cell Biol 26:2399–2407
237. Kotlyarov A, Neininger A, Schubert C et al (1999) MAPKAP kinase 2 is essential for LPS-induced TNF-alpha biosynthesis. Nat Cell Biol 1:94–97
238. Miyazawa K, Mori A, Miyata H, Akahane M, Ajisawa Y, Okudaira H (1998) Regulation of interleukin-1beta-induced interleukin-6 gene expression in human fibroblast-like synoviocytes by p38 mitogen-activated protein kinase. J Biol Chem 273:24832–24838
239. Ridley SH, Dean JL, Sarsfield SJ, Brook M, Clark AR, Saklatvala J (1998) A p38 MAP kinase inhibitor regulates stability of interleukin-1-induced cyclooxygenase-2 mRNA. FEBS Lett 439:75–80
240. Sirenko OI, Lofquist AK, DeMaria CT, Morris JS, Brewer G, Haskill JS (1997) Adhesion-dependent regulation of an A + U-rich element-binding activity associated with AUF1. Mol Cell Biol 17:3898–3906
241. Winzen R, Gowrishankar G, Bollig F, Redich N, Resch K, Holtmann H (2004) Distinct domains of AU-rich elements exert different functions in mRNA destabilization and stabilization by p38 mitogen-activated protein kinase or HuR. Mol Cell Biol 24: 4835–4847
242. Frevel MA, Bakheet T, Silva AM, Hissong JG, Khabar KS, Williams BR (2003) p38 Mitogen-activated protein kinase-dependent and -independent signaling of mRNA stability of AU-rich element-containing transcripts. Mol Cell Biol 23:425–436
243. Neininger A, Kontoyiannis D, Kotlyarov A et al (2002) MK2 targets AU-rich elements and regulates biosynthesis of tumor necrosis factor and interleukin-6 independently at different post-transcriptional levels. J Biol Chem 277:3065–3068
244. Maitra S, Chou CF, Luber CA, Lee KY, Mann M, Chen CY (2008) The AU-rich element mRNA decay-promoting activity of BRF1 is regulated by mitogen-activated protein kinase-activated protein kinase 2. RNA 14:950–959
245. Zhao W, Liu M, D'Silva NJ, Kirkwood KL (2011) Tristetraprolin Regulates Interleukin-6 Expression Through p38 MAPK-Dependent Affinity Changes with mRNA 3' Untranslated Region. J Interferon Cytokine Res 31:629–637
246. Otkjaer K, Holtmann H, Kragstrup TW et al (2010) The p38 MAPK regulates IL-24 expression by stabilization of the 3' UTR of IL-24 mRNA. PLoS One 5:e8671
247. Sandler H, Stoecklin G (2008) Control of mRNA decay by phosphorylation of tristetraprolin. Biochem Soc Trans 36:491–496
248. Dhanasekaran DN, Johnson GL (2007) MAPKs: function, regulation, role in cancer and therapeutic targeting. Oncogene 26:3097–3099
249. Lasa M, Mahtani KR, Finch A, Brewer G, Saklatvala J, Clark AR (2000) Regulation of cyclooxygenase 2 mRNA stability by the mitogen-activated protein kinase p38 signaling cascade. Mol Cell Biol 20:4265–4274
250. Stoecklin G, Stubbs T, Kedersha N et al (2004) MK2-induced tristetraprolin:14–3-3 complexes prevent stress granule association and ARE-mRNA decay. EMBO J 23: 1313–1324
251. Chang L, Karin M (2001) Mammalian MAP kinase signalling cascades. Nature 410:37–40
252. Carballo E, Cao H, Lai WS, Kennington EA, Campbell D, Blackshear PJ (2001) Decreased sensitivity of tristetraprolin-deficient cells to p38 inhibitors suggests the involvement of tristetraprolin in the p38 signaling pathway. J Biol Chem 276:42580–42587

253. Chrestensen CA, Schroeder MJ, Shabanowitz J et al (2004) MAPKAP kinase 2 phosphorylates tristetraprolin on in vivo sites including Ser178, a site required for 14–3-3 binding. J Biol Chem 279:10176–10184
254. Mahtani KR, Brook M, Dean JL, Sully G, Saklatvala J, Clark AR (2001) Mitogen-activated protein kinase p38 controls the expression and posttranslational modification of tristetraprolin, a regulator of tumor necrosis factor alpha mRNA stability. Mol Cell Biol 21:6461–6469
255. Cao H, Deterding LJ, Venable JD et al (2006) Identification of the anti-inflammatory protein tristetraprolin as a hyperphosphorylated protein by mass spectrometry and site-directed mutagenesis. Biochem J 394:285–297
256. Johnson BA, Stehn JR, Yaffe MB, Blackwell TK (2002) Cytoplasmic localization of tristetraprolin involves 14–3-3-dependent and -independent mechanisms. J Biol Chem 277:18029–18036
257. Brook M, Tchen CR, Santalucia T et al (2006) Posttranslational regulation of tristetraprolin subcellular localization and protein stability by p38 mitogen-activated protein kinase and extracellular signal-regulated kinase pathways. Mol Cell Biol 26:2408–2418
258. Ming XF, Kaiser M, Moroni C (1998) c-jun N-terminal kinase is involved in AUUUA-mediated interleukin-3 mRNA turnover in mast cells. EMBO J 17:6039–6048
259. Chen CY, Gherzi R, Andersen JS et al (2000) Nucleolin and YB-1 are required for JNK-mediated interleukin-2 mRNA stabilization during T-cell activation. Genes Dev 14:1236–1248
260. Pages G, Berra E, Milanini J, Levy AP, Pouyssegur J (2000) Stress-activated protein kinases (JNK and p38/HOG) are essential for vascular endothelial growth factor mRNA stability. J Biol Chem 275:26484–26491
261. Lahti A, Jalonen U, Kankaanranta H, Moilanen E (2003) c-Jun NH2-terminal kinase inhibitor anthra(1,9-cd)pyrazol-6(2H)-one reduces inducible nitric-oxide synthase expression by destabilizing mRNA in activated macrophages. Mol Pharmacol 64: 308–315
262. Esnault S, Malter JS (2002) Extracellular signal-regulated kinase mediates granulocyte-macrophage colony-stimulating factor messenger RNA stabilization in tumor necrosis factor-alpha plus fibronectin-activated peripheral blood eosinophils. Blood 99:4048–4052
263. Esnault S, Malter JS (2003) Hyaluronic acid or TNF-alpha plus fibronectin triggers granulocyte macrophage-colony-stimulating factor mRNA stabilization in eosinophils yet engages differential intracellular pathways and mRNA binding proteins. J Immunol 171:6780–6787
264. Headley VV, Tanveer R, Greene SM, Zweifach A, Port JD (2004) Reciprocal regulation of beta-adrenergic receptor mRNA stability by mitogen activated protein kinase activation and inhibition. Mol Cell Biochem 258:109–119
265. Shen ZJ, Esnault S, Malter JS (2005) The peptidyl-prolyl isomerase Pin1 regulates the stability of granulocyte-macrophage colony-stimulating factor mRNA in activated eosinophils. Nat Immunol 6:1280–1287
266. Zhai B, Yang H, Mancini A, He Q, Antoniou J, Di Battista JA (2010) Leukotriene B(4) BLT receptor signaling regulates the level and stability of cyclooxygenase-2 (COX-2) mRNA through restricted activation of Ras/Raf/ERK/p42 AUF1 pathway. J Biol Chem 285:23568–23580
267. Bermudez O, Jouandin P, Rottier J, Bourcier C, Pages G, Gimond C (2011) Post-transcriptional regulation of the DUSP6/MKP-3 phosphatase by MEK/ERK signaling and hypoxia. J Cell Physiol 226:276–284
268. Taylor GA, Thompson MJ, Lai WS, Blackshear PJ (1995) Phosphorylation of tristetraprolin, a potential zinc finger transcription factor, by mitogen stimulation in intact cells and by mitogen-activated protein kinase in vitro. J Biol Chem 270:13341–13347
269. Cheng JQ, Lindsley CW, Cheng GZ, Yang H, Nicosia SV (2005) The Akt/PKB pathway: molecular target for cancer drug discovery. Oncogene 24:7482–7492
270. Testa JR, Bellacosa A (2001) AKT plays a central role in tumorigenesis. Proc Natl Acad Sci U S A 98:10983–10985

271. Fayard E, Tintignac LA, Baudry A, Hemmings BA (2005) Protein kinase B/Akt at a glance. J Cell Sci 118:5675–5678
272. Woodgett JR (2005) Recent advances in the protein kinase B signaling pathway. Curr Opin Cell Biol 17:150–157
273. Alessi DR, James SR, Downes CP et al (1997) Characterization of a 3-phosphoinositide-dependent protein kinase which phosphorylates and activates protein kinase Balpha. Curr Biol 7:261–269
274. Gherzi R, Trabucchi M, Ponassi M et al (2006) The RNA-binding protein KSRP promotes decay of beta-catenin mRNA and is inactivated by PI3K-AKT signaling. PLoS Biol 5:e5
275. Ruggiero T, Trabucchi M, Ponassi M et al (2007) Identification of a set of KSRP target transcripts upregulated by PI3 K-AKT signaling. BMC Mol Biol 8:28
276. Pei Y, Zhu P, Dang Y et al (2008) Nuclear export of NF90 to stabilize IL-2 mRNA is mediated by AKT-dependent phosphorylation at Ser647 in response to CD28 costimulation. J Immunol 180:222–229
277. Lopez de Silanes I, Lal A, Gorospe M (2005) HuR: post-transcriptional paths to malignancy. RNA Biol 2:11–13
278. Altomare DA, Testa JR (2005) Perturbations of the AKT signaling pathway in human cancer. Oncogene 24:7455–7464
279. Gouble A, Grazide S, Meggetto F, Mercier P, Delsol G, Morello D (2002) A new player in oncogenesis: AUF1/hnRNPD overexpression leads to tumorigenesis in transgenic mice. Cancer Res 62:1489–1495
280. Abdelmohsen K, Lal A, Kim HH, Gorospe M (2007) Posttranscriptional orchestration of an anti-apoptotic program by HuR. Cell Cycle 6:1288–1292
281. Carrick DM, Blackshear PJ (2007) Comparative expression of tristetraprolin (TTP) family member transcripts in normal human tissues and cancer cell lines. Arch Biochem Biophys 462:278–285
282. Brennan SE, Kuwano Y, Alkharouf N, Blackshear PJ, Gorospe M, Wilson GM (2009) The mRNA-destabilizing protein tristetraprolin is suppressed in many cancers, altering tumorigenic phenotypes and patient prognosis. Cancer Res 69:5168–5176
283. Sanduja S, Kaza V, Dixon DA (2009) The mRNA decay factor tristetraprolin (TTP) induces senescence in human papillomavirus-transformed cervical cancer cells by targeting E6-AP ubiquitin ligase. Aging (Albany NY) 1:803–817
284. Young LE, Sanduja S, Bemis-Standoli K, Pena EA, Price RL, Dixon DA (2009) The mRNA binding proteins HuR and tristetraprolin regulate cyclooxygenase 2 expression during colon carcinogenesis. Gastroenterology 136:1669–1679
285. Kanies CL, Smith JJ, Kis C et al (2008) Oncogenic Ras and transforming growth factor-beta synergistically regulate AU-rich element-containing mRNAs during epithelial to mesenchymal transition. Mol Cancer Res 6:1124–1136
286. Planel S, Salomon A, Jalinot P, Feige JJ, Cherradi N (2010) A novel concept in antiangiogenic and antitumoral therapy: multitarget destabilization of short-lived mRNAs by the zinc finger protein ZFP36L1. Oncogene 29:5989–6003
287. Soussi T (2007) p53 alterations in human cancer: more questions than answers. Oncogene 26:2145–2156
288. Vilborg A, Wilhelm MT, Wiman KG (2010) Regulation of tumor suppressor p53 at the RNA level. J Mol Med 88:645–652
289. Abbas T, Dutta A (2009) p21 in cancer: intricate networks and multiple activities. Nat Rev Cancer 9:400–414

Alternative Pre-mRNA Splicing, Cell Death, and Cancer

Kong Ruirui, Payal Ray, Mengxue Yang, Pushuai Wen, Li Zhu, Jianghong Liu, Kazuo Fushimi, Amar Kar, Ying Liu, Rongqiao He, David Kuo and Jane Y. Wu

Abstract

Alternative splicing is one of the most powerful mechanisms for generating functionally distinct products from a single genetic loci and for fine-tuning gene activities at the post-transcriptional level. Alternative splicing plays important roles in regulating genes critical for cell death. These cell death genes encode death ligands, cell surface death receptors, intracellular death regulators, signal transduction molecules, and death executor enzymes such as caspases and nucleases. Alternative splicing of these genes often leads to the formation of functionally different products, some of which have antagonistic effects that are either cell death-promoting or cell death-preventing. Differential alternative splicing can affect expression, subcellular distribution, and functional activities of the gene products. Molecular defects in splicing regulation of cell death genes have been associated with cancer development and resistance to treatment. Studies using molecular, biochemical, and systems-based approaches have begun to reveal mechanisms underlying the regulation of alternative splicing of cell death genes. Systematic studies have begun to uncover the multi-level interconnected networks that regulate alternative splicing. A global picture of the complex mechanisms that regulate cell death genes at the pre-mRNA splicing level has thus begun to emerge.

K. Ruirui · M. Yang · P. Wen · L. Zhu (✉) · J. Liu · Y. Liu · R. He
State Key Laboratory of Brain and Cognitive Science, Institute of Biophysics, Chinese Academy of Science, Beijing, China
e-mail: lzhu2000@gmail.com

P. Ray · K. Fushimi · A. Kar · D. Kuo · J. Y. Wu (✉)
Department of Neurology, Robert H. Lurie Comprehensive Cancer Center, Center for Genetic Medicine, Northwestern University Feinberg School of Medicine, 303 E. Superior, Chicago, IL 60611, USA
e-mail: jane-wu@northwestern.edu

J. Y. Wu (ed.), *RNA and Cancer*, Cancer Treatment and Research,
DOI: 10.1007/978-3-642-31659-3_8,

Keywords
Programmed cell death · Apoptosis · Necrosis · Pyroptosis · Autophagy · Alternative splicing regulation

Contents

1 Introduction

Although the major mechanism of programmed cell death (PCD) has been characterized by activation of caspases and packaging of cells into apoptotic bodies, several types of cell death have been described with distinct features: apoptosis, necrosis, pyroptosis, and autophagic cell death [15, 47]. Prominent morphological features of apoptosis include cell shrinkage, nuclear condensation, nuclear fragmentation, chromatin condensation, membrane blebbing, retention of intact organelles, vacuole formation, and DNA fragmentation [83, 189]. Necrosis, now recognized as an alternate form of programmed cell death, often involves prominent immune responses. Recent studies suggest that by initiating inflammatory and reparative responses, necrosis may also serve to maintain tissue homeostasis and organismal integrity (reviewed in [178, 203]). In addition, autophagy plays important roles in cell death signaling in both promotional and inhibitory manners (for reviews: [55, 176]). Cell death can also be induced by microbial and viral infection. Infection induced cell death, termed "pyroptosis", involves an inflammatory response with neighboring cells [15].

A common feature of cell death is the activation of proteases followed by DNA degradation. Similar to the activation of caspases during apoptosis, other types of PCD are triggered by specific proteases. Cells undergoing necrotic death activate cathepsins and calpains, whereas pyroptotic cells activate caspase-1 and caspase-7. Furthermore, many downstream DNases have been discovered, such as Caspase-activated DNase (CAD), EndoG, LEI/L-DNase II, and Granzyme A-activated DNase (GAAD). PCD is a complex phenomenon that engages more than 400 proteins with diverse functions ranging from PCD receptors to the execution proteins.

Regulated cell death processes are critical for the development and homeostasis of multi-cellular organisms. Disruption of cell death regulation plays an important role in the pathogenesis of a wide spectrum of human diseases. Cell death regulation occurs at multiple levels and involves many different PCD associated proteins (for recent reviews, [15, 33, 60, 176]). One important step of this regulation occurs during pre-mRNA splicing because many cell death genes are expressed as functionally distinct or even antagonistic isoforms as a result of alternative splicing. Genes implicated in autophagy have been reported to undergo alternative splicing, including autophagosome markers (reviewed in [188]), although the functional significance remains to be investigated.

In this chapter, we review recent molecular and biochemical studies on alternative splicing of genes involved in regulating PCD and illustrate the current PCD paradigms. These genes range from extracellular signals and death receptors to the intracellular components of the PCD machinery. It is possible that alternative splicing profoundly contributes to the life-or-death decision of cells. Because of the large number of different PCD genes that undergo alternative splicing, it is difficult to cover all relevant aspects of these genes within this short chapter. We will describe selected examples to illustrate the extreme complexity of alternative splicing in cell death regulation and its impact on cancer pathogenesis and treatment.

2 Pre-mRNA Splicing and Alternative Splicing Regulation

In mammals, nascent transcripts (messenger RNA precursor, or pre-mRNAs) produced from the vast majority of protein-encoding genes contain intervening sequences or introns, that must be accurately removed to form functional messenger RNAs. In addition, it is now estimated that more than 90 % of human protein-coding genes undergo alternative splicing to generate distinct transcripts [114, 142], providing a robust post-transcriptional mechanism for increasing genetic diversity. Mammalian gene regulation is a highly complex process, involving multiple interconnected networks of regulation [184]. Disruption of such a regulated process leads to a wide range of diseases including cancer [36, 165].

Alternative splicing is regulated by intricate interactions between cis-regulatory elements and splicing machinery. There are four types of cis-acting regulatory sequence elements: splicing enhancers (SE) in introns (ISE) or exons (ESE) and splicing silencers (SS) in introns (ISS) or exons (ESS) [177]. Splicing enhancers recruit splicing activators to the spliceosome to stimulate splicing, whereas splicing silencers block the interaction between the spliceosome and the corresponding splice site. Multiple families of splicing factors have been identified with characteristic sequences such as the RNA-recognition motifs (RRM) and serine/arginine-rich (SR) proteins among others [124].

3 Alternative Splicing Regulation of Cell Death Genes

Cell death is a tightly regulated process. The components of the cell death machinery that control and execute this process are under strict regulation as well. At the post-transcriptional level, alternative splicing is one of the most powerful and diverse mechanisms that regulate the expression and function of many PCD genes. A large number of players function together in a carefully orchestrated manner to control cell death.

3.1 Alternative Splicing Isoforms of Genes Encoding Caspases and Other PCD-Related Proteases

Caspases are a family of cysteine proteases that play important roles in cell death regulation and cytokine secretion. Activation of pro-apoptotic caspase (caspase 2, 3, 6, 7, 8, 9, and 10) is a central pathway for different death signals (for reviews; [104, 156]). Each caspase has different sets of isoforms as a result of alternative splicing ([74, 75, 76, 95, 128], for reviews see [185, 190]). Many caspase genes produce pro- and anti-PCD isoforms as a result of alternative splicing, further support that alternative splicing is a common mechanism for regulating caspase gene expression [74, 85].

Caspase-1 is also known as IL-1β converting enzyme (ICE) that processes pro-inflammatory cytokine precursors pro-IL-1β and pro-IL-18. Recent studies show that caspase-1 also activates pro-apoptotic caspase-7 by processing pro-caspase-7 ([3, 105], for review [55]). Caspase-1 is activated by various cell death stimuli, such as bacterial toxin, LPS, microbial/viral nucleic acids, viral infection, reactive oxygen species (ROS), and asbestos. Five splicing isoforms of caspase-1 (caspase $1\alpha - 1\varepsilon$) have been reported. Among these, caspase-1δ and -1ε display an anti-apoptotic effect [6, 52].

Alternative splicing of caspase-2 generates five splicing isoforms: caspase-2L, caspase-2S, caspase-2β, caspase-2L-Pro, and caspase-2S-Pro. Caspase-2β, a possible negative regulator of caspase-2 activity, contains a deletion downstream of the first potential aspartic proteolytic cleavage site between the large and small subunits [5]. In addition, caspase-2S has anti-apoptotic activity [14, 46]. Interestingly, caspase-2S is abundant in the developing brain, suggesting that caspase-2 alternative splicing is developmentally regulated [14].

In caspase-8, retention of intron 8 results in the formation of caspase-8L mRNA and the caspase-8L protein that lacks the C-terminal half of the proteolytic domain. Patients with systemic lupus erythematosus (SLE) also display alternative splicing of caspase-8 [76]. Overexpression of caspase-8L inhibits Fas-mediated apoptosis, suggesting dominant negative effects of caspase-8L [75].

In addition to caspase genes, other protease genes involved in cell death also undergo alternative splicing. Calpains are Ca^{2+}-regulated proteases important for apoptotic, necrotic, and pyroptotic cell death. M- and μ-calpain are expressed ubiquitously and share the regulatory small subunit called calpain 4. Cells lacking calpain 4 exhibit resistance against certain PCD stimuli. In addition, an intrinsic calpain inhibitor, calpastatin, has at least eight splicing isoforms, some of which exhibit tissue-specific expression [66]. The role of alternative splicing in regulating calpains and calpastatin remains to be further characterized.

Cathepsins are a family of lysosomal proteases participating in the hydrolysis of macro-molecules in lysosomes. Cathepsins are released into the cytosol by various cell death signals and activate downstream PCD signaling. For example, Bid, a pro-apoptotic Bcl-2 family member, is cleaved by cathepsins released from lysosomes and translocates from the cytosol to the mitochondria, inducing mitochondrial death. Cathepsins activate other PCD associated DNases. Cathepsin leakage from lysosomes is observed during necrosis and pyroptosis as well [192].

The cathepsin B gene generates at least 3 splicing isoforms. Exon 2, which is an alternative cassette exon located at the 5′ untranslated region (UTR) of cathepsin B full-length mRNA, down-regulates cathepsin B expression [203]. On the other hand, alternative splicing also modulates the subcellular localization of cathepsin B. Exclusion of exons 2 and 3 results in a protein with a different N-terminus that serves as a mitochondrial targeting sequence [135]. This isoform contains a catalytic domain but does not have protease activity possibly because of misfolding. Overexpression of this isoform changes the mitochondrial morphology and induces cell death. Therefore, alternative splicing may trigger cell death by changing the cellular localization of cathepsin B.

3.2 Bcl-2 Superfamily

The Bcl-2 gene family of proteins mediates a complex network of interactions among different pro- and anti-apoptotic proteins as well as downstream molecules [99, 112]. They play important roles in controlling mitochondrial permeability, cytochrome C release, and caspase activation. The human Bcl-2 family has multiple members including pro- and anti-apoptotic genes. Prototypical anti-apoptotic members including Bcl-2, Bcl-w, Bfl-1/A1, Mcl-1, and Boo/DIVA usually contain four Bcl2-homology (BH) (BH1-4) domains. Pro-apoptotic members, on the other hand, contain two or more BH domains (BH1-3) (Bax, Bak, Bok/Mtd, Bcl-G, Boo/Diva, and Bfk) or only the BH3 domain (BH3-only protein family). The list of BH3-only protein family members has continuously grown (Bad, Bid, Bik, Bim, Blk, Hrk, Noxa, BNIP1, BNIP3, BNIP3L, Bmf, and Beclin-1). Furthermore, many proteins containing BH3-like domains have been reported (APO L1, APO L6, BRCC2, HER2, HER4, MAP-1, MULE, SPHK2, Rad9, and TGM2). These proteins have death inducing activity as well as the ability to interact with the anti-apoptotic Bcl-2 family as well as BH3-only proteins. Beclin-1, for example, is a critical effecter of autophagy. Bad and Bik can induce autophagic cell death.

The role of alternative splicing in the Bcl-2 family gene regulation has not yet been fully elucidated. Several genes of this superfamily including Bcl-x, Bak, Mcl-1, and Bid encode for anti-apoptotic (Bcl-xL, N-Bak, Mcl-1L, BidS) and pro-apoptotic (Bcl-xS, Bak, Mcl-1S, Bid) isoforms as a result of alternative splicing [10, 18, 154]. Bid is a prominent member of the BH3-only family that bridges the death receptor signaling pathway to the mitochondrial signaling pathway, which is mediated by other Bcl-2 family member proteins. Alternative splicing of *Bid* pre-mRNA generates isoforms lacking proteolytic cleavage sites (BidES, lacking all cleavage sites; BidS, lacking the granzyme B cleavage site) [110, 117]. In addition, some of Bcl-2 family proteins have a transmembrane domain that can be removed by alternative splicing, leading to differential subcellular distribution. Therefore, alternative splicing regulation of Bcl-2-related proteins has a considerable impact on cell death signaling pathway.

3.3 Death Ligands and Death Receptors

Death ligands and their receptors have been studied since the discovery of FAS, a member of the TNF (Tumor Necrosis Factor) superfamily. TNF-α, TNFSF1/Lynphotoxin-α, TNFSF3/Lynphotoxin-α, TRAIL, VEGI, TWEAK, and LIGHT proteins mediate apoptosis. TRAIL (*TNF-related apoptosis-inducing ligand*) has three splicing isoforms: TRAIL-α, β, and γ. TRAIL-α, the full-length form, contains five exons and promotes apoptosis. In contrast, apoptotic activity is not observed when exon 3 (TRAIL-β) or exons 2 and 3 (TRAIL-γ) are skipped [100]. In addition to TRAIL, splicing isoforms of TNFSF1 and VEGI are reported [26, 170]. In naïve T cell lymphocytes, TNF-α transcripts do not undergo splicing and are instead stored as pre-mRNA. TNF-α pre-mRNA splicing is initiated to produce TNF-α protein following the engagement of T cell receptors [195].

In addition to the TNF superfamily, other ligands, such as growth factors, neurotrophic factors, and cytokines participate in cell death regulation. Several neurotrophic factor genes of the TGF-β superfamily contain introns in their prodomains, including persephin, neurturin (NTN), and glial cell line–derived neurotrophic factor (GDNF). The GDNF gene produces a short isoform by removing 78 bases at the end of exon 1. The short isoform GDNFΔ78 accumulates in the Golgi apparatus and secretion of GDNFΔ78 is repressed [182]. It is conceivable that activation of this splicing event occurs in response to certain stimuli, providing an efficient post-transcriptional mechanism controlling the production of functional mRNAs for trophic factors such as NTN and GDNF.

Alternative splicing of transmembrane receptors may lead to the formation and secretion of the soluble receptors of cell death related ligands. In fact, many transmembrane receptors have splicing isoforms that encode soluble proteins capable of modifying the downstream ligand effects in antagonistic or agonistic manners [108]. For example, FAS has multiple alternative splicing isoforms lacking the transmembrane domain [25, 145]. Alternative splicing of Fas exon 6 produces a soluble (lacking exon 6) or a membrane-bound (containing exon 6) protein product. Soluble FAS proteins suppress PCD induced by FAS ligand and participate in T cell regulation, immune diseases, and cancer development. A membrane-bound form of the FAS receptor found in thymocytes lacks exon 7 and is missing the death domain (DD) due to the frame shift caused by exon 6 retention. This FAS alternative splicing isoform acts as a FAS decoy receptor (FDR) because it blocks PCD induced by FAS ligands as well as soluble FAS.

Other death receptors have multiple splicing variants: tumor necrosis factor receptor 1 (TNF-R1), lymphocyte-associated receptor of death (LARD, also named as DR3, Apo-3 or TRAMP), death receptor-4 (DR4), and TRAIL receptor inducer of cell killing-2 (TRICK-2) [101]. Additionally, many cytokine receptor genes are alternatively spliced to generate functionally diverse receptor isoforms. For example, alternative splicing generates truncated interleukin 7 (IL-7) receptor isoforms associated with leukemia [180]. Therefore, alternative splicing modulates the expression and function of genes encoding both death ligands and death receptors.

PCD signals from extracellular ligands are often transduced by proteins containing death domains (DDs) and death effector domains (DEDs). DD and DED are homophilic protein interaction motifs that allow association between different proteins containing DDs or DEDs. For example, FAS recruits FADD through an interaction between their respective DDs. The DED of FADD in turn recruits caspase 8 via interaction between DEDs of the FADD and caspase 8. In addition, some DD and/or DED containing proteins modulate cell death signaling. Two DEDs are located at N terminus of caspase 8 and 10. Viral proteins named v-FLIPs have been found in equine herpesvirus-2, bovine herpesvirus-4, herpesvirus saimili human herpesvirus-8, and human poxvirus. These v-FLIP proteins show homology to the N-terminus of caspase 8/10 but lack the cysteine protease domain. Viral-FLIP proteins bind to FADD and/or caspase 8/10 and interfere with their recruitment to Fas-FADD receptor complex. Cellular FLIP (c-FLIP, also known as Casper/I-FLICE/FLAM/CASH/CLARP/MRIT/usurpin) was discovered based on viral protein sequence information. The *c-FLIP* gene generates three splicing isoforms—$FLIP_L$, $FLIP_S$, and $FLIP_R$ by alternative splicing [44, 65]. The sequence of $FLIP_L$ protein is similar to caspase 8, including the two aspartic acid residues at the autocleavage site, although it lacks caspase enzymatic activity. $FLIP_S$ and $FLIP_R$ lack a cysteine protease-like region, similar to v-FLIP. $FLIP_L$ is expressed in many tissues, whereas $FLIP_S$ is detectable mainly in T lymphocytes. $FLIP_S$ expression in T cells activated by CD3 and CD28 has been shown to correlate with the cellular resistance against FAS-mediated apoptosis [94]. On the other hand, IL-2 upregulates FAS expression and represses the transcription and expression of $FLIP_S$ in T cells, sensitizing T cells to apoptosis [152]. These results suggest important roles of $FLIP_S$ in activation-induced cell death (AICD) and self-tolerance. A similar expression pattern of $FLIP_R$ and $FLIP_S$ in CD3 and CD28-activated T cells has been reported [65]. Although the anti-apoptotic effects of $FLIP_L$ and $FLIP_S$ are reported, $FLIP_L$ also stimulates apoptosis under certain conditions. $FLIP_L$ can activate caspase 8 after the formation of a heterodimer on FADD and death receptor complexes. It has been proposed that activation of caspase 8 by $FLIP_L$ results in partial autocleavage of caspase 8 into the p43/41 and p12 subunits. This mechanism tethers caspase 8 on the death-induced signaling complex (DISC) by FADD and processes receptor-interacting kinase (RIP) within the FAS-signaling complex [125]. $FLIP_L$ may generate proliferation signals from DISC by processing DISC-proximal substrates, as a result of activation of ERK and NFkB by $FLIP_L$ in T cells [91].

The caspase activation and recruitment domain/caspase recruitment domain (CARD) is engaged in homophilic interactions with CARD containing caspases. TUCAN/CARD8/CARDINAL, cloned as an anti-apoptotic CARD containing protein, is overexpressed in colon cancer [147]. TUCAN can interact with caspase-9 via the CARD domains and interfere with the binding between Apaf-α and caspase-9. Interestingly, TUCAN also induces cell death when overexpressed in MCF7 and VERO cells. A TUCAN splicing isoform, TUCAN-54, has been recently reported as a cancer-specific protein expressed in gastric, colon, and breast cancer tissues. TUCAN-54 exhibits anti-apoptotic activity by inhibiting caspase-9 and caspase-8 activation. TUCAN along with caspase-9 and DRAL (a LIM domain protein) are recruited by the Shh receptor, Patched, to enhance cell death [127]. Therefore, TUCAN alternative splicing regulation may be important both in normal development and in cancer pathogenesis.

MAPK-activating death domain-containing protein (MADD) is a Rab3 GTP/GDP exchange protein containing a DD motif. There are six reported isoforms: IG20pa, MADD, IG20-SV2, DENN-SV, KIAA0358, and IG20-SV4 [111]. IG20pa render cells more susceptible to PCD by TNF-α, TRAIL, γ-irradiation, and cancer drugs; however, DENN-SV has an opposite effect, promoting cancer cell suvival [7, 48, 49, 102, 136, 137].

3.4 Intrinsic Cell Death Signals

The death domain mediates not only receptor-mediated cell death signals, but also intrinsic cell death signals. PIDD (P53-Induced Protein with Death Domain), which is induced by p53, interacts with caspase 2 by RAIDD bridging, and activates caspase-2, forming a protein complex known as PIDDosome. Binding between PIDD and RAIDD is mediated by a homophilic interaction of their DDs. Caspase 2 is recruited via an interaction between the CARDs of caspase 2 and RAIDD. Among the five reported splicing isoforms of PIDD, isoform 2 (also known as LRDD) counteracts the pro-apoptotic activity of full-length PIDD isoform 1 [35]. Similarly, Apaf-1 recruits caspase 9 with cytochrome C and dATP and forms apoptosome. Apaf-*1* gene also generates pro- and anti- apoptotic splicing isoforms [140].

Similar to PIDDosome, NALP1 (NACHT leucine-rich-repeat protein 1) interacts with caspase 1 via ASC (Apoptosis-associated speck-like protein containing a CARD). The PYD motifs of NALP1 and ASC and the CARD motifs of ASC and caspase 1 interact together to comprise inflammasomes. The NALP family is composed of at least 14 genes (NALP1-14). NALP proteins consist of PYD, NACHT domain, and leucine-rich repeats (LRRs). The NACHT domain has a predicted P-loop NTPase sequence and is extracted across different proteins: NAIP (Neural Apoptosis Inhibitory Peptide), CIITA (class II transactivator), HET-E (incompatibility locus protein from Podospora anserine), and TP1 (telomerase-associated protein). Interestingly, NACHT domain shares homology with the dATP binding domain of Apaf-1. The LRRs of NALPs are thought to be able to sense various microbial molecules in intracellular space to form inflammasomes. Many members of NALP family have multiple alternative splicing isoforms (JYW, unpublished data).

PYD (pyrin domain) containing proteins and caspase 1 are involved in processing pro-IL-1/18 and pro-apoptotic caspase 7. PYD is a homophilic adapter domain as well as for DD and DED. Familial Mediterranean fever (MEFV) encodes PYD containing proteins interacting with ASC. The human *MEFV* gene produces multiple isoforms including full-length (MEFV-fl) and MEFV-d2 [42]. MEFV-fl encodes a cytoplasmic protein, whereas MEFV-d2 protein is concentrated in the nucleus [144]. Multiple components of inflammasome, including TUCAN, have distinct alternative splicing isoforms [2]. Alternative splicing may regulate the pyroptotic cell death signaling.

3.5 Inhibitor of Apoptosis Proteins (IAPs)

IAPs, first identified in baculovirus, contain 1–3 BIR motifs and one RING domain. BIR domains bind caspases and inhibit protease activity and RING domains recruit E2 ubiquitin conjugating enzyme and transfer ubiquitins onto itself or binding partners. Survivin, a member of the IAP family, contains a BIR domain but lacks a RING domain. Interestingly, Survivin still retains anti-apoptotic activity (for reviews, [141]). The Survivin gene generates several splicing isoforms. Among them, Survivin 2α and 2β uniquely display pro-apoptotic activity. Survivin 2β splicing is upregulated by Wilms Tumor 1 associated protein (WTAP) [169]. The alternative splicing pattern of Survivin pre-mRNA changes dynamically in cancer. Survivin alternative splicing has been considered as a diagnostic marker and therapeutic target (reviewed in [158]).

Two different splicing isoforms of livin, another member of the IAP family, livin α and β, have different tissue expression patterns and show distinct properties in inhibiting apoptosis induced by different signals [9].

3.6 Cell Death-Related DNases and Their Regulators

Caspase-activated DNases (CAD) are critical nucleases in PCD. Other notable DNAses are Endo G, LEI/L-DNase II, and GAAD. ICAD/DFF45 is a chaperonin for Caspase-activated DNase (CAD/DFF40) and inhibits the CAD/DFF40 activity. ICAD/DFF45 is one of substrates for capsases. Cleavage of ICAD/DFF45 by caspases releases CAD/DFF40 from the ICAD/DFF45-CAD/DFF40 complex and activates CAD/DFF40 DNase activity. There are at least two splicing isoforms encoded by the ICAD/DFF45 gene. The short isoform is generated by the retention of intron 5 which contains an in-frame stop codon. Although ICAD/DFF45 (ICAD-L) is necessary for CAD/DFF40 peptide to be folded properly, the short isoform ICAD-S/DFF35 does not have the ability to function as a chaperonin. However, ICAD-S binds to CAD/DFF40 more strongly than ICAD/DFF45 and can inhibit the DNase activity of CAD/DFF40. ICAD/DFF45 contains a nuclear localization signal and is expressed in nuclei whereas ICAD-S/DFF35 is also distributed to the cytosol. Aberrant splicing products of CAD/DFF40 have been detected in human hepatoma cells, but biological functions of those isoforms have not yet been characterized [78].

Endonuclease G (Endo G) is another DNase that is released from the mitochondria during PCD. Because the yeast orthologue of Endo G participates in caspase independent PCD, Endo G is thought to contribute to caspase independent PCD in mammalian cells [23, 34]. LEI/L-DNase II and GAAD also contribute to caspase independent PCD. There are many predicted alternative splicing isoforms for Endo G, LEI/L-DNase II, and GAAD isoforms; however, their biological roles and splicing regulation are still unclear.

3.7 Mitochondrial Cell Death Proteins

Since the discovery of the role of cytochrome C in apoptosis, many other mitochondrial factors have been reported to regulate cell death, such as Smac, Omi, and AIF.

Initially identified as an inhibitor of IAPs, Smac/DIABLO has a number of splicing isoforms including Smac-β (Smac S), γ, δ, and Smac 3 [56, 172]. As a result of alternative splicing, Smac-β lacks the mitochondrial targeting sequence at its N terminus and displays a distinct distribution in cells, rather than the mitochondrial localization. Although Smac-β does not interact with IAPs, Smac-β is pro-apoptotic. Smac 3 is missing exon 4, but still contains the mitochondria targeting sequence and IAPs binding domain. Smac 3 disrupts caspase 9 binding to XIAP, promotes caspase 3 activation, and accelerates the auto-ubiquitination of XIAP, whereas the full-length Smac does not accelerate XIAP auto-ubiquitination. Smac 3 localizes to the mitochondria and is released into the cytosol following apoptosis signaling [56].

AIF induces cell death after being released from mitochondria. However, AIF induced cell death does not show oligonucleosome fragmentation, a hallmark of caspase-dependent cell death induced by CAD activation. In fact, cathepsins and calpains can release AIF from the mitochondria to trigger necrotic cell death [37]. Human AIF gene generates multiple alternative splicing isoforms: AIF, AIF-exB, AIFsh, AIFsh2, and AIFsh3 [38, 39]. AIFsh retains pro-apoptotic activity and is expressed in the cytosol due to a missing mitochondria targeting sequence caused by alternative splicing. Therefore, alternative splicing may induce cell death by producing cytosolic AIFsh.

3.8 Autophagy, Cell Death, and Alternative Splicing of Autophagy Regulatory Genes

Autophagy is an essential cellular process mediating the degradation of damaged or degenerated cellular materials. During this process, an isolated membrane sequesters unwanted macromolecules and organelles, such as aggregation-prone proteins and malfunctioning mitochondria. The formed double-membraned vacuoles are called autophagosomes, which in turn fuse with lysosomes forming autolysosomes to degrade their contents [96, 107]. The autophagy pathway is highly conserved from yeast to humans, playing important roles in cellular homeostasis [11, 153]. Under physiological conditions, autophagy degrades altered proteins and organelles, eliminating from the cell malfunctioning components and simultaneously recycling molecular components for the regeneration of new organelles. During nutrient deprivation, autophagy plays critical roles in the adaptation of organisms to new environmental conditions, providing nutrients from degraded cellular contents to maintain cellular metabolism [129].

In addition to cell survival, autophagy mediates cell death, although the underlying molecular mechanisms remain to be elucidated. The phenomenon of autophagic cell death (also known as type II programmed cell death) was observed in the 1960s. At the ultrastructural level, autophagic cell death is characterized primarily by the formation of numerous autophagic vacuoles in dying cells [27, 160, 161]. Autophagy genes Atg7 and Beclin1 are required for cell death in certain types of cells [197, 198]. However, the role of autophagy in regulating cell death remains unclear.

The mammalian target of rapamycin (mTOR) is a kinase that plays important roles in cellular metabolism, cell growth, cell proliferation, and autophagy [41, 43, 71, 188]. mTOR is initially inhibited during starvation, which triggers autophagy. A recent study shows that the mTOR signaling can be reactivated by prolonged starvation, which in turn forms an evolutionarily conserved cycle that maintains energetic homeostasis during cellular starvation [199]. Two splicing isoforms of mTOR have been identified: mTORα (the full-length protein) and mTORβ. mTORβ is capable of regulating cell cycle and cell proliferation. Notably, mTORβ may act as a proto-oncogene, because overexpression of mTORβ leads to immortalization of cells and is tumorigenic in nude mice [143]. However, the role of mTORβ in autophagy remains to be investigated.

Microtubule-associated protein light chain 3 (LC3), a mammalian homologue of yeast Atg8, is another essential component of autophagy [88]. LC3-I can be converted to LC3-II and then processed to bind tightly to the autophagosomal membrane. In rats, two alternative splicing isoforms of LC3 are produced, LC3A and LC3B, which generate proteolytic II forms from precursor I forms and colocalize with LC3. In different rat tissues LC3A, LC3B, and LC3 show different expression patterns, suggesting possible regulation of LC3 by alternative splicing [186].

Tumor protein 53-induced nuclear protein 1, TP53INP1, shows sequence similarity to TP53INP2, a protein essential for autophagy in mammalian cells by interacting with VMP1 and recruiting LC3 and/or LC3-related proteins to initiate the autophagosome [139]. Alternative splicing of TP53INP2 appears to be important for cell invasion, although its role in autophagy remains unclear [134].

Many other autophagy regulatory genes have splicing isoforms. For instance, ULK (uncoordinated-51 like kinase) protein is the mammalian counterpart of yeast Atg1, a Ser/Thr protein kinase involved in the initial step of autophagosome formation in collaboration with its regulators, Atg13, Atg17, Atg29, and Atg31 [61, 86]. Human ULK2 has two alternatively spliced transcript variants that differ in the 3′ UTR that may have different mRNA stability. However, the functional difference among the splicing variants is still unknown. Further studies are necessary to understand the role of alternative splicing in regulating autophagy.

4 Alternative Splicing: A Versatile Mechanism for Regulating Expression and Function of Cell Death Genes

Emerging evidence, some of which is summarized above, supports that a wide range of cell death genes undergo alternative splicing that impact their activities in regulating programmed cell death. Many of these PCD genes express alternative splicing isoforms in a tissue- or development stage-specific manner. In naïve T lymphocytes, TNF-α transcripts do not undergo splicing and are stored as pre-mRNA. TNF-α pre-mRNA splicing is only initiated to produce TNF-α protein following the engagement of T cell receptors [194]. In na B and T cells, LARD-1 (lymphocyte-associated receptor of death 1) is expressed as alternative isoforms with very little full-length mRNA [163]. The full-length LARD-1 becomes the predominant product after T cell activation.

Bcl-x pre-mRNA is alternatively spliced to produce two isoforms with opposing functions. The two isoforms are produced by using different 5′ splice sites (ss) in exon 2. The use of the upstream 5′ ss produces a shorter product, Bcl-xS and the downstream site gives rise to Bcl-xL. Bcl-xS is pro-apoptotic while the longer form is anti-apoptotic. Adult neurons predominantly express the Bcl-xL mRNA; whereas immature thymocytes express a relatively high level of Bcl-xS transcript [18]. Adding further to the complexity, several critical PCD regulators have been found to use alternative splicing to generate gene products that have antagonistic activities in cell death. The mechanism by which alternative splicing may regulate function of these PCD genes can be summarized in at least three aspects:

- regulating subcellular localization of PCD gene products
- modulating functional activity of PCD gene products
- influencing stability of mRNA and/or translational control

4.1 Regulation of Subcellular Localization

Many cell death genes, including the death receptor family, Bcl-2 superfamily, and cell death associated proteases, have both membrane associated as well as soluble isoforms (see review [185]). Alternative splicing of these cell death genes produce proteins that contain or lack their transmembrane domains, thus generating gene products with different subcellular localization. These different isoforms may have distinct functions in PCD. For example, several Fas splicing variant mRNAs encode soluble proteins that block Fas-mediated apoptosis induced by the agonistic antibody [25] and by the Fas ligand [145]. Another Fas isoform, Fas-EX08Del, is generated by exon 8 skipping. This isoform contains a premature termination codon and thus lacks the entire intracytoplasmic death domain. Fas-EX08Del is only expressed in resistant tumor clones [25]. It is likely that different alternative splicing products of the death receptor may have distinct roles in the propagation of the cell death or survival signals.

Genes from the Bcl-2 superfamily undergo alternative splicing to generate different isoforms with distinct intracellular localization (reviewed in [4]). For example, both membrane-bound and soluble isoforms of Bcl-2 gene members are produced as a result of alternative splicing. As described previously, different splicing isoforms of mitochondrial cell death proteins lacking or containing their mitochondrial targeting sequences may have distinct function in cell death. Finally, alternative splicing may regulate the terminal events in cell death such as chromosome fragmentation and DNA degradation. For example, the nuclear localized ICAD-L and cytoplasmic ICAD-S are generated by alternative splicing which removes the nuclear localization signal in ICAD-L to form ICAD-S [157]. ICAD-L and ICAD-S may have different regulatory activities in cell death.

4.2 Modulating Functional Activities

Interestingly, many PCD associated genes generate splicing isoforms that have antagonistic activities, such as caspase-2L versus caspase-2S [31, 59]. Recent analyses indicate that a majority of the known caspase family members have alternative splicing at or near the regions encoding peptide sequences contributing to their active sites for enzyme activity [74]. Alternative splicing events that generate truncated peptides provide an additional mechanism to quantitatively regulate gene expression. The delicate balance of different pro-apoptotic and anti-apoptotic products of these PCD genes likely plays a critical role in determining cellular susceptibility to death signals. Alternative splicing can regulate each step of cell death induction or execution by generating distinct gene products with different or even antagonistic activities in cell death.

4.3 Altering mRNA Stability or Translational Efficiency

Alternative splicing can generate mRNAs with differential turnover rates or with differential properties in translational control (reviewed in [79]). A large number of alternative splicing events occur at 5′ or 3′ untranslated regions of cell death genes. For example, exon 2 of cathepsin B is an alternative exon and encodes the 5′ UTR regulating the protein expression level [135]. Caspase-2 mRNA undergoes nonsense-mediated decay (NMD) under certain conditions, and its protein expression may be tightly regulated by combination of alternative splicing and NMD [29]. A conserved AU-rich element has been identified in the 3′ UTR of Bcl-2 mRNA. This element interacts with AU-rich binding proteins and is associated with bcl-2-down-regulation during apoptosis [45, 159]. IL-1RI-associated kinase-1 (IRAK1) is a serine-threonine kinase important for IL-1 signaling and has different splicing isoforms. The IRAK1b isoform is kinase inactive and more stable than IRAK1 isoform. It is conceivable that different splicing isoforms of critical cell death genes that contain distinct elements for controlling their mRNA or protein stability could have a significant impact on the expression and function of these cell death genes.

5 Molecular Mechanisms Regulating Alternative Splicing of Cell Death Genes

5.1 Splicing Signals, Splicing Machinery, and Alternative Splicing Regulators

With combined approaches, significant progress has been made in identifying the molecular components of splicing machinery and in understanding the mechanisms that control alternative splicing [17, 24, 73, 123, 132, 133, 166]. Through highly dynamic RNA–RNA, protein-RNA, and protein–protein interactions, components of the splicing machinery assemble onto the pre-mRNA and form the catalytically active spliceosome in which biochemical reactions of splicing take place.

The basic splicing signals include the 5′ splice site, branch site, and polypyrimidine track-AG at the 3′ splice site. These signals are initially recognized by the U1 snRNP, U2 snRNP, and U2 snRNP Auxiliary Factor (U2AF), respectively. In mammals, these basic splicing signals tend to be degenerate and are not sufficient by themselves to confer the specificity required to achieve accurate splice site selection. A number of other factors also contribute to splice site recognition and influence splicing efficiency. These include the distance between two splice sites, exon size, as well as local secondary structures in the pre-mRNAs. In addition, various types of exonic and intronic elements have been identified that modulate the usage of nearby splice sites. For example, exonic or intronic splicing enhancers (ESEs or ISEs) and exonic or intronic splicing silencers (ESEs or ISEs and ESSs or ISSs respectively) in different genes have been described (for reviews see Hertel et al. 2008; [70, 183]). These splicing enhancers or silencers can promote or inhibit the use of either upstream 3′ splice sites or downstream 5′ splice sites. Many splicing enhancer elements function by interacting with different members or combinations of SR proteins and hnRNP proteins. A general theme has begun to emerge that the alternative splicing events of a given gene are regulated by a number of different splicing activators and repressors. In most cases, precise molecular mechanisms underlying the splicing inhibition remain to be elucidated.

The specific recognition of splice sites and proper association between authentic 5′ and 3′ splice sites is the central issue for pre-mRNA splicing and alternative splicing regulation. Spliceosomal snRNPs including U1 (or U11), U2 (or U12), U4/U6 (or U4atac/U6atac), and U5 play important roles in splice site recognition and association. In addition to the snRNPs, several families of accessory proteins are also important in regulating alternative splicing. These factors include heteronuclear ribonucleoproteins family (hnRNP proteins), proteins containing serine-arginine-rich sequences (SR proteins) and other RNA-binding proteins ([16, 187]; see Chap. 3). In many cases, SR proteins function as splicing activators by binding enhancer sequences, whereas hnRNP proteins often function as splicing respressors by binding splicing silencer sequences [113]. Other splicing regulators include KH-domain-containing proteins, CUGBP proteins, and proteins containing other sequence motifs (for example, helicase, RGG, zinc finger) [87]. There are also a number of proteins that can act as either splicing activators or splicing repressors depending on the splicing substrates and their binding sites [186, 187].

Aberrant pre-mRNA splicing has been implicated in human diseases associated with either excessive or insufficient cell death, although underlying molecular mechanisms remain to be elucidated (for reviews, [17, 89, 123, 149, 168, 183].

5.2 Mechanisms Underlying Alternative Splicing Regulation of PCD Genes

In recent years, a number of cell death genes have been characterized in detail for mechanisms underlying their alternative splicing regulation. Only a few examples are shown here, including FAS, Bcl-x, and caspase-2. As discussed before, alternative splicing of FAS exon 6 leads to the formation of the membrane-bound full-length FAS-L isoform and exon 6-skipped soluble FAS-s isoform. Two related splicing regulators TIA1 and TIAR stimulate exon 6 inclusion by binding to a U-rich sequence downstream of the 5′ splice site of exon 6 and promoting U1 snRNP interaction with this 5′ splice site [53, 54]. A protein kinase, Fas-activated serine/threonine kinase (FAST K) synergizes with TIA1 and TIAR to enhance FAS exon 6 inclusion [83]. On the other hand, Polypyrimidine Tract Binding protein (PTB), promotes exon 6 skipping by binding to an exonic splicing silencer [82]. RNA binding protein SPF45, which has a U2AF homology motif (UHM), interacts with the SF3b155 ULM (UHM-ligand motif) domain to enhance inclusion of Fas exon 6. This binding plays a critical role in FAS exon 6 inclusion [30]. During the early stages of apoptosis, U2AF65 is cleaved and the N-terminal fragment of U2AF65 has a dominant negative effect on FAS exon 6 splicing [81] thus leading to formation of the Fas-s isoform. Hu antigen R (HuR) binds to the ESS on FAS pre-mRNA and inhibits the association of U2AF65 with the 3′ss [84]. RBM5 excludes exon 6 of FAS pre-mRNA. Interestingly, RBM5 does not affect U1 and U2 snRNP assembly on FAS pre-mRNA but inhibits the transition from pre-spliceosome to mature spliceosome via interaction between U4/5/6 trisnRNP and the OCRE domain of RBM5 [20].

The production of anti- and pro-apoptotic isoforms of Bcl-x involves alternative selection of two competing 5′ splice sites. Both exonic and intronic elements have been identified in Bcl-x that regulate its alternative splicing [109, 120]. Trans-acting factors involved include SAP155, Sam68, hnRNA A1, hnRNP F/H, SRp30c, and RBM25 [28, 62, 146, 201]. An apoptotic agent Ro-31-8220 inhibits PKC and activates JNK, and concomitantly, Bcl-xL splicing is inhibited. This effect is repressed by okadaic acid, an inhibitor against PP1 and PP2A. Okadaic acid splicing regulation is mediated via a 16-nt G-tract element (Gt16) on pre-mRNAs [69]. Emetine, a protein synthesis inhibitor, also upregulates Bcl-xS splicing. However, emetine upregulation is blocked by calyculin A by inhibiting PP1 and PP2A [21]. Various stimuli are reported to change Bcl-xL/Bcl-xS ratio. For example, IL-6, GM-CSF, and TPA all upregulate Bcl-xL splicing in erythroleukemia and glioma. The Bcl-xS isoform is induced by S-adenosylmethionine (SAMe), whose synthesis is impaired by liver injury. β-adrenergic receptor activation upregulates Bcl-xS and induces cell death of cardiomyocytes. Consistently, β-blockers inhibit Bcl-xS induction. Ceramide responsive elements CRCE1 and 2 have been identified in Bcl-x pre-mRNA. Ceramide appears to regulate Bcl-x splicing via SAP155 which binds to CRCE1 [121, 122]. Although Bcl-x splicing responds to a number of stimuli, it still remains unclear how these signals transduce to the splicing machinery. A recent study using genomic siRNA screening for Bcl-x splicing regulators has uncovered a complex network of splicing regulators that link cell cycle and cell death controls [133].

In the case of caspase-2, several splicing factors have been identified to regulate the formation of anti-apoptotic (caspase-2S) and pro-apoptotic (caspase-2L) splicing isoforms. Interestingly, SR proteins including SC35 and ASF/SF2 promote exon skipping to produce caspase-2L, whereas, hnRNPA1 facilitates exon inclusion to produce caspase-2S [85]. The effects of these SR proteins and of hnRNP A1 on caspase-2 splicing are opposite to their effects on other model splicing substrates. A caspase-2 mini-gene model system has been used to dissect the cis-elements and trans-acting factors involved in caspase-2 alternative splicing ([85, 32]). An evolutionarily conserved 100 nt intronic element, In100, has been identified as an intronic splicing silencer element responsible for exon 9 exclusion between exon 9 and 10. The In100 element contains two domains: an upstream decoy 3′ splice site and a downstream PTB binding domain 32. The decoy 3′ splice site engages the 5′ splice site of the alternative exon 9 in a non-productive manner, effectively suppressing the use of this 5′ splice site without reducing U1 snRNP binding. PTB plays a role in regulating alternative splicing of a number of other genes (reviewed in [16, 171, 181]). The regulatory mechanism of PTB in caspase-2 alternative splicing appears to be distinct from that involved in other genes. Furthermore, our recent survey of human genome suggests that In100-like (Intron 100-like) intronic elements (i.e., decoy 3′ splice site juxtaposed to PTB binding domains) may represent a general intronic splicing regulatory motif and that such elements may play a role in the regulation alternative splicing of other cell death genes [74]. Recently, we reported that caspase 2 splicing is regulated by RBM5, which is frequently deleted in lung cancer [59]. RBM5 binds to the U/C-rich region immediately upstream of In100. These results suggest that splicing regulation plays an important role in cancer development via PCD-related gene products. However, crucial questions still remain unanswered. How does splicing machinery differentially recognize the decoy 3′ splice site inside In100 as a regulatory element as opposed to a true 3′ splice site? How are splicing regulators and cis-elements coordinated to regulate alternative splicing? Molecular dissection of cis-acting elements and trans-acting splicing regulators involved in caspase-2 alternative splicing has provided a good beginning point to understand the mechanisms underlying the complex regulation of alternative splicing of important PCD genes. The involvement of such a pseudo- or decoy splice site in alternative splicing regulation may provide an explanation for the phylogenic conservation of sequences containing pseudo-splicing signals in mammalian introns. Further studies are necessary to test whether pseudo-splice sites proximal to splicing repressor binding sites represent general splicing regulatory motifs.

5.3 Complex Networks Linking Alternative Splicing, Cell Death, and Other Processes

Recent efforts using systems biology approaches have begun to reveal the complex networks that link splicing regulation, cell death, and other important cellular processes [133]. Genome-wide analyses of splicing patterns can help identify specific gene products that are tumorigenic as well as involved in other cellular pathways. Gene regulation by alternative splicing plays critical roles in cellular differentiation, cell proliferation, and cell death. Therefore, imbalance in the splicing pathway can lead to tumorigenic events [63]. High-throughput microarray analyses and next-generation sequencing assays have been used to identify alternative splicing events or factors involved in specific pathways [191]. Such studies will help to decipher the splicing codes that dictate normal cell development and subsequently, how mutations affect these events to give rise to cancer. Given the importance of alternative splicing in generating antagonistic isoforms of pro- or anti-apoptotic proteins, it is hopeful to target alternative splicing machinery for future cancer therapeutics.

6 Cell Death Regulation, Pre-mRNA Splicing, and Cancer

Mounting evidence supports that alternative splicing of genes involved in cell cycle control, cell proliferation, apoptosis, angiogenesis, motility, and invasion are associated with tumor progression and metastasis [116, 200]. In cancer, aberrant alternative splicing has been associated with mutations affecting cis-elements that regulate splicing. Such mutations may alter the abundance, localization, or post-translationally modify trans-acting factors that determine splice site selection [123]. The precise mechanisms by which alternative splicing controls expression of genes related to cancer remain poorly understood.

6.1 Splicing Factors, Splicing Variants, and Cancer

A number of factors regulating alternative splicing of cell death genes show oncogenic properties [68]. Splicing factors, such as hnRNP A1 [22], hnRNP A2, hnRNP B1, polypyrimidine tract binding protein (PTB), [148] and HuR, are frequently overexpressed in tumors. Splicing factor overexpression can trigger malignant transformation.

In addition, cancer-related splicing factor isoforms could alter function of these splicing factors, resulting in aberrant alternative splicing. Depletion of splicing factors prevents the generation of cancer-associated isoforms, suggesting splicing factors as potential therapeutic targets for cancer therapies. Tumor-specific variations in splicing may also generate new epitopes that can serve as anticancer agents.

6.2 Death Receptors and Cancer

Fas (Apo-1/CD95), a transmembrane death receptor, has a soluble isoform (sFas) generated by alternative splicing of Fas mRNA. sFas lacks the transmembrane domain and antagonizes cell-surface Fas function. sFas is detected in patients with different types of leukemia and solid tumors [90, 126], such as adult T cell leukemia (ATL), large granular lymphocyte (LGL), leukemia and renal cell carcinoma.

TNF-related apoptosis-inducing ligand (TRAIL) and its receptors, namely DR4, DR5, DcR1, and DcR2 have become attractive targets for anti-cancer therapies, because they seem to trigger apoptosis selectively in cancer cells but not in normal cells. Thus far, several compounds and biologics (such as agonistic TRAIL antibodies) have gained attention due to their anti-tumor efficacy [131, 151, 196].

In addition, c-FLIP modulates the activation of procaspase-8 and thereby prevents induction of apoptosis mediated by death receptors. There is evidence for increased c-FLIP expression in various types of tumor cells, including colorectal cancer [97], gastric cancer [138], Hodgkin's lymphoma [138], and ovarian cancer [1]. Thus, downregulating c-FLIP induced by pharmacological agents, such as proteasome inhibitors, protein or RNA synthesis inhibitors [57], or chemotherapeutic agents [103], may have therapeutic value for these types of cancer.

6.3 BCL-2 Family and Cancer

The Bcl-2 family of proteins are crucial players in regulation of apoptosis. Aberrant expression of members of this family has been associated with different cancers. Over-expression of Bcl-2 was originally observed in B cell lymphomas ([130]; reviewed in [98]). Bcl-2 overexpression has since been detected in other solid tumors in the lung, kidney, stomach, and brain [67, 119]. Interestingly, the relationship between Bcl-2 expression levels and cancer prognosis is cell type-dependent. For example, high levels of Bcl-2 were correlated with poor prognosis in certain lymphomas; however, low Bcl-2 expression as correlated with a poor prognosis in breast cancer. Experiments using knockout mice have advanced our understanding of the role of Bcl-2 family members in tumorigenesis. *Bad*-knockout mice develop B cell lymphoblastic leukemia/lymphoma when exposed to sub-lethal doses of γ-irradiation, whereas Bid-knockout mice show chromosomal aberrations and develop leukemia [202].

Furthermore, the imbalances between apoptosis-promoting and apoptosis-inhibiting members of the Bcl-2 family are also common in various human cancers. Myeloid cell leukemia-1 (MCL-1) has three splicing variants: anti-apoptotic MCL-1L and pro-apoptotic MCL-1S and MCL-1ES. There is an imbalance between the expression levels of MCL-1L, MCL-1S, and MCL-1ES in the skin basal cell carcinoma (BCC) cell line [167] and renal cancer [92]. Bcl-x mRNAs encoding a long isoform, Bcl-xL, predominates in various types of malignant lymphomas and may be involved in lymphomagenesis [190]. Bcl-xL was also expressed in human hepatoma cell lines at high levels and its down-regulation activated apoptosis [173]. Another Bcl-x alternative splicing product is Bcl-xAK, which contains the Bcl-2 homology domains, BH2 and BH4, as well as the transmembrane domain but lacks BH1 and BH3. Bcl-xAK is expressed in melanoma and other tumor cells and its overexpression results in significant induction of apoptosis in melanoma cells [77]. Another Bcl-2 family member, Bfk undergoes alternative splicing to produce four isoforms, out of which two are pro-apoptotic. In the transition from normal tissue to tumor, pro-apoptotic Bfk isoform expression is substantially reduced in tumors isolated from the human gastrointestinal tract [40].

6.4 Caspase Alternative Splicing and Cell Death Regulation in Cancer

Caspases play important roles in the regulation of physiological cell death, therefore, the disturbance of the caspases expression or function may contribute to the cancer formation. Caspase-9 initiates apoptosis and has two distinct protein isoforms generated as a result of alternative pre-mRNA splicing: pro-apoptotic caspase-9a and anti-apoptotic caspase-9b. A recent study demonstrated that hnRNP family member L (hnRNP L) is specifically phosphorylated in non–small cell lung cancer cells (NSCLC cells) and also associated with caspase-9 pre-mRNA. The interaction of hnRNP L with caspase-9 pre-mRNA in NSCLC cells promotes preferential expression of the 9b isoform of caspase-9, which is anti-apoptotic, and promotes tumor growth [64].

Another example is the caspase-2 tumor suppressor, which is alternatively spliced to generate multiple isoforms (discussed in Sect. 3.1). RBM5, by virtue of binding to the U/C-rich region in In100 splicing repressor element (see Sect. 5.2), promotes production of the proapoptotic caspase-2L isoform and regulates the ratio of caspase-2 isoforms in HeLa cells [59, 155]. Fas can lead to cell death and also be alternatively spliced to produce shorter isoforms. Exclusion of exon 6 in Fas pre-mRNA generates FasDelE6 which can inhibit Fas-mediated cell death. Recently, RBM5 [20] and HuR [81] have been identified to play an important role in Fas exon 6 inclusion.

Caspase-8L, generated by alternative splicing of caspase-8, can suppresses caspase 8-dependent apoptosis. The imbalanced expression of the caspase-8L splicing isoform has been associated with cancer. Suppressing the formation of caspase-8L splice variant renders cells more sensitive to apoptosis-induced neuroblastoma cell death [128]. In addition, a splice variant of IG20 gene regulating the activation of caspase-8 was implicated during tumorigenesis [111, 137].

6.5 IAPS and Cancer

Survivin, a member of the IAPS (inhibitor of apoptosis proteins) family, functions as a key regulator of mitosis and programmed cell death. It regulates cell death by interrupting multiple cell cycle-related proteins, such as INCENP and Aurora B kinase. Studies have shown survivin overexpression results from several polymorphisms in the survivin gene promoter [19, 150], which also correlate with tumorigenesis and prognosis [115, 172]. Therefore, survivin has become a target for cancer therapeutics [174].

Livin, an IAPS-related protein, has two different functional splicing variants that are characterized as anti-apoptotic [9]. Livin interacts with downstream caspases, such as caspase-3, caspase-7, and caspase-9, leading to their inactivation and degradation. Aberrant expression of Livin has been reported to be associated with tumorigenesis in many different cancer types including melanoma [179], breast cancer [193], and lung cancer [72]. Therefore, Livin is believed to be a new target for immunotherapy and gene therapy for treatment of cancer.

6.6 Cell Death-Related DNases and Their Regulators

Previous studies have demonstrated that the activity of alkaline (DNase I; EC 3.1.21.1) and acidic DNases (DNase II; EC 3.1.22.1) was inhibited in non-necrotic cells in malignant tumors. In subsequent studies, vitamin C and K3 administration reactivated these DNases to induce cancer cell death [175].

Endonuclease G (EndoG) cleaves chromatin DNA into nucleosomal fragments in the nucleus and participates in the caspase independent apoptotic pathway [80]. As a pro-apoptotic protein, decreased expression of EndoG has been found in several cancers, such as hepatocellular carcinomas and breast cancer [12].

6.7 Mitochondrial Cell Death Proteins and Cancer

Apoptosis can be activated through two pathways: the extrinsic pathway (mediated by death receptors) or the intrinsic pathway (mediated by mitochondria). As mentioned previously, mitochondrial factors such as Smac and AIF can adhere to IAPs and inhibit their caspase-binding activity, thereby regulating cell death and tumorigenesis. For example, in a malignant glioma xenograft mice model, co-administration of Smac/DIABLO peptides and TRAIL sensitized glioma cells lead to apoptotic death and induced malignant glioma regression [58]. Furthermore, several Smad analogs can induce cancer cell death and have shown potential as cancer therapies [106, 164].

6.8 Defective Autophagy and Cancer

Autophagy is an evolutionarily conserved mechanism for protein degradation and maintains homeostasis. Studies have implicated autophagy in tumorigenesis and tumor progression. Autophagy deficiency predisposes cells to tumor development. To this end, haploinsufficiency of autophagy genes increased tumor formation in mouse [118]. Conversely, once tumors were established, autophagy may enable cancer cell survival. For example, autophagy increases cancer drug resistance to Imatinib in chronic myeloid leukemia [13] and facilitates resistance trastuzumab for HER2 positive breast cancer cells [178]. Conversely, autophagy abrogation by autophagy inhibitors re-sensitizes the resistant cancer cells to the chemotherapy or radiation [8, 13].

7 Concluding Remarks

Many genes involved in PCD undergo alternative splicing to produce multiple isoforms with distinct functional activities. Alternative splicing not only generates products with different subcellular localization (membrane associated versus soluble proteins; nuclear versus cytoplasmic) but also produces proteins with different, and often antagonistic functional activities. Molecular analyses of these cell death genes suggest fundamental importance of alternative splicing in regulating PCD. However, molecular mechanisms controlling the alternative splicing of these PCD genes remain unclear. Recent studies using model systems have initiated molecular dissection of the link between alternative splicing and PCD regulation. These studies are only the beginning, given the wide variety of functionally distinct proteins generated by alternative splicing. A global landscape of alternative splicing patterns as well as molecular mechanisms involved in cell death regulation await further investigation using multidimensional and combinatorial approaches. Due to the complex regulatory networks that work in harmony to control cell fate and cell differentiation, mutations affecting one pathway can have far reaching consequences at the cellular, multicellular, and tissue levels. Therefore, elucidating regulatory mechanisms underlying functionally important alternative splicing events will not only help us understand pathogenetic mechanisms of human diseases caused by splicing defects but also provide molecular insights into designing new cancer therapies by targeting aberrant or defective splicing.

Acknowledgments We apologize to our colleagues for not being able to cite their original research articles due to the space limit. The authors' work was supported by grants from the NIH to Wu JY, a Scholar Award from the Leukemia Society of America. We would like to thank members of Wu lab for critical reading of the manuscript.

References

1. Abedini MR, Qiu Q, Yan X, Tsang BK (2004) Possible role of FLICE-like inhibitory protein (FLIP) in chemoresistant ovarian cancer cells in vitro. Oncogene 23(42):6997–7004
2. Agostini L, Martinon F, Burns K, McDermott MF, Hawkins PN, Tschopp J (2004) NALP3 forms an IL-1beta-processing inflammasome with increased activity in Muckle-Wells autoinflammatory disorder. Immunity 20(3):319–325
3. Akhter A, Gavrilin MA, Frantz L, Washington S, Ditty C, Limoli D, Day C, Sarkar A, Newland C, Butchar J, Marsh CB, Wewers MD, Tridandapani S, Kanneganti TD, Amer AO (2009) Caspase-7 activation by the Nlrc4/Ipaf inflammasome restricts Legionella pneumophila infection. PLoS Pathog 5(4):e1000361
4. Akgul C, Moulding DA, Edwards SW (2004) Alternative splicing of Bcl-2-related genes: functional consequences and potential therapeutic applications. Cell Mol Life Sci 61(17):2189–2199
5. Alnemri ES (1997) Mammalian cell death proteases: a family of highly conserved aspartate specific cysteine proteases. J Cell Biochem 64:33–42
6. Alnemri ES, Fernandes-Alnemri T, Litwack G (1995) Cloning and expression of four novel isoforms of human interleukin-1 beta converting enzyme with different apoptotic activities. J Biol Chem 270(9):4312–4317
7. Al-Zoubi AM, Efimova EV, Kaithamana S, Martinez O, El-Idrissi M-A, Dogan RE, Prabhakar BS (2001) Contrasting effects of IG20 and its splice isoforms, MADD and DENN-SV, on tumor necrosis factor alpha-induced apoptosis and activation of caspase-8 and -3. J Biol Chem 276(50):47202–47211
8. Apel A, Herr I, Schwarz H, Rodemann HP, Mayer A (2008) Blocked autophagy sensitizes resistant carcinoma cells to radiation therapy. Cancer Res 68(5):1485–1494
9. Ashhab Y, Alian A, Polliack A, Panet A, Ben Yehuda D (2001) Two splicing variants of a new inhibitor of apoptosis gene with different biological properties and tissue distribution pattern. FEBS Lett 495(1–2):56–60
10. Bae J, Leo CP, Hsu SY, Hsueh AJ (2000) MCL-1S, a splicing variant of the antiapoptotic BCL-2 family member MCL-1, encodes a proapoptotic protein possessing only the BH3 domain. J Biol Chem 275(33):25255–25261

11. Baehrecke EH (2002) How death shapes life during development. Nat Rev Mol Cell Biol 3:779–787
12. Basnakian AG, Apostolov EO, Yin X, Abiri SO, Stewart AG, Singh AB, Shah SV (2006) Endonuclease G promotes cell death of non-invasive human breast cancer cells. Exp Cell Res 312(20):4139–4149
13. Bellodi C, Lidonnici MR, Hamilton A, Helgason GV, Soliera AR, Ronchetti M, Galavotti S, Young KW, Selmi T, Yacobi R, Van Etten RA, Donato N, Hunter A, Dinsdale D, Tirrò E, Vigneri P, Nicotera P, Dyer MJ, Holyoake T, Salomoni P, Calabretta B (2009) Targeting autophagy potentiates tyrosine kinase inhibitor-induced cell death in Philadelphia chromosome-positive cells, including primary CML stem cells. J Clin Invest 119(5):1109–1123
14. Bergeron L, Perez GI, Macdonald G, Shi L, Sun Y, Jurisicova A, Varmuza S, Latham KE, Flaws JA, Salter JC, Hara H, Moskowitz MA, Li E, Greenberg A, Tilly JL, Yuan J (1998) Defects in regulation of apoptosis in caspase-2-deficient mice. Genes Dev 12(9):1304–1314
15. Bergsbaken T, Fink SL, Cookson BT (2009) Pyroptosis: host cell death and inflammation. Nat Rev Microbiol 7(2):99–109
16. Black DL (2003) Mechanisms of alternative pre-messenger RNA splicing. Annu Rev Biochem 72:291–336
17. Blencowe BJ (2006) Alternative splicing: new insights from global analyses. Cell 126:37–47
18. Boise LH, González-García M, Postema CE, Ding L, Lindsten T, Turka LA, Mao X, Nuñez G, Thompson CB (1993) bcl-x, a bcl-2-related gene that functions as a dominant regulator of apoptotic cell death. Cell 74(4):597–608
19. Borbély AA, Murvai M, Szarka K, Kónya J, Gergely L, Hernádi Z, Veress G (2007) Survivin promoter polymorphism and cervical carcinogenesis. J Clin Pathol 60(3):303–306
20. Bonnal S, Martinez C, Forch P, Bachi A, Wilm M, Valcarcel J (2008) RBM5/Luca-15/H37 regulates Fas alternative splice site pairing after exon definition. Mol Cell 32:81–95
21. Boon-Unge K, Yu Q, Zou T, Zhou A, Govitrapong P, Zhou J (2007) Emetine regulates the alternative splicing of Bcl-x through a protein phosphatase 1-dependent mechanism. Chem Biol 14(12):1386–1392
22. Boukakis G, Patrinou-Georgoula M, Lekarakou M, Valavanis C, Guialis A (2010) Deregulated expression of hnRNP A/B proteins in human non-small cell lung cancer: parallel assessment of protein and mRNA levels in paired tumour/non-tumour tissues. BMC Cancer 10:434
23. Büttner S, Eisenberg T, Carmona-Gutierrez D, Ruli D, Knauer H, Ruckenstuhl C, Sigrist C, Wissing S, Kollroser M, Fröhlich KU, Sigrist S, Madeo F (2007) Endonuclease G regulates budding yeast life and death. Mol Cell 25(2):233–246
24. Cartegni L, Chew SL and Krainer AR (2002) Listening to silence and understanding nonsense: exonicmutations that affect splicing. Nat Rev Genet 3:285–298
25. Cascino I, Papoff G, Eramo A, Ruberti G (1996) Soluble Fas/Apo-1 splicing variants and apoptosis. Front Biosci 1:d12–d18
26. Chew LJ, Pan H, Yu J, Tian S, Huang WQ, Zhang JY, Pang S, Li LY (2002) A novel secreted splice variant of vascular endothelial cell growth inhibitor. FASEB J 16(7):742–744
27. Clarke PG (1990) Developmental cell death: morphological diversity and multiple mechanisms. Anat Embryol (Berl) 181:195–213
28. Cloutier P, Toutant J, Shkreta L, Goekjian S, Revil T, Chabot B (2008) Antagonistic effects of the SRp30c protein and cryptic 5′ splice sites on the alternative splicing of the apoptotic regulator Bcl-x. J Biol Chem 283(31):21315–21324
29. Corcos L, Solier S (2005) Alternative mRNA splicing, pathology and molecular therapeutics. Med Sci (Paris) 21(3):253–260
30. Corsini L, Bonnal S, Basquin J, Hothorn M, Scheffzek K, Valcárcel J, Sattler M (2007) U2AF-homology motif interactions are required for alternative splicing regulation by SPF45. Nat Struct Mol Biol 14(7):620–629

31. Côté J, Dupuis S and Wu JY (2001) Polypyrimidine track-binding protein binding downstream of caspase-2 alternative exon 9 represses its inclusion. J Biol Chem 276:8535–8543
32. Coté J, Dupuis S, Jiang Z, and Wu JY (2001) Caspase-2 pre-mRNA alternative splicing: Identification ofan intronic element containing a decoy 3' acceptor site. Proc Nat Acad Sci USA 98:938–943
33. Cotter TG (2009) Apoptosis and cancer: the genesis of a research field. Nat Rev Cancer 9(7):501–507
34. Cregan SP, Dawson VL, Slack RS (2004) Role of AIF in caspase-dependent and caspase-independent cell death. Oncogene 23(16):2785–2796
35. Cuenin S, Tinel A, Janssens S, Tschopp J (2008) p53-induced protein with a death domain (PIDD) isoforms differentially activate nuclear factor-kappaB and caspase-2 in response to genotoxic stress. Oncogene 27(3):387–396
36. David CJ, Manley JL (2010) Alternative pre-mRNA splicing regulation in cancer: pathways and programs unhinged. Genes Dev 24:2343–2364
37. Delavallée L, Cabon L, Galán-Malo P, Lorenzo HK, Susin SA (2011) AIF-mediated caspase-independent necroptosis: a new chance for targeted therapeutics. IUBMB Life 63(4):221–232
38. Delettre C, Yuste VJ, Moubarak RS, Bras M, Lesbordes-Brion JC, Petres S, Bellalou J, Susin SA (2006) AIFsh, a novel apoptosis-inducing factor (AIF) pro-apoptotic isoform with potential pathological relevance in human cancer. J Biol Chem 281(10):6413–6427
39. Delettre C, Yuste VJ, Moubarak RS, Bras M, Robert N, Susin SA (2006) Identification and characterization of AIFsh2, a mitochondrial apoptosis-inducing factor (AIF) isoform with NADH oxidase activity. J Biol Chem 281(27):18507–18518
40. Dempsey CE, Dive C, Fletcher DJ, Barnes FA, Lobo A, Bingle CD, Whyte MK, Renshaw SA (2005) Expression of pro-apoptotic Bfk isoforms reduces during malignant transformation in the human gastrointestinal tract. FEBS Lett 579(17):3646–3650
41. Dennis PB, Jaeschke A, Saitoh M, Fowler B, Kozma SC, Thomas G (2001) Mammalian TOR: a homeostatic ATP sensor. Science 294:1102–1105
42. Diaz A, Hu C, Kastner DL, Schaner P, Reginato AM, Richards N, Gumucio DL (2004) Lipopolysaccharide-induced expression of multiple alternatively spliced MEFV transcripts in human synovial fibroblasts: a prominent splice isoform lacks the C-terminal domain that is highly mutated in familial Mediterranean fever. Arthritis Rheum 50(11):3679–3689
43. Diaz-Troya S, Perez–Perez ME, Florencio FJ, Crespo JL (2008) The role of TOR in autophagy regulation from yeast to plants and mammals. Autophagy 4:851–865
44. Djerbi M, Darreh-Shori T, Zhivotovsky B, Grandien A (2001) Characterization of the human FLICE-inhibitory protein locus and comparison of the anti-apoptotic activity of four different flip isoforms. Scand J Immunol 54(1–2):180–189
45. Donnini M, Lapucci A, Papucci L, Witort E, Tempestini A, Brewer G, Bevilacqua A, Nicolin A, Capaccioli S, Schiavone N (2001) Apoptosis is associated with modifications of bcl-2 mRNA AU-binding proteins. Biochem Biophys Res Commun 287(5):1063–1069
46. Droin N, Beauchemin M, Solary E, Bertrand R (2000) Identification of a caspase-2 isoform that behaves as an endogenous inhibitor of the caspase cascade. Cancer Res 60(24):7039–7047
47. Edinger AL, Thompson CB (2004) Death by design: apoptosis, necrosis and autophagy. Curr Opin Cell Biol 16(6):663–669
48. Efimova E, Martinez O, Lokshin A, Arima T, Prabhakar BS (2003) IG20, a MADD splice variant, increases cell susceptibility to gamma-irradiation and induces soluble mediators that suppress tumor cell growth. Cancer Res 63(24):8768–8776
49. Efimova EV, Al-Zoubi AM, Martinez O, Kaithamana S, Lu S, Arima T, Prabhakar BS (2004) IG20, in contrast to DENN-SV, (MADD splice variants) suppresses tumor cell survival, and enhances their susceptibility to apoptosis and cancer drugs. Oncogene 23(5):1076–1087
50. Eisenberg-Lerner A, Bialik S, Simon HU, Kimchi A (2009a) Life and death partners: apoptosis, autophagy and the cross-talk between them. Cell Death Differ 16(7):966–975

51. Eisenberg-Lerner A, Kimchi A (2009b) The paradox of autophagy and its implication in cancer etiology and therapy. Apoptosis 14(4):376–391
52. Feng Q, Li P, Leung PC, Auersperg N (2004) Caspase-1zeta, a new splice variant of the caspase-1 gene. Genomics 84(3):587–591
53. Forch P, Puig O, Kedersha N, Martinez C, Granneman S, Seraphin B, Anderson P, Valcarcel J (2000) The apoptosis-promoting factor TIA-1 is a regulator of alternative pre-mRNA splicing. Mol Cell 6(5):1089–1098
54. Forch P, Valcarcel J (2001) Molecular mechanisms of gene expression regulation by the apoptosis-promoting protein TIA-1. Apoptosis 6(6):463–468
55. Franchi L, Eigenbrod T, Muñoz-Planillo R, Nuñez G (2009) The inflammasome: a caspase-1-activation platform that regulates immune responses and disease pathogenesis. Nat Immunol 10(3):241–247
56. Fu J, Jin Y, Arend LJ (2003) Smac3, a novel Smac/DIABLO splicing variant, attenuates the stability and apoptosis-inhibiting activity of X-linked inhibitor of apoptosis protein. J Biol Chem 278(52):52660–52672
57. Fulda S, Meyer E, Debatin K-M (2000) Metabolic Inhibitors Sensitize for CD95 (APO-1/Fas)-inducedApoptosis by Down-Regulating Fas-associated Death Domain-like Interleukin 1-Converting EnzymeInhibitory Protein Expression. Cancer Res 60:3947–3956
58. Fulda S, Wick W, Weller M, Debatin KM (2002) Smac agonists sensitize for Apo2L/TRAIL- or anticancer drug-induced apoptosis and induce regression of malignant glioma in vivo. Nat Med 8(8):808–815
59. Fushimi K, Ray P, Kar A, Wang L, Sutherland LC, Wu JY (2008) Up-regulation of the proapoptotic caspase 2 splicing isoform by a candidate tumor suppressor, RBM5. Proc Natl Acad Sci U S A 105:15708–15713
60. Galluzzi L, Blomgren K, Kroemer G (2009) Mitochondrial membrane permeabilization in neuronal injury. Nat Rev Neurosci 10(7):481–494
61. Ganley IG, du Lam H, Wang J, Ding X, Chen S, Jiang X (2009) ULK1.ATG13.FIP200 complex mediates mTOR signaling and is essential for autophagy. J Biol Chem 284:12297–12305
62. Garneau D, Revil T, Fisette JF, Chabot B (2005) Heterogeneous nuclear ribonucleoprotein F/H proteins modulate the alternative splicing of the apoptotic mediator Bcl-x. J Biol Chem 280(24):22641–22650
63. Germann S, Gratadou L, Dutertre M, Auboeuf D (2012) Splicing programs and cancer. J Nucleic Acids 2012:269570
64. Goehe RW, Shultz JC, Murudkar C, Usanovic S, Lamour NF, Massey DH, Zhang L, Camidge DR, Shay JW, Minna JD et al (2010) hnRNP L regulates the tumorigenic capacity of lung cancer xenografts in mice via caspase-9 pre-mRNA processing. J Clin Invest 120:3923–3939
65. Golks A, Brenner D, Fritsch C, Krammer PH, Lavrik IN (2005) c-FLIPR, a new regulator of death receptor-induced apoptosis. J Biol Chem 280(15):14507–14513
66. Goll DE, Thompson VF, Li H, Wei W, Cong J (2003) The calpain system. Physiol Rev 83(3):731–801
67. Groeger AM, Esposito V, De Luca A, Cassandro R, Tonini G, Ambrogi V, Baldi F, Goldfarb R, MineoTC, Baldi A, et al. (2004) Prognostic value of immunohistochemical expression of p53, bax, Bcl-2 andBcl-xL in resected non-small-cell lung cancers. Histopathology 44:54–63
68. Grosso AR, Martins S, Carmo-Fonseca M (2008) The emerging role of splicing factors in cancer. EMBO Rep 9:1087–1093
69. Hai Y, Cao W, Liu G, Hong SP, Elela SA, Klinck R, Chu J, Xie J (2008) A G-tract element in apoptotic agents-induced alternative splicing. Nucleic Acids Res 36(10):3320–3331
70. Han J, Xiong J, Wang D, Fu XD (2011) Pre-mRNA splicing: where and when in the nucleus. Trends Cell Biol 21(6):336–343
71. Harris TE, Lawrence JC Jr (2003) TOR signaling. Sci STKE 2003, re15

72. Hariu H, Hirohashi Y, Torigoe T, Asanuma H, Hariu M, Tamura Y, Aketa K, Nabeta C, Nakanishi K, Kamiguchi K, Mano Y, Kitamura H, Kobayashi J, Tsukahara T, Shijubo N, Sato N (2005) Aberrant expression and potency as a cancer immunotherapy target of inhibitor of apoptosis protein family, Livin/ML-IAP in lung cancer. Clin Cancer Res 11(3):1000–1009
73. Hastings ML, Krainer AR (2001) Pre-mRNA splicing in the new millennium. Curr Opin Cell Biol 13:302–309
74. Havlioglu N, Wang J, Fushimi K, Vibranovski MD, Kan Z, Gish W, Fedorov A, Long M, Wu JY (2007) An intronic signal for alternative splicing in the human genome. PLoS One 2(11):e1246
75. Himeji D, Horiuchi T, Tsukamoto H, Hayashi K, Watanabe T, Harada M (2002) Characterization of caspase-8L: a novel isoform of caspase-8 that behaves as an inhibitor of the caspase cascade. Blood 99(11):4070–4078
76. Horiuchi T, Himeji D, Tsukamoto H, Harashima S, Hashimura C, Hayashi K (2000) Dominant expression of a novel splice variant of caspase-8 in human peripheral blood lymphocytes. Biochem Biophys Res Commun 272(3):877–881
77. Hossini AM, Geilen CC, Fecker LF, Daniel PT, Eberle J (2006) A novel Bcl-x splice product, Bcl-xAK, triggers apoptosis in human melanoma cells without BH3 domain. Oncogene 25(15):2160–2169
78. Hsieh SY, Liaw SF, Lee SN, Hsieh PS, Lin KH, Chu CM, Liaw YF (2003) Aberrant caspase-activated DNase (CAD) transcripts in human hepatoma cells. Br J Cancer 88(2):210–216
79. Hughes TA (2006) Regulation of gene expression by alternative untranslated regions. Trends Genet 22(3):119–122
80. Ishihara Y, Shimamoto N (2006) Involvement of endonuclease G in nucleosomal DNA fragmentation under sustained endogenous oxidative stress. J Biol Chem 281(10): 6726–6733
81. Izquierdo JM (2008) Hu antigen R (HuR) functions as an alternative pre-mRNA splicing regulator of Fasapoptosis-promoting receptor on exon definition. J Biol Chem 283: 19077–19084
82. Izquierdo JM, Majós N, Bonnal S, Martínez C, Castelo R, Guigó R, Bilbao D, Valcárcel J (2005) Regulation of Fas alternative splicing by antagonistic effects of TIA-1 and PTB on exon definition. Mol Cell 19(4):475–484
83. Izquierdo JM, Valcárcel J (2007) Fas-activated serine/threonine kinase (FAST K) synergizes with TIA-1/TIAR proteins to regulate Fas alternative splicing. J Biol Chem 282(3):1539–1543
84. Izquierdo JM (2008) Fas splicing regulation during early apoptosis is linked to caspase-mediated cleavage of U2AF65. Mol Biol Cell 19(8):3299–3307
85. Jiang ZH, Zhang WJ, Rao Y, Wu JY (1998) Regulation of Ich-1 pre-mRNA alternative splicing and apoptosis by mammalian splicing factors. Proc Natl Acad Sci USA 95:9155–9160
86. Jung CH, Jun CB, Ro SH, Kim YM, Otto NM, Cao J, Kundu M, Kim DH (2009) ULK-Atg13-FIP200 complexes mediate mTOR signaling to the autophagy machinery. Mol Biol Cell 20:1992–2003
87. Jurica MS, Moore MJ (2003) Pre-mRNA splicing: awash in a sea of proteins. Mol Cell 12(1):5–14
88. Kabeya Y, Mizushima N, Ueno T, Yamamoto A, Kirisako T, Noda T, Kominami E, Ohsumi Y, Yoshimori T (2000) LC3, a mammalian homologue of yeast Apg8p, is localized in autophagosome membranes after processing. EMBO J 19:5720–5728
89. Kalsotra A, Cooper TA (2011) Functional consequences of developmentally regulated alternative splicing. Nat Rev Genet 12(10):715–729
90. Kamihira S, Yamada Y, Tomonaga M, Sugahara K, Tsuruda K (1999) Discrepant expression of membrane and soluble isoforms of Fas (CD95/APO-1) in adult T-cell

leukaemia: soluble Fas isoform is an independent risk factor for prognosis. Br J Haematol 107(4):851–860
91. Kataoka T, Tschopp J (2004) N-terminal fragment of c-FLIP(L) processed by caspase 8 specifically interacts with TRAF2 and induces activation of the NF-kappaB signaling pathway. Mol Cell Biol 24(7):2627–2636
92. Kempkensteffen C, Hinz S, Johannsen M, Krause H, Magheli A, Christoph F, Köllermann J, Schrader M, Schostak M, Miller K, Weikert S (2009) Expression of Mcl-1 splicing variants in clear-cell renal cancer and their correlation with histopathological parameters and prognosis. Tumour Biol 30(2):73–79
93. Kerr JF, Wyllie AH, Currie AR (1972) Apoptosis: a basic biological phenomenon with wide-ranging implications in tissue kinetics. Br J Cancer 26(4):239–257
94. Kirchhoff S, Müller WW, Krueger A, Schmitz I, Krammer PH (2000) TCR-mediated up-regulation of c-FLIPshort correlates with resistance toward CD95-mediated apoptosis by blocking death-inducing signaling complex activity. J Immunol 165(11):6293–6300
95. Kisenge RR, Toyoda H, Kang J, Tanaka S, Yamamoto H, Azuma E, Komada Y (2003) Expression of short-form caspase 8 correlates with decreased sensitivity to Fas-mediated apoptosis in neuroblastoma cells. Cancer Sci 94(7):598–605
96. Klionsky DJ, Emr SD (2000) Autophagy as a regulated pathway of cellular degradation. Science 290:1717–1721
97. Korkolopoulou P, Saetta AA, Levidou G, Gigelou F, Lazaris A, Thymara I, Scliri M, Bousboukea K, Michalopoulos NV, Apostolikas N, Konstantinidou A, Tzivras M, Patsouris E (2007) c-FLIP expression in colorectal carcinomas: association with Fas/FasL expression and prognostic implications. Histopathology 51(2):150–156
98. Korsmeyer SJ (1999) Programmed cell death and the regulation of homeostasis. Harvey Lect 1999–2000(95):21–41
99. Korsmeyer SJ, Gross A, Harada H, Zha J, Wang K, Yin XM, Wei M, Zinkel S (1999) Death and survival signals determine active/inactive conformations of pro-apoptotic BAX, BAD, and BID molecules. Cold Spring Harb Symp Quant Biol 64:343–50
100. Krieg A, Krieg T, Wenzel M, Schmitt M, Ramp U, Fang B, Gabbert HE, Gerharz CD, Mahotka C (2003) TRAIL-beta and TRAIL-gamma: two novel splice variants of the human TNF-related apoptosis-inducing ligand (TRAIL) without apoptotic potential. Br J Cancer 88(6):918–927
101. Krieg A, Schulte am Esch J 2nd, Ramp U, Hosch SB, Knoefel WT, Gabbert HE, Mahotka C. (2006) TRAIL-R4-beta: a new splice variant of TRAIL-receptor 4 lacking the cysteine rich domain 1. Biochem Biophys Res Commun.349(1):115–121
102. Kurada BR, Li LC, Mulherkar N, Subramanian M, Prasad KV, Prabhakar BS (2009) MADD, a splice variant of IG20, is indispensable for MAPK activation and protection against apoptosis upon tumor necrosis factor-alpha treatment. J Biol Chem 284(20):13533–13541
103. Lacour S, Micheau O, Hammann A, Drouineaud V, Tschopp J, Solary E, Dimanche-Boitrel MT (2003) Chemotherapy enhances TNF-related apoptosis-inducing ligand DISC assembly in HT29 human colon cancer cells. Oncogene 22(12):1807–1816
104. Lamkanfi M, Festjens N, Declercq W, Vanden Berghe T, Vandenabeele P (2007) Caspases in cell survival, proliferation and differentiation. Cell Death Differ 14(1):44–55
105. Lamkanfi M, Kanneganti TD, Van Damme P, Vanden Berghe T, Vanoverberghe I, Vandekerckhove J, Vandenabeele P, Gevaert K, Núñez G.(2008). Targeted peptidecentric proteomics reveals caspase-7 as a substrate of the caspase-1 inflammasomes. Mol Cell Proteomics 7(12):2350–2363
106. Lecis D, Drago C, Manzoni L, Seneci P, Scolastico C, Mastrangelo E, Bolognesi M, Anichini A, Kashkar H, Walczak H, Delia D (2010) Novel SMAC-mimetics synergistically stimulate melanoma cell death in combination with TRAIL and Bortezomib. Br J Cancer 102(12):1707–1716
107. Levine B, Klionsky DJ (2004) Development by self-digestion: molecular mechanisms and biological functions of autophagy. Dev Cell 6:463–477

108. Levine SJ (2008) Molecular mechanisms of soluble cytokine receptor generation. J Biol Chem 283(21):14177–14181
109. Li CY, Chu JY, Yu JK, Huang XQ, Liu XJ, Shi L, Che Y C, Xie J Y (2004) Regulation ofalternative splicing of Bcl-x by IL-6, GM-CSF and TPA. Cell Res 14:473–479
110. Li H, Zhu H, Xu CJ, Yuan J (1998) Cleavage of BID by caspase 8 mediates the mitochondrial damage in the Fas pathway of apoptosis. Cell 94(4):491–501
111. Li LC, Sheng JR, Mulherkar N, Prabhakar BS, Meriggioli MN (2008) Regulation of apoptosis and caspase-8 expression in neuroblastoma cells by isoforms of the IG20 gene. Cancer Res 68(18):7352–7361
112. Lomonosova E, Chinnadurai G (2008) BH3-only proteins in apoptosis and beyond: an overview. Oncogene Suppl 1:S2–S19
113. Long JC, Caceres JF (2009) The SR protein family of splicing factors: master regulators of gene expression. Biochem J 417(1):15–27
114. Lopez-Bigas N, Audit B, Ouzounis C, Parra G, Guigo R (2005) Are splicing mutations the most frequent cause of hereditary disease? FEBS Lett 579:1900–1903
115. Lu H, Gan M, Zhang G, Zhou T, Yan M, Wang S (2010) Expression of survivin, caspase-3 and p53 in cervical cancer assessed by tissue microarray: correlation with clinicopathology and prognosis. Eur J Gynaecol Oncol 31(6):662–666
116. Luan XY, Liu XB (2010) Comparison the inhibitory effects of human bone marrow mesenchymal stem cells and human placenta mesenchymal stem cells on T cell proliferation. Xi Bao Yu Fen Zi Mian Yi Xue Za Zhi 26: 849–851
117. Luo X, Budihardjo I, Zou H, Slaughter C, Wang X (1998) Bid, a Bcl2 interacting protein, mediates cytochrome c release from mitochondria in response to activation of cell surface death receptors. Cell 94(4):481–490
118. Mariño G, Salvador-Montoliu N, Fueyo A, Knecht E, Mizushima N, López-Otín C (2007) Tissuespecificautophagy alterations and increased tumorigenesis in mice deficient in Atg4C/ autophagin-3. J Biol Chem 282:18573–18583
119. Martin S, Toquet C, Oliver L, Cartron PF, Perrin P, Meflah K, Cuillère P, Vallette FM (2001)Expression of bcl-2, bax and bcl-xl in human gliomas: a re-appraisal. J Neurooncol 52:129–139
120. Massiello A, Salas A, Pinkerman RL, Roddy P, Roesser JR, Chalfant CE (2004) Identification oftwo RNA cis-elements that function to regulate the 5' splice site selection of Bcl-x pre-mRNA in response toceramide. J Biol Chem 279:15799–15804
121. Massiello A, Chalfant CE (2006) SRp30a (ASF/SF2) regulates the alternative splicing of caspase-9 pre-mRNA and is required for ceramide-responsiveness. J Lipid Res 47:892–897
122. Massiello A, Roesser JR, Chalfant CE (2006) SAP155 Binds to ceramide-responsive RNA cis-element 1 and regulates the alternative 5′ splice site selection of Bcl-x pre-mRNA. FASEB J 20(10):1680–1682
123. Matlin AJ, Clark F, Smith CW (2005) Understanding alternative splicing: towards a cellular code. Nat Rev Mol Cell Biol 6:386–398
124. Matlin AJ, Moore MJ (2007) Spliceosome assembly and composition. Adv Exp Med Biol 623:14–35
125. Micheau O, Thome M, Schneider P, Holler N, Tschopp J, Nicholson DW, Briand C, Grütter MG (2002) The long form of FLIP is an activator of caspase-8 at the Fas death-inducing signaling complex. J Biol Chem 277(47):45162–45171
126. Midis GP, Shen Y, Owen-Schaub LB (1996) Elevated soluble Fas (sFas) levels in nonhematopoietic human malignancy. Cancer Res 56(17):3870–3874
127. Mille F, Thibert C, Fombonne J, Rama N, Guix C, Hayashi H, Corset V, Reed JC, Mehlen P (2009) The Patched dependence receptor triggers apoptosis through a DRAL-caspase-9 complex. Nat Cell Biol 11(6):739–746
128. Miller MA, Karacay B, Zhu X, O'Dorisio MS, Sandler AD (2006) Caspase 8L, a novel inhibitory isoform of caspase 8, is associated with undifferentiated neuroblastoma. Apoptosis 11(1):15–24

129. Mizushima N (2007) Autophagy: process and function. Genes Dev 21:2861–2873
130. Monni O, Joensuu H, Franssila K, Klefstrom J, Alitalo K, Knuutila S (1997) BCL2 overexpression associated with chromosomal amplification in diffuse large B-cell lymphoma. Blood 90(3):1168–1174
131. Moon DO, Park SY, Choi YH, Ahn JS, Kim GY (2011) Guggulsterone sensitizes hepatoma cells to TRAIL-induced apoptosis through the induction of CHOP-dependent DR5: involvement of ROS-dependent ER-stress. Biochem Pharmacol 82(11):1641–1650
132. Moore MJ, Silver PA (2008) Global analysis of mRNA splicing. RNA (New York, N.Y.) 14(2):197–203
133. Moore MJ, Wang Q, Kennedy CJ, Silver PA (2010) An alternative splicing network links cell-cycle control to apoptosis. Cell 142:625–636
134. Moran-Jones K, Grindlay J, Jones M, Smith R, Norman JC (2009) hnRNP A2 regulates alternative mRNA splicing of TP53INP2 to control invasive cell migration. Cancer Res 69:9219–9227
135. Müntener K, Zwicky R, Csucs G, Baici A (2003) The alternative use of exons 2 and 3 in cathepsin B mRNA controls enzyme trafficking and triggers nuclear fragmentation in human cells. Histochem Cell Biol 119(2):93–101
136. Mulherkar N, Ramaswamy M, Mordi DC, Prabhakar BS (2006) MADD/DENN splice variant of the IG20 gene is necessary and sufficient for cancer cell survival. Oncogene 25(47):6252–6261
137. Mulherkar N, Prasad KV, Prabhakar BS (2007) MADD/DENN splice variant of the IG20 gene is a negative regulator of caspase-8 activation. Knockdown enhances TRAIL-induced apoptosis of cancer cells. J Biol Chem 282(16):11715–11721
138. Nam SY, Jung GA, Hur GC, Chung HY, Kim WH, Seol DW, Lee BL (2003) Upregulation of FLIP(S) by Akt, a possible inhibition mechanism of TRAIL-induced apoptosis in human gastric cancers. Cancer Sci 94(12):1066–1073
139. Nowak J, Archange C, Tardivel-Lacombe J, Pontarotti P, Pebusque MJ, Vaccaro MI, Velasco G, Dagorn JC, Iovanna JL (2009) The TP53INP2 protein is required for autophagy in mammalian cells. Mol Biol Cell 20:870–881
140. Ogawa T, Shiga K, Hashimoto S, Kobayashi T, Horii A, Furukawa T (2003) APAF-1-ALT, a novel alternative splicing form of APAF-1, potentially causes impeded ability of undergoing DNA damage-induced apoptosis in the LNCaP human prostate cancer cell line. Biochem Biophys Res Commun 306(2):537–543
141. Ouhtit A, Matrougui K, Bengrine A, Koochekpour S, Zerfaoui M, Yousief Z (2007) Survivin is not only a death encounter but also a survival protein for invading tumor cells. Front Biosci 12:1260–1270
142. Pan Q, Shai O, Lee LJ, Frey BJ, Blencowe BJ (2008) Deep surveying of alternative splicing complexity in the human transcriptome by high-throughput sequencing. Nat Genet 40:1413–1415
143. Panasyuk G, Nemazanyy I, Zhyvoloup A, Filonenko V, Davies D, Robson M, Pedley RB, Waterfield M, Gout I (2009) mTORbeta splicing isoform promotes cell proliferation and tumorigenesis. J Biol Chem 284:30807–30814
144. Papin S, Duquesnoy P, Cazeneuve C, Pantel J, Coppey-Moisan M, Dargemont C, Amselem S (2000) Alternative splicing at the MEFV locus involved in familial Mediterranean fever regulates translocation of the marenostrin/pyrin protein to the nucleus. Hum Mol Genet 9(20):3001–3009
145. Papoff G, Cascino I, Eramo A, Starace G, Lynch DH, Ruberti G (1996) An N-terminal domain shared by Fas/Apo-1 (CD95) soluble variants prevents cell death in vitro. J Immunol 156:4622–4630
146. Paronetto MP, Achsel T, Massiello A, Chalfant CE, Sette C (2007) The RNA-binding protein Sam68 modulates the alternative splicing of Bcl-x. J Cell Biol 176(7):929–939

147. Pathan N, Marusawa H, Krajewska M, Matsuzawa S, Kim H, Okada K, Torii S, Kitada S, Krajewski S, Welsh K, Pio F, Godzik A, Reed JC (2001) TUCAN, an antiapoptotic caspase-associated recruitment domain family protein overexpressed in cancer. J Biol Chem 276(34):32220–32229
148. Pautz A, Linker K, Hubrich T, Korhonen R, Altenhofer S, Kleinert H (2006) The polypyrimidine tract-binding protein (PTB) is involved in the post-transcriptional regulation of human inducible nitric oxide synthase expression. J Biol Chem 281:32294–32302
149. Pio R, Blanco D, Pajares MJ, Aibar E, Durany O, Ezponda T, Agorreta J, Gomez-Roman J, Anton MA, Rubio A et al (2010) Development of a novel splice array platform and its application in the identification of alternative splice variants in lung cancer. BMC Genomics 11:352
150. Porebska I, Sobańska E, Kosacka M, Jankowska R (2010) Apoptotic regulators: P53 and survivin expression in non-small cell lung cancer. Cancer Genomics Proteomics 7(6):331–335
151. Prasad S, Yadav VR, Kannappan R, Aggarwal BB (2011) Ursolic acid, a pentacyclin triterpene, potentiates TRAIL-induced apoptosis through p53-independent up-regulation of death receptors: evidence for the role of reactive oxygen species and JNK. J Biol Chem 286(7):5546–5557
152. Refaeli Y, Van Parijs L, London CA, Tschopp J, Abbas AK (1998) Biochemical mechanisms of IL-2-regulated Fas-mediated T cell apoptosis. Immunity 8(5):615–623
153. Reggiori F, Klionsky DJ (2002) Autophagy in the eukaryotic cell. Eukaryot Cell 1:11–21
154. Renshaw SA, Dempsey CE, Barnes FA, Bagstaff SM, Dower SK, Bingle CD, Whyte MK (2004) Three novel Bid proteins generated by alternative splicing of the human Bid gene. J Biol Chem 279(4):2846–2855
155. Rintala-Maki ND, Sutherland LC (2004) LUCA-15/RBM5, a putative tumour suppressor, enhances multiple receptor-initiated death signals. Apoptosis 9(4):475–484
156. Salvesen GS, Abrams JM (2004) Caspase activation—stepping on the gas or releasing the brakes? Lessons from humans and flies Oncogene 23:2774–2784
157. Samejima K, Earnshaw WC (2000) Differential localization of ICAD-L and ICAD-S in cells due toremoval of a C-terminal NLS from ICAD-L by alternative splicing. Exp Cell Res 255:314–320
158. Sampath J, Pelus LM (2007) Alternative splice variants of survivin as potential targets in cancer. Curr Drug Discov Technol 4(3):174–191
159. Schiavone N, Rosini P, Quattrone A, Donnini M, Lapucci A, Citti L, Bevilacqua A, Nicolin A, Capaccioli S (2000) A conserved AU-rich element in the 3′ untranslated region of bcl-2 mRNA is endowed with a destabilizing function that is involved in bcl-2 down-regulation during apoptosis. FASEB J 14(1):174–184
160. Schin KS, Clever U (1965) Lysosomal and free acid phosphatase in salivary glands of chironomus tentans. Science 150:1053–1055
161. Schin KS, Clever U (1968) Ultrastructural and cytochemical studies of salivary gland regression in Chironomus tentans. Z Zellforsch Mikrosk Anat 86:262–279
162. Schwerk C, Schulze-Osthoff K (2005) Regulation of apoptosis by alternative pre-mRNA splicing.Mol Cell 19(1):1–13
163. Screaton GR, Xu XN, Olsen AL, Cowper AE, Tan R, McMichael AJ, Bell JI (1997) LARD: a new lymphoid-specific death domain containing receptor regulated by alternative pre-mRNA splicing. Proc Nat Acad Sci USA 94:4615–4619
164. Servida F, Lecis D, Scavullo C, Drago C, Seneci P, Carlo-Stella C, Manzoni L, Polli E, Lambertenghi Deliliers G, Delia D, Onida F (2011) Novel second mitochondria-derived activator of caspases (Smac) mimetic compounds sensitize human leukemic cell lines to conventional chemotherapeutic drug-induced and death receptor-mediated apoptosis. Invest New Drugs 29(6):1264–1275
165. Shankarling G, Lynch KW (2010) Living or dying by RNA processing: caspase expression in NSCLC. J Clin Invest 120:3798–3801

166. Sharma S, Black DL (2006) Maps, codes, and sequence elements: can we predict the protein outputfrom an alternatively spliced locus? Neuron 52:574–576
167. Shieh JJ, Liu KT, Huang SW, Chen YJ, Hsieh TY (2009) Modification of alternative splicing of Mcl-1 pre-mRNA using antisense morpholino oligonucleotides induces apoptosis in basal cell carcinoma cells. J Invest Dermatol 129(10):2497–2506
168. Singh RK, Cooper TA (2012) Pre-mRNA splicing in disease and therapeutics. Trends Mol Med 18(8):472–482
169. Smirnova AS, Ferreira-Silva KC, Mine KL, Andrade-Oliveira V, Shulzhenko N, Gerbase-DeLima M, Morgun A (2008) Differential expression of new LTA splice variants upon lymphocyte activation. Mol Immunol 45(1):295–300
170. Solier S, Logette E, Desoche L, Solary E, Corcos L (2005) Nonsense-mediated mRNA decay among human caspases: the caspase-2S putative protein is encoded by an extremely short-lived mRNA. Cell Death Differ 12(6):687–689
171. Spellman R, Rideau A, Matlin A, Gooding C, Robinson F, McGlincy N, Grellscheid SN, Southby J,Wollerton M, Smith CWJ (2005) Regulation of alternative splicing by PTB and associated factors.Biochem Soc Trans 33:457–460
172. Stenner M, Weinell A, Ponert T, Hardt A, Hahn M, Preuss SF, Guntinas-Lichius O, Klussmann JP (2010) Cytoplasmic expression of survivin is an independent predictor of poor prognosis in patients with salivary gland cancer. Histopathology 57(5):699–706
173. Takehara T, Liu X, Fujimoto J, Friedman SL, Takahashi H (2001) Expression and role of Bcl-xL in human hepatocellular carcinomas. Hepatology 34(1):55–61
174. Talbot DC, Ranson M, Davies J, Lahn M, Callies S, André V, Kadam S, Burgess M, Slapak C, Olsen AL, McHugh PJ, de Bono JS, Matthews J, Saleem A, Price P (2010) Tumor survivin is downregulated by the antisense oligonucleotide LY2181308: a proof-of-concept, first-in-human dose study. Clin Cancer Res 16(24):6150–6158
175. Taper HS, Jamison JM, Gilloteaux J, Summers JL, Calderon PB (2004) Inhibition of the development of metastases by dietary vitamin C:K3 combination. Life Sci 75(8):955–967
176. Tsuchihara K, Fujii S, Esumi H (2009) Autophagy and cancer: dynamism of the metabolism of tumor cells and tissues. Cancer Lett 278(2):130–138
177. van Alphen RJ, Wiemer EA, Burger H, Eskens FA (2009) The spliceosome as target for anticancer treatment. Br J Cancer 100:228–232
178. Vazquez-Martin A, Oliveras-Ferraros C, Menendez JA (2009) Autophagy facilitates the development of breast cancer resistance to the anti-HER2 monoclonal antibody trastuzumab. PLoS One 4(7):e6251
179. Vucic D, Stennicke HR, Pisabarro MT, Salvesen GS, Dixit VM (2000) ML-IAP, a novel inhibitor of apoptosis that is preferentially expressed in human melanomas. Curr Biol 10(21):1359–1366
180. Vudattu NK, Magalhaes I, Hoehn H, Pan D, Maeurer MJ (2009) Expression analysis and functional activity of interleukin-7 splice variants. Genes Immun 10(2):132–140
181. Wagner EJ, Garcia-Blanco MA (2001) Polypyrimidine tract binding protein antagonizes exon definition.Mol Cell Biol 21:3281–3288
182. Wang Y, Geng Z, Zhao L, Huang SH, Sheng AL, Chen ZY (2008) GDNF isoform affects intracellular trafficking and secretion of GDNF in neuronal cells. Brain Res 1226:1–7
183. Wang Z, Burge CB (2008) Splicing regulation: from a parts list of regulatory elements to an integrated splicing code. RNA 14(5):802–813
184. Ward AJ, Cooper TA (2010) The pathobiology of splicing. J Pathol 220:152–163
185. Wu JY, Tang H, avlioglu N (2003) Alternative pre-mRNA splicing and regulation of programmed celldeath. Prog Mol Subcell Biol 31:153–185
186. Wu J, Dang Y, Su W, Liu C, Ma H, Shan Y, Pei Y, Wan B, Guo J, Yu L (2006) Molecular cloning and characterization of rat LC3A and LC3B–two novel markers of autophagosome. Biochem Biophys Res Commun 339:437–442
187. Wu JY, Yuan L, Havlioglu N (2004) Alternatively spliced genes. In Meyers RA (ed.) Encyclopedia of Molecular CellBiology and Molecular Medicine. Wiley-VCH, pp. 125–177

188. Wullschleger S, Loewith R, Hall MN (2006) TOR signaling in growth and metabolism. Cell 124:471–484
189. Wyllie AH, Kerr JF, Currie AR (1980) Cell death: the significance of apoptosis. Int Rev Cytol 68:251–306
190. Xerri L, Parc P, Brousset P, Schlaifer D, Hassoun J, Reed JC, Krajewski S, Birnbaum D (1996)Predominant expression of the long isoform of Bcl-x (Bcl-xL) in human lymphomas. Brit J Haematol 92:900–906
191. Xiao X, Lee JH (2010) Systems analysis of alternative splicing and its regulation. Wiley Interdiscip Rev Syst Biol Med 2(5):550–556
192. Yamashima T, Oikawa S (2009) The role of lysosomal rupture in neuronal death. Prog Neurobiol 89(4):343–358
193. Yagihashi A, Ohmura T, Asanuma K, Kobayashi D, Tsuji N, Torigoe T, Sato N, Hirata K, Watanabe N (2005) Detection of autoantibodies to survivin and livin in sera from patients with breastcancer. Clinica chimica acta; Int J Clin Chem 362:125–130
194. Yang Y, Chang JF, Parnes JR, Fathman CG (1998) T cell receptor (TCR) engagement leads to activation-induced splicing of tumor necrosis factor (TNF) nuclear pre-mRNA. J Exp Med 188(2):247–254
195. Yang G, Huang SC, Wu JY, Benz EJ Jr (2005) An erythroid differentiation-specific splicing switch in protein 4.1R mediated by the interaction of SF2/ASF with an exonic splicing enhancer. Blood 105:2146–2153
196. Yano K, Horinaka M, Yoshida T, Yasuda T, Taniguchi H, Goda AE, Wakada M, Yoshikawa S, Nakamura T, Kawauchi A, Miki T, Sakai T (2011) Chetomin induces degradation of XIAP and enhances TRAIL sensitivity in urogenital cancer cells. Int J Oncol 38(2):365–374
197. Yu L, Alva A, Su H, Dutt P, Freundt E, Welsh S, Baehrecke EH, Lenardo MJ (2004) Regulation of an ATG7-beclin 1 program of autophagic cell death by caspase-8. Science 304:1500–1502
198. Yu L, Lenardo MJ, Baehrecke EH (2004) Autophagy and caspases: a new cell death program. Cell Cycle 3:1124–1126
199. Yu L, McPhee CK, Zheng L, Mardones GA, Rong Y, Peng J, Mi N, Zhao Y, Liu Z, Wan F et al (2010) Termination of autophagy and reformation of lysosomes regulated by mTOR. Nature 465:942–946
200. Zhang T, Huang XH, Dong L, Hu D, Ge C, Zhan YQ, Xu WX, Yu M, Li W, Wang X et al (2010) PCBP-1 regulates alternative splicing of the CD44 gene and inhibits invasion in human hepatoma cell line HepG2 cells. Mol Cancer 9:72
201. Zhou A, Ou AC, Cho A, Benz EJ Jr, Huang SC (2008) Novel splicing factor RBM25 modulates Bcl-x pre-mRNA 5′ splice site selection. Mol Cell Biol 28:5924–5936
202. Zinkel SS, Hurov KE, Ong C, Abtahi FM, Gross A, Korsmeyer SJ (2005) A role for proapoptotic BID in the DNA-damage response. Cell 122(4):579–591
203. Zwicky R, Müntener K, Csucs G, Goldring MB, Baici A (2003) Exploring the role of 5′ alternative splicing and of the 3′-untranslated region of cathepsin B mRNA. Biol Chem 384(7):1007–1018

Oligonucleotide Therapeutics in Cancer

Jing Wan, John A. Bauman, Maria Anna Graziewicz, Peter Sazani and Ryszard Kole

Abstract

Alterations in pre-mRNA splicing can have profound effects on gene expression and lead to cellular transformation. Oligonucleotide therapeutics are drugs that manipulate gene expression and improve the disease state. Antisense oligonucleotides hybridize with a target mRNA to downregulate gene expression via an RNase H-dependent mechanism. Additionally, RNase H-independent splice switching oligonucleotides (SSO) modulate alternative or aberrant splicing, to favor the therapeutically relevant splicing product. This chapter summarizes the progress made in the application of these oligonucleotide drugs in the treatment of cancer.

Keywords

Alternative RNA splicing · Modulation of RNA splicing · Bcl-x (bcl2l1) · Splice switching oligonucleotides (sso)

Contents

J. Wan · J. A. Bauman · M. A. Graziewicz · P. Sazani · R. Kole (✉)
AVI Biopharma, 3450 Monte Villa Parkway, Bothell, WA 98021, USA
e-mail: kole@med.unc.edu

J. Y. Wu (ed.), *RNA and Cancer*, Cancer Treatment and Research,
DOI: 10.1007/978-3-642-31659-3_9, © Springer-Verlag Berlin Heidelberg 2013

1 Introduction

Recent estimates state that over 90 % of the approximately 26,000 human genes undergo alternative splicing [1–3], yielding a vast protein diversity from a limited number of genes. However, dysregulation of this process can affect cellular events such as induction of apoptosis and proliferation, which may contribute to the development of cancer. In addition, several cancer-associated genes are naturally alternatively spliced and, in cancer, splicing is shifted in favor of the anti-apoptotic form [4, 5]. Antisense oligonucleotides can be used to target the transcripts generated from oncogenes for destruction via RNase H, constituting a gene-specific treatment for cancer. In a more powerful approach, alternative or aberrant splicing can be manipulated by RNase H-independent, steric blocking antisense molecules, termed splice switching oligonucleotides (SSO), resulting in the upregulation of favorable splice variants, and the simultaneous downregulation of the detrimental forms, thus providing potentially greater clinical benefits [6–10]. In this chapter, we review oligonucleotide drugs, used for the manipulation of alternative/aberrant splicing and gene downregulation, as cancer therapeutics.

2 Splice Switching Oligonucleotides

SSO are a class of antisense compounds that are used to manipulate alternative splicing to yield a therapeutic benefit. In general, SSOs can: (1) restore correct splicing of an aberrantly spliced transcript, (2) manipulate alternative splicing, yielding upregulation of one splicing isoform, with simultaneous downregulation of another, and (3) generate a novel splice variant protein that is not naturally present, but has therapeutic value in a disorder, including malignancy.

Alternative splicing and its regulation have been extensively reviewed elsewhere [11–14]. In general, splice site selection is guided by loosely conserved sequences, namely 5′ and 3′ splice sites, branch points and polypyrimidine tracts as well as sequence elements within exons and introns such as exonic splicing enhancers (ESE), exonic splicing silencers (ESS), intronic splicing enhancers (ISE), and intronic splicing silencers (ISS) [15–17]. Selection of alternative splice sites is determined by competition between the above splice elements for splicing factors during assembly of spliceosome, a splicing complex composed of up to 100 proteins, and five small nuclear RNAs [18–20].

SSOs bind with high affinity to specific splice elements within the pre-mRNA (e.g., splice site or ESE) and therefore compete with splicing factors for access to elements, that help define exons and introns. Thus, the spliceosome is redirected to the other accessible splice elements and in consequence, the manner in which the pre-mRNA is spliced is altered. Upon blocking of a splice element by SSOs, several alternative splicing events may take place, including exon skipping, exon inclusion, intron retention, or selection of alternative 5′ or 3′ splice sites (see Chap. 3).

Early work by Dominski and Kole on aberrant splicing of human thalassemic pre-mRNA led to initial discovery that blocking an active splice site with an SSO does not lead to the complete shutdown of splicing in that transcript, but simply forces the spliceosome to select an alternative splicing pathway [6].

The SSO technology has been applied to a number of pre-mRNAs in cell culture, in animal models, and most recently in patients. Non-cancer genes that have been targeted, included β-globin, for the treatment of β-thalassemia [7, 8], SMN2 for the treatment of spinal muscular atrophy [21], tau for the treatment of dementia [22, 23], and dystrophin for the treatment of muscular dystrophy [24, 25]. In addition, morpholino (PMO) SSO targeted to the dystrophin pre-mRNA was tested in a clinical trial for the treatment of patients with Duchenne Muscular Dystrophy [26].

As described in the following section, to be useful as an SSO, an oligonucleotide must be composed of highly modified nucleotides, with biochemical characteristics distinct from classical antisense compounds.

3 Oligonucleotide Chemistry

3.1 RNAse H-Competent Chemistries (First Generation)

Classical antisense oligonucleotides (ASO) form double-stranded hybrids in which RNA is digested by RNase H (Fig. 1b*1*, an enzyme that catalyses endonucleolytic breakdown of the RNA strand in an RNA/DNA heteroduplex [27–30]. A typical antisense oligonucleotide molecule is 17–25 nucleotides (nt) in length [31–35], and since a specific 17nt sequence occurs only once within the human genome, exhibits exquisite target specificity [36]. Natural phosphodiester oligonucleotides have poor biodistribution, are quickly degraded by endogenous nucleases, and are of limited clinical use. Therefore, the "1st generation" phosphorothioate backbone modification (Fig. 1a*1*, in which one of non-bridging oxygen atoms of the phosphodiester linkage is replaced with a sulfur atom, was introduced to improve the therapeutic efficacy of antisense compounds [30, 32].

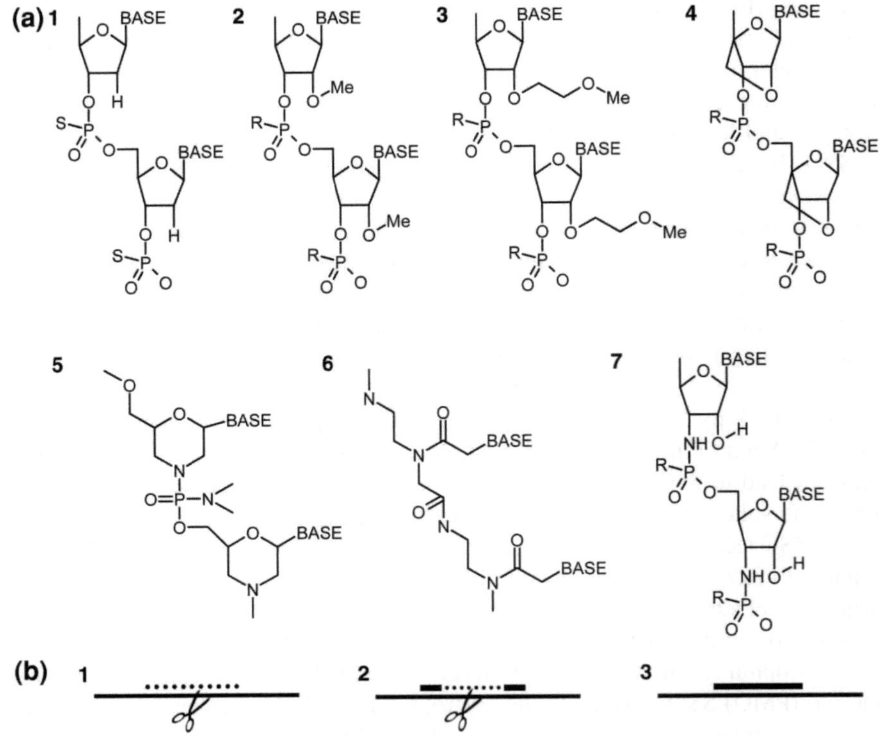

Fig. 1 **a** Oligonucleotide structures: *1* DNA phosphorothioate, *2* 2'-O-methyl-oligoribonucleotide (*2'OMe*), *3* 2′-O-methoxyethyl oligoribonucleotide (*2′MOE*), *4* locked nucleic acid (*LNA*), *5* phosphorodiamidate morpholino oligomer (*PMO*), *6* peptide nucleic acid (*PNA*), 7 phosphoroamidate oligoribonucleotide. R = O or S. **b** Antisense oligonucleotide strategies. *1* Traditional antisense oligonucleotides utilize RNase H-competent chemistries to mediate degradation of the RNA in oligonucleotide-mRNA duplex, *2* antisense gapmer oligonucleotides utilize an RNase H-competent core flanked by more potent and stable RNase H non-competent ends, *3* potent RNase H-resistant oligonucleotide chemistries are used to sterically block access to RNA without leading to its degradation. Compounds that block access to pre-mRNA by splicing factors modulate splicing as splice switching oligomers (*SSO*). Compounds that block access of ribosomes to mRNA inhibit translation as translation suppressing oligomers (*TSO*)

3.2 RNAse H Non-Competent Chemistries (Second Generation)

Other modifications that improve oligonucleotide performance in vivo, but that do not support RNase H activation, may also be used as so-called "2nd generation" gapmers, in which a core of RNase H competent DNA-phosphorothioates are flanked by more highly modified nucleotides (Figs. 1b2 and 1a2–*4*). Importantly, fully modified second generation oligonucleotides are ideal for use as SSO (Fig. 1b*3*). Thus, these second generation chemistries, developed over the past 20–30 years benefit both the antisense and SSO fields.

In contrast to ASOs that downregulate expression of the genes by leading to target RNA degradation, the SSOs must be sufficiently modified, such that RNase H does not recognize the RNA:SSO duplex and destroy the pre-mRNA before it can be spliced. To ensure RNase H non-competence, modified nucleotides must be included such that not more than three contiguous deoxynucleotides are present in the SSO; this is in contrast to gapmers, which use modified nucleotides to provide stability and high target affinity by flanking up to 10 nucleotide long RNase H competent core.

The SSO must also form very stable duplexes with its pre-mRNA targets, a feature that allows successful competition with natural splicing factors for specific binding sequences. It must also have a significant therapeutic window, be resistant to enzymatic degradation in the cellular environment and demonstrate preferable tissue distribution and pharmacodynamics in the organism [37]. The following second generation chemistries have thus far shown the above characteristics.

3.2.1 Locked Nucleic Acids

Locked nucleic acids (LNA) contain a methylene group that links the 2′-O and 4′ position of the ribose ring (Fig. 1a*4*). The furanose ring is locked into the N-type conformation, which favors RNA binding, and importantly LNA:RNA duplexes do not activate RNase H [38, 39]. SSOs containing a uniform phosphorothioate backbone and alternating LNA/DNA sugars have been shown to be both potent and persistent modulators of splicing in vivo, especially in the liver, small intestine, and colon [40]. LNA are sometimes referred to as third generation modifications.

3.2.2 Substitutions at 2′ Carbohydrate

Substitutions at the 2′-positition of deoxyribose with an O-alkyl groups or Fluorine renders RNA-oligonucleotide duplexes RNase H non-competent [41]. 2′-O-alkylated oligonucleotides, such as the common 2′-O-methyl (2′OMe) (Fig. 1a*2*), have higher affinity toward their targets and are resistant to nuclease degradation [41]. The 2′-O-methoxyethyl (MOE) oligonucleotides (Fig. 1a*3*) have demonstrated significant target affinity and high efficiency as ASO and SSO in cell culture [21, 42], in mice [43, 44], and in patients with familial cholesterolemia [45].

3.2.3 Morpholino Oligomers

Morpholino oligomers (PMO) are RNA-based molecules, in which the ribose is replaced with a 6-membered morpholine ring, and which contain phosphorodiamidate linkages that eliminate backbone charge [46] (Fig. 1a*5*). PMOs are highly nuclease resistant and have good affinity, which results in effective blocking of AUG start codons in eukaryotic cells [47], in zebrafish [48], in bacteria-infected mice [49, 50], and in cynomolgus monkeys where PMO-based drugs eliminated infection by deadly hemorrhagic Ebola and Marburg viruses [51]. PMOs also act as potent SSOs, yielding significant increases in β-globin production in erythropoietic progenitor cells in thalassemic mice in vivo [8], and restoring dystrophin in humans [26] and muscle function and strength in a mouse model of muscular dystrophy [25].

3.2.4 Peptide Nucleic Acids

The bases of peptide nucleic acids (PNAs) are connected by a non-cyclic peptide-like backbone (Fig. 1a*6*). They have high affinity toward their mRNA targets, are neutral, do not activate RNase H and are both peptidase and nuclease resistant. PNAs can be used both as gene expression inhibitors, as transcription and translation blocking agents, and as SSOs; their splice correction efficiency was significantly improved by placing positively charged amino acid modifications at the 3′ end [44, 52].

3.2.5 Phosphoramidates

In a N3′-P5′ phosphoramidate oligonucleotide the 3′ oxygen linking the ribose to the phosphorus is replaced by a nitrogen [53] (Fig. 1a*7*). This modification renders the compound RNase H and nuclease resistant [54] and allows formation of stable duplexes with target RNA [53]. Oligonucleotides were shown to have a good bioavailability and biodistribution, while being non-toxic in mice [55]. However, there is no evidence that they are effective in modulating splicing in vivo.

4 Positive Readout Assay for Antisense Oligonucleotide Activity

The assay, developed in Kole laboratory, is based on a transgenic mouse that ubiquitously expresses the coding sequence for enhanced green fluorescence protein (EGFP) interrupted by an aberrantly spliced intron 2 of human *β*-globin, such that basal expression of EGFP protein is essentially zero [44]. The aberrant splicing is induced by a thalassemic IVS2-654 mutation. Delivery to the nuclei of the cells of SSO targeting the 654 mutation (SSO-654) results in correctly spliced mRNA with restored EGFP reading frame, which renders the cells fluorescent and provides a positive readout of nuclear oligonucleotide activity.

Development of EGFP-654 transgenic mouse allowed efficacy comparison in vivo of SSO-654 with different oligonucleotide chemistries: 2′OMe, MOE, morpholino, PNA, and LNA [40, 44]. We found that MOE and PNA were active in vivo in several tissues, with highest activity in the liver and small intestine. LNA were potent in the liver, small intestine, and colon. Interestingly, in contrast to MOE and PNA, LNA functional distribution was limited to these organs.

5 Splice Switching Oligonucleotide Targets in Cancer

5.1 Bcl-x (BCL2L1)

Bcl-x is a member of the Bcl-2 family of genes involved in regulating apoptosis, which has been a major focus of cancer research [56]. The bcl-x pre-mRNA undergoes alternative splicing giving rise to two protein isoforms with opposing functions (Fig. 2a). The longer, anti-apoptotic bcl-xL, and the shorter,

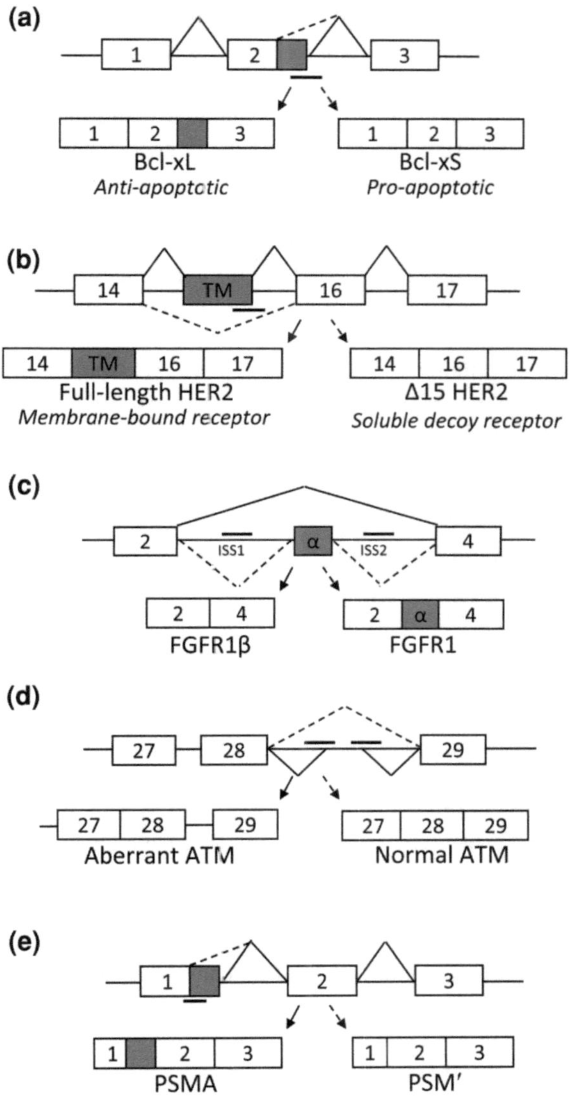

Fig. 2 Applications of SSOs in cancer. **a** Manipulation of Bcl-x alternative splicing switches production from anti-apoptotic Bcl-xL to pro-apoptotic Bcl-xS. **b** Modification of Her2 splicing leads to the production of a novel splice variant, Δ15HER2, that acts as a dominant-negative soluble decoy receptor. **c** Blocking intronic splicing silencer elements switches mRNA splicing from aberrant FGFR1β, a variant expressed predominantly in malignant tissues, to the normal FGFR variant that encodes the α exon. See text for details. **d** Correction of aberrant splicing in the ATM gene leads to production of functional protein ATM protein. **e** Modification of PSMA splicing switches production from membrane-bound PSMA protein, which is expressed predominantly in malignant prostate tissue, to PSM′, a variant that lacks the transmembrane domain but retains enzymatic activity and is expressed predominantly in normal prostate epithelium. See text for details

pro-apoptotic bcl-xS are produced by splicing at the proximal 5′ splice site of exon two, while bcl-xS is produced by splicing at the distal (upstream) 5′ splice site of exon 2 [57]. Bcl-xL promotes cell survival by sequestering the pro-apoptotic molecules Bak and Bax. Bcl-xS is thought to promote apoptosis by interacting with Bcl-xL, as well as the anti-apoptotic Bcl-2 protein, thereby freeing Bax and Bak to carry out their apoptotic function [58–60]. Overexpression of bcl-xL enables tumor cells to escape apoptosis and leads to resistance to chemotherapeutic agents [61]. Not surprisingly, bcl-xL overexpression is common in numerous cancers including multiple myeloma [62], small cell lung carcinoma

[63], breast cancer [64], prostate cancer [65], and hepatocellular carcinoma [66]. Recent data show that bcl-xL is essential for survival of a large fraction of all cancers [67]. Furthermore, bcl-xL expression has correlated with reduced sensitivity to chemotherapeutic agents [61] and in some cases is actually induced by chemotherapy, protecting residual cancer cells and setting the stage for re-emergence of metastatic cancer [68].

Bcl-x is an attractive target for SSOs because for each molecule of pre-mRNA that is affected, an anti-apoptotic Bcl-xL is replaced with a pro-apoptotic Bcl-xS. The resulting pool of bcl-xS protein is then capable of counteracting bcl-xL and bcl-2 [65, 69, 70]. Previous studies have validated bcl-x as an appropriate cancer target for ASOs that activate RNase H-mediated degradation [71–73]. However, by simultaneously upregulating one pro-apoptotic bcl-xS protein and downregulating one bcl-xL protein for each pre-mRNA affected, an SSO approach was predicted to be more potent than traditional downregulating ASOs. SSOs were designed to the proximal 5′ splice site of bcl-x pre-mRNA to block splicing at this site and induce splicing at the distal 5′ site. Treatment of various cancer cell lines with these SSOs caused a decrease in bcl-xL mRNA and protein, and a concomitant increase in bcl-xS mRNA and protein [65]. These effects were both dose-dependent and sequence specific.

Bcl-x SSO was also more effective than classical ASOs at inducing apoptosis, particularly in PC3 cells [65]. Similarly, bcl-x SSO sensitized MCF7 and A159 cells to apoptosis induced by chemotherapeutic agents or UV radiation [65, 69, 74]. Of note, the potency of bcl-x SSOs correlated with the level of bcl-xL expression, indicating that the therapeutic effects of the SSO are more profound in those cells overexpressing bcl-xL [69].

SSO-induced shift from Bcl-xL to Bcl-xS was recently shown to reduce tumor burden in vivo in a mouse model of melanoma lung metastases. Bcl-x SSO was systemically delivered using a lipid nanoparticles and was evidently taken up by B16F10 tumor xenografts that were lodged in the lungs after i.v. injection. Nanoparticle alone or formulated with a control SSO had no effect. This was the first demonstration of SSO efficacy in tumors in vivo [70].

5.2 HER2

HER2 is a member of the epidermal growth factor receptor (EGFR) family of receptor tyrosine kinases. EGFR family members are comprised of three functional domains: an extracellular ligand-binding domain, a transmembrane domain, and an intracellular tyrosine kinase domain. Ligand-binding to a monomeric receptor promotes homo- or hetero-dimerization, which leads to auto- or trans-phosphorylation in the cytoplasmic domain and downstream signaling, primarily through mitogen-activated protein kinase (MAPK) and phosphatidylinositol 3-kinase (PI3K)/protein kinase B (Akt) pathways [75]. Therefore, EGFR receptors play critical roles in cell proliferation, differentiation and survival, and deregulation of EGFR receptors has been implicated in numerous types of tumors. HER2 is amplified and/or overexpressed in many human malignancies, including 25–30 % breast cancers [76].

The transmembrane domain of HER2 is encoded by a single exon, exon 15 (TM, Fig. 2b). Screening a series of MOE SSOs identified SSO111 that induced exon 15 skipping in a sequence-specific, dose-dependent manner, thereby downregulating full-length HER2 while producing a novel splice variant lacking the transmembrane domain, Δ15HER2 [77]. In SK-BR-3 human breast cancer cells, which highly express HER2, SSO111-induced splice switching potently inhibited cell growth and induced apoptosis. This effect was less pronounced in MCF7 cells, in which HER2 expression is 100-fold lower, despite the fact that splice switching was still observed, confirming that SSO111-induced growth inhibition was HER2-dependent. This was consistent with the previously reported correlation of SSO potency with increased target gene expression [69]. It also indicates that tumors highly expressing HER2 would be more sensitive to SSO treatment than surrounding healthy tissue. It was further demonstrated that His-tagged Δ15HER2 protein potently downregulated HER2 protein expression and inhibited HER3 activation in dose-dependent manner in SK-BR-3 cells [77].

5.3 FGFR1

Fibroblast growth factor receptor 1 (FGFR1) belongs to a family of tyrosine kinases that bind FGFs play a role in cellular proliferation and differentiation. FGFR1 is one of the most frequently amplified genes in large number of cancers [67]. Alternative splicing of FGFR1 leads to numerous splicing isoforms with different ligand affinities. FGFR1β, produced by skipping of the α-exon, exhibits increased ligand affinity and altered subcellular localization. Upregulation of FGFR1β is associated with pancreatic cancer [78], breast cancer [79], and glioblastoma [80]. In FGFR1 pre-mRNA, the α-exon is flanked on either side by ISS sequences, ISS1 and ISS2 [81]. A recent report sought to block recruitment of *trans*-splicing factors. Morpholino SSOs targeted to either ISS resulted in α-exon inclusion in a dose-dependent, sequence-specific manner in various cell lines (Fig. 2c). Interestingly, simultaneous targeting of SSOs to ISS1 and ISS2 had no additive effect, suggesting these splicing elements contribute to a common mechanism. SSO treatment had no effect on cell viability of U251 glioblastoma cells although it did result in upregulation of activated caspase-3 and caspase-7 [82].

5.4 ATM

Ataxia telangiectasia (AT) is a progressive autosomal recessive disease resulting from mutations in the ATM gene. ATM encodes a serine-threonine kinase involved in cell cycle checkpoint control, DNA damage repair and apoptosis, and is a potent tumor suppressor [83]. In addition to neurological symptoms, AT patients are predisposed to leukemia and lymphomas [84]. Heterozygote carriers, although generally asymptomatic, also have increased risk of breast cancer [85]. Most AT patients do not express detectable levels of active ATM protein, due to point mutations, half of which disrupt proper pre-mRNA splicing. A subset of patients with low levels (5–20 %) of wild type ATM exhibit milder phenotypes, suggesting that even a modest increase in ATM protein expression could have a therapeutic effect [86].

Approximately 50 % of ATM mutations affect splicing, usually altering less conserved sequences surrounding splice sites or creating novel splice sites [87]. A recent report utilized SSOs to correct splicing in cell lines carrying three types of splicing mutations: an exonic 5′ cryptic splice site in TAT[C] cells, an exonic 3′ splice site in IRAT9 cells, and a pseudoexon inclusion in AT203LA cells [88]. Treatment of each cell line with 25-mer morpholino SSOs targeted to mutation-activated cryptic splice sites restored correct splicing of ATM 20–55 % in a dose-dependent and sequence-specific manner (Fig. 2d). Furthermore, SSO treatment resulted in the expression of kinase-active ATM protein [88].

5.5 PSMA

Prostate-specific membrane antigen (PSMA) is a type II glycoprotein encoded by the folate hydrolase (FOLH1) gene. PSMA has been extensively studied because it is highly expressed in cancerous prostate tissue and non-prostate tumor neovasculature. SSOs targeted to *FOLH*1 pre-mRNA were used to shift splicing from the full-length PSMA to three different splice variants: the cytoplasmic PSM′ alternatively spliced at exon 1 (Fig. 2e), and two other isoforms, PSMAΔ6 and PSMAΔ18, which lack exons six and eight respectively [89]. While the PSM′ isoform was demonstrated to retain enzymatic activity, PSMAΔ6 and PSMAΔ18 were inactive. Although the role of PSMA in prostate cancer is unclear, the presence of the cytoplasmic MXXXL internalization motif and demonstrated ability to internalize in response to ligand binding suggest PSMA may act as a receptor or transport protein [90, 91].

6 Other Applications of SSO Technology

6.1 ESSENCE

Point mutations that affect splicing frequently result in exon exclusion, which is not always amenable to correction by antisense SSOs alone [92]. Exon-specific splicing enhancement by small chimeric effectors (ESSENCE) is a PNA oligonucleotide-based approach designed to enhance the inclusion of a targeted, alternatively or aberrantly spliced exon into the spliced mRNA. This technology is based on manipulating the function of ESEs [93]. An ESSENCE PNA oligonucleotide contains a covalently bound peptide RS domain at the 3′ end designed to mimic SR proteins known to bind ESEs. This oligonucleotide bound internally to the exon targeted for inclusion is expected to promote SR-protein-mediated exon definition and enhance exon inclusion into mature mRNA.

ESSENCE was used to correct splicing BRCA1 exon 18, which requires recognition of an intact ESE by the SR protein SF2/ASF. A point mutation, present in some breast and ovarian cancers, disrupts the ESE in exon 18 of BRCA1, causing its exclusion from the mature mRNA transcript [94, 95]. Using ESSENCE, Cartegni and Kramer corrected splicing of BRCA1 exon 18 in a specific, dose-dependent manner, restoring splicing to wild type levels [96]. Interestingly, oligonucleotide alone also induced an intermediate level of exon inclusion, albeit at lower levels than when the tethered splicing enhancer was included.

ESSENCE has also been applied to modify the splicing of bcl-x [97]. A PNA oligonucleotide was conjugated to an eight-amino acid SR domain and targeted to a region of bcl-x pre-mRNA that does not encode splicing regulatory sequences. Bcl-x ESSENCE caused a dose-dependent increase in the bcl-xS:bcl-xL ratio in HeLa cells. In addition, treatment of HeLa cells with bcl-x ESSENCE triggered apoptosis as indicated by Annexin V staining.

6.2 TOSS

Targeted oligonucleotide silencers of splicing (TOSS) take advantage of the specificity of oligonucleotides-based approaches combined with the interfering capacity of protein or complexes bound near splice sites. This strategy employs an oligonucleotide with a 5′ or 3′ extension that is recognized by hnRNP A1/A2 proteins, which strongly inhibits splicing at the targeted splice site [98].

TOSS was first used to alter splicing of bcl-x in favor of the pro-apoptotic bcl-xS [98]. In cell culture, an oligonucleotide targeted just upstream of the proximal, -xL 5′ splice site, alone did not alter splicing. Delivery of TOSS, containing the consensus-binding sequence for hnRNP A1, resulted in a dose-dependent increase in the ratio of bcl-xS to bcl-xL. Of note, hnRNP A1/A2 proteins are typically highly expressed in tumor cells as opposed to normal cells, a feature that could be exploited by TOSS in cancer therapy [99].

7 RNA Interference

RNA interference (RNAi) is the oligonucleotide-based strategy of targeting mRNA for degradation with short double-stranded RNA molecules [100–102]. In this process exogenous double-stranded RNA molecules are processes by Dicer, a protein complex containing endonuclease, into 21–22 nucleotide double-stranded small interfering RNA (siRNA) [103–105]. The siRNAs themselves may also be directly delivered to the cytoplasm of cells, or expressed as short hairpin RNA, or shRNA that is processed to an siRNA and integrated into the RNA-induced silencing complex (RISC). Subsequently, RISC cleaves the target mRNA [102, 105, 106], which as a result, is silenced.

Numerous studies in cultured mammalian cell lines focused on the use of siRNA in treating cancer and other diseases [107–110]. Additionally, several pre-clinical studies using siRNA against cancer targets have been reported. ALN-VSP01 was developed for the treatment of liver cancers and potentially other solid tumors (www.alnylam.com). With a liposomal formulation, ALN-VSP01 is comprised of two siRNAs, targeting vascular endothelial growth factor (VEGF), and kinesin spindle protein (KSP), respectively. These two genes are involved in distinct pathways of tumor pathology, cell proliferation, and angiogenesis in a broad range of cancers. ALN-VSP01 delivered to the liver caused silencing of both VEGF and KSP expression in the liver, and stopped cancer cell growth in vitro. Importantly, RNAi is being used as a tool for the discovery and validation of cancer gene targets [111].

Because naked siRNA is quickly degraded by serum nucleases in vivo, many groups have focused on improving siRNA delivery [112]. CALAA-01 is an experimental therapeutic comprised of siRNA targeted to ribonucleotide reductase subunit 2 (RRM2) formulated in a targeted nanoparticle [113]. A Phase I clinical trial with CALAA-01 was initiated in 2008. An interim analysis of the trial indicated that CALAA-01 demonstrated a true RNAi mechanism in humans for the first time [114].

RNAi technology has also entered clinical trials for the treatment of Respiratory Syncytial Virus, and promising studies in non-human primates show that siRNAs may be effective cholesterol lowering agents, by targeting APOB100 [115].

8 Inhibition of Translation Initiation and Other Antisense Approaches

Several types of oligonucleotide analogs have been used to inhibit translation initiation, and thus downregulate expression of the target gene. PMO oligomers that span the AUG start codon have been effectively used to downregulate therapeutic gene targets, including c-myc [47] and TNF-α [116], by preventing ribosomal assembly on the mRNA. Phosphoramidates have also proven to be effective translation inhibitors, yielding downregulation of the cancer targets c-myc and bcl-2 in cell culture and in mice [55, 117–119].

Downregulation of gene expression via RNA degradation can be also achieved by direct application of protein ribonucleases, such as onconase and bovine seminal-RNase, or ribozymes and DNazymes. These strategies have been extensively reviewed by Tafech and colleagues [120].

9 Antisense-Based Therapeutics in Cancer Clinical Trials

To date, only RNase H competent first and second generation ASO have entered clinical trials for the treatment of cancer. Below is a summary of these compounds. Note that although the first generation oligonucleotides have reached Phase III clinical trials in some instances, it appears that the second generation molecules, with their superior chemistry, are poised to outperform the first generation phosphorothioates as therapeutics.

9.1 First Generation: Phosphorothioate DNA Oligonucleotides

9.1.1 Oblimersen Sodium (G3139, Genasense, from Genta)

Oblimersen Sodium is a clinically advanced first generation 18-mer phosphorothioate oligonucleotide [121], that is complementary to the first six codons of bcl-2, a well-characterized oncogene [122, 123]. Between July 2000 and February 2003, the largest randomized phase III trial in advanced melanoma was conducted, in which 771 patients with irresectable stage III or stage IV melanoma were randomly assigned to receive dacarbazine alone or preceded by Oblimersen treatment [124]. The combination of Oblimersen/dacarbazine slightly improved survival compared to the dacarbazine alone (median, 9.0 *vs.* 7.8 months; $P = .077$), and improved secondary end points. Importantly, patients with normal LDH level exhibited significantly improved multiple clinical outcomes to the addition of Oblimersen compared to patients with elevated LDH.

Recently, results of a randomized phase III trial of chemotherapy (fludarabine plus cyclophosphamide) with or without Oblimersen in 241 patients with relapsed or refractory chronic lymphocytic leukemia (CLL) were reported [125]. Addition of Oblimersen to chemotherapy increased CR/nPR from 7 to 17 % ($P = .025$). Overall, this trial met its intent-to-treat primary endpoint, and demonstrated that Oblimersen can improve the outcomes of standard CLL chemotherapy.

9.1.2 Trabedersen (AP 12009, From Antisense Pharma)

Trabedersen is a PS ASO targeted to the cytokine transforming growth factor-β, the overexpression of which is a hallmark of various cancers, including pancreatic carcinoma, malignant glioma, metastatic melanoma, and metastatic colorectal carcinoma. In randomized, open-label, dose-finding phase IIb study, Trabedersen was administered intratumorally by convection-enhanced delivery in patients with recurrent/refractory high-grade glioma. Median survival of patients treated with 10 μM Trabedersen following recurrence was 39.1 months compared 21.7 months for those treated with chemotherapy standard of care; however, this difference was no statistically significant [126]. A randomized, controlled international Phase III study was initiated in March 2009 and will compare trabedersen 10 microM versus conventional alkylating chemotherapy in patients with recurrent or refractory anaplastic astrocytoma after standard radio- and chemotherapy [127]. (Table 1)

9.2 Second Generation: Phosphorothioate Gapmers

Antisense drugs that incorporate second generation chemistries have more promise of success than first generation compounds clinically. Below is a summary of these second generation drugs.

Table 1 Clinical evaluation of other first generation antisense oligonucleotides

Drug name	Drug target	Clinical phase	Company
Oblimersen	Bcl-2	III	Genta
Trabedersen	TGF-β	III	Antisense pharma
LOR-2040	Ribonucleotide reductase	II	Lorus therapeutics
Archexin	AKT-1	II	Rexahn pharmaceuticals

9.2.1 OGX-011 (from OncoGeneX/ISIS)

OGX-011 is a second generation (i.e. phosphorothioate backbone with 2′-MOE modifications on the four nucleotides at the 3′ and 5′ end) 21-mer gapmer ASO targeting the translation-initiation site of clusterin, a cell survival gene associated with the development of hormone and drug resistance [128]. In phase II study of OGX-011in combination with docetaxel/prednisone in patients with metastatic prostate cancer OGX-011 treatment resulted in 26 % decline in target clusterin versus 0.9 % increase without the drug. Although the treatment translated into significant reduction in PSA, the declines were similar in treatment and control groups (50 and 54 % respectively). More encouraging results were observed, however, in patient survival. Progression-free survival was extended by 20 % (6.1–7.3 months) and overall survival by 41 % (16.9–23.8 months). Overall, the treatment with OGX-011 and docetaxel was well-tolerated and sufficiently promising to warrant further studies [129].

9.2.2 SPC2996 (from Santaris Pharma)

SPC2996 is a second generation ASO gapmer with LNA modifications at the 3′ and 5′ end. By targeting Bcl-2, SPC2996 showed strong induction of apoptosis and inhibition of proliferation in vitro and exhibited tumor growth inhibition both as a single agent and in combination with chemotherapy in mouse models. SPC2996 is currently in phase I/II clinical study for CLL. Preliminary results have shown evidence of efficacy, including decreased lymphocyte count, decreased bcl-2 expression in lymphocytes, and a beneficial effect on lymph nodes and tumors (www.santaris.com).

9.2.3 LY2181308 (from Eli Lilly/ISIS)

LY2181308 is a second generation 2′-MOE ASO gapmer that potently downregulates Survivin, an inhibitor of apoptosis protein (IAP), in a broad range of human tumor cells [130]. Survivin is generally not expressed in normal tissues, but has been detected at a high level in a broad range of human cancers [131], and elevated Survivin expression level in cancer patients is associated with lower apoptotic index in tumor cells and poor prognosis [132]. Phase I trials for LY2181308 have been initiated against a broad range of human cancers. One phase IB/II study of

Table 2 Clinical evaluation of other second generation antisense oligonucleotides

Drug name	Drug target	Chemistry	Clinical phase	Company
Custirsen	Clusterin	2′-O-MOE gapmer	II	ISIS pharmaceuticals
LY2181308	Survivin	2′-O-MOE gapmer	II	Eli Lily/ISIS
AEG35156	X-IAP	2′-OMe gapmer	II	Aegera therapeutics
OGX-427	Heat shock protein 27	2′-O-MOE gapmer	I	OncoGeneX
LY2275796	eIF-4E	2′-O-MOE gapmer	I	Eli Lily/ISIS
SPC2996	Bcl-2	LNA gapmer	I	Santaris pharmaceuticals
EZN2968	Hypoxia inducing factor 1-α	LNA gapmer	I	Enzon pharmaceuticals
EZN3042	Survivin	LNA gapmer	I	Enzon pharmaceuticals
CALAA-01	Ribonucleotide reductase	siRNA/ nanoparticle	I	Colando pharmaceuticals

LY2181308 in patients with advanced hepatocellular carcinoma began in 2007. (Table 2)

References

1. Graveley BR (2001) Alternative splicing: increasing diversity in the proteomic world. Trends Genet 17:100–107
2. Johnson JM, Castle J, Garrett-Engele P, Kan Z, Loerch PM, Armour CD, Santos R, Schadt EE, Stoughton R, Shoemaker DD (2003) Genome-wide survey of human alternative pre-mRNA splicing with exon junction microarrays. Science 302:2141–2144
3. Modrek B, Lee C (2002) A genomic view of alternative splicing. Nat Genet 30:13–19
4. Kalnina Z, Zayakin P, Silina K, Line A (2005) Alterations of pre-mRNA splicing in cancer. Genes Chromosomes Cancer 42:342–357
5. Wang ET, Sandberg R, Luo S, Khrebtukova I, Zhang L, Mayr C, Kingsmore SF, Schroth GP, Burge CB (2008) Alternative isoform regulation in human tissue transcriptomes. Nature 456:470–476
6. Dominski Z, Kole R (1993) Restoration of correct splicing in thalassemic pre-mRNA by antisense oligonucleotides. Proc Natl Acad Sci U S A 90:8673–8677
7. Suwanmanee T, Sierakowska H, Lacerra G, Svasti S, Kirby S, Walsh C, Fucharoen S, Kole R (2002) Restoration of human beta-globin gene expression in murine and human Ivs2-654 thalassemic erythroid cells by free uptake of antisense oligonucleotides. Mol Pharmacol 62:545–553

8. Svasti S, Suwanmanee T, Fucharoen S, Moulton HM, Nelson MH, Maeda N, Smithies O, Kole R (2009) RNA repair restores hemoglobin expression in IVS2-654 thalassemic mice. Proc Natl Acad Sci U S A 106:1205–1210
9. Garcia-Blanco MA, Baraniak AP, Lasda EL (2004) Alternative splicing in disease and therapy. Nat Biotechnol 22:535–546
10. Faustino NA, Cooper TA (2003) Pre-mRNA splicing and human disease. Genes Dev 17:419–437
11. Pajares MJ, Ezponda T, Catena R, Calvo A, Pio R, Montuenga LM (2007) Alternative splicing: an emerging topic in molecular and clinical oncology. Lancet Oncol 8:349–357
12. Matlin AJ, Clark F, Smith CW (2005) Understanding alternative splicing: towards a cellular code. Nat Rev Mol Cell Biol 6:386–398
13. Cartegni L, Chew SL, Krainer AR (2002) Listening to silence and understanding nonsense: exonic mutations that affect splicing. Nat Rev Genet 3:285–298
14. Spellman R, Rideau A, Matlin A, Gooding C, Robinson F, McGlincy N, Grellscheid SN, Southby J, Wollerton M, Smith CW (2005) Regulation of alternative splicing by PTB and associated factors. Biochem Soc Trans 33:457–460
15. Cartegni L, Wang J, Zhu Z, Zhang MQ, Krainer AR (2003) ESE finder: a web resource to identify exonic splicing enhancers. Nucleic Acids Res 31:3568–3571
16. Zhang XH, Heller KA, Hefter I, Leslie CS, Chasin LA (2003) Sequence information for the splicing of human pre-mRNA identified by support vector machine classification. Genome Res 13:2637–2650
17. Fairbrother WG, Yeh RF, Sharp PA, Burge CB (2002) Predictive identification of exonic splicing enhancers in human genes. Science 297:1007–1013
18. Wang Y, Selvakumar M, Helfman D (1997) In: Krainer A (ed) Eukaryotic mRNA processing. Oxford University Press, New York, pp 242–278
19. Wang YC, Selvakumar M, Helfman D (1997) Alternative pre-mRNA splicing. In: Eukaryotic mRNA processing. Oxford University Press, New York, pp 242–279
20. Herbert A, Rich A (1999) RNA processing and the evolution of eukaryotes. Nat Genet 21:265–269
21. Hua Y, Sahashi K, Hung G, Rigo F, Passini MA, Bennett CF, Krainer AR (2010) Antisense correction of SMN2 splicing in the CNS rescues necrosis in a type III SMA mouse model. Genes Dev 24:1634–1644
22. Donahue CP, Muratore C, Wu JY, Kosik KS, Wolfe MS (2006) Stabilization of the tau exon 10 stem loop alters pre-mRNA splicing. J Biol Chem 281:23302–23306
23. Kalbfuss B, Mabon SA, Misteli T (2001) Correction of alternative splicing of tau in front temporal dementia and parkinsonism linked to chromosome 17. J Biol Chem 276:42986–42993
24. Lu QL, Rabinowitz A, Chen YC, Yokota T, Yin H, Alter J, Jadoon A, Bou-Gharios G, Partridge T (2005) Systemic delivery of antisense oligoribonucleotide restores dystrophin expression in body-wide skeletal muscles. Proc Natl Acad Sci U S A 102:198–203
25. Goyenvalle A, Babbs A, Powell D, Kole R, Fletcher S, Wilton SD, Davies KE (2010) Prevention of dystrophic pathology in severely affected dystrophin/utrophin-deficient mice by morpholino-oligomer-mediated exon-skipping. Mol Ther 18:198–205
26. Kinali M, Arechavala-Gomeza V, Feng L, Cirak S, Hunt D, Adkin C, Guglieri M, Ashton E, Abbs S, Nihoyannopoulos P et al (2009) Local restoration of dystrophin expression with the morpholino oligomer AVI-4658 in Duchenne muscular dystrophy: a single-blind, placebo-controlled, dose-escalation, proof-of-concept study. Lancet Neurol 8:918–928
27. Crooke S (2001) Antisense drug technology. Marcel Dekker, New York
28. Sazani P, Kole R (2003) Therapeutic potential of antisense oligonucleotides as modulators of alternative splicing. J Clin Invest 112:481–486
29. Koch T, Orum H (2008) In: Crooke ST (ed) Antisense drug technology, 2nd edn. CRC Press, Boca Raton
30. Lee LK, Roth CM (2003) Antisense technology in molecular and cellular bioengineering. Curr Opin Biotechnol 14:505–511
31. Friedrich I, Shir A, Klein S, Levitzki A (2004) RNA molecules as anti-cancer agents. Semin Cancer Biol 14:223–230

32. Jason TL, Koropatnick J, Berg RW (2004) Toxicology of antisense therapeutics. Toxicol Appl Pharmacol 201:66–83
33. Kurreck J (2003) Antisense technologies. Improvement through novel chemical modifications. Eur J Biochem 270:1628–1644
34. Pirollo KF, Rait A, Sleer LS, Chang EH (2003) Antisense therapeutics: from theory to clinical practice. Pharmacol Ther 99:55–77
35. Stahel RA, Zangemeister-Wittke U (2003) Antisense oligonucleotides for cancer therapy-an overview. Lung Cancer 41(Suppl 1):S81–S88
36. Gleave ME, Monia BP (2005) Antisense therapy for cancer. Nat Rev Cancer 5:468–479
37. Sazani P, GM, Kole R (2007) Antisense drug technology. CRC Press Taylor & Francis Group, Boca Raton, FL USA, pp 89–114
38. Orum H, Wengel J (2001) Locked nucleic acids: a promising molecular family for gene-function analysis and antisense drug development. Curr Opin Mol Ther 3:239–243
39. Torigoe H, Hari Y, Sekiguchi M, Obika S, Imanishi T (2001) 2'-O,4′-C-methylene bridged nucleic acid modification promotes pyrimidine motif triplex DNA formation at physiological pH. Thermodynamic and kinetic studies. J Biol Chem 276:2354–2360
40. Roberts J, Palma E, Sazani P, Orum H, Cho M, Kole R (2006) Efficient and persistent splice switching by systemically delivered Lna oligonucleotides in mice. Mol Ther 14:471–475
41. Manoharan M (1999) 2′-carbohydrate modifications in antisense oligonucleotide therapy: importance of conformation, configuration and conjugation. Biochim Biophys Acta 1489:117–130
42. Sazani P, Astriab-Fischer A, Kole R (2003) Effects of base modifications on antisense properties of 2′-O-methoxyethyl and PNA oligonucleotides. Antisense Nucleic Acid Drug Dev 13:119–128
43. Zhang H, Cook J, Nickel J, Yu R, Stecker K, Myers K, Dean NM (2000) Reduction of liver Fas expression by an antisense oligonucleotide protects mice from fulminant hepatitis. Nat Biotechnol 18:862–867
44. Sazani P, Gemignani F, Kang SH, Maier MA, Manoharan M, Persmark M, Bortner D, Kole R (2002) Systemically delivered antisense oligomers upregulate gene expression in mouse tissues. Nat Biotechnol 20:1228–1233
45. Raal FJ, Santos RD, Blom DJ, Marais AD, Charng MJ, Cromwell WC, Lachmann RH, Gaudet D, Tan JL, Chasan-Taber S et al (2010) Mipomersen, an apolipoprotein B synthesis inhibitor, for lowering of LDL cholesterol concentrations in patients with homozygous familial hypercholesterolemia: a randomized, double-blind, placebo-controlled trial. Lancet 375:998–1006
46. Summerton J (1999) Morpholino antisense oligomers: the case for an RNase H-independent structural type. Biochim Biophys Acta 1489:141–158
47. Hudziak RM, Summerton J, Weller DD, Iversen PL (2000) Antiproliferative effects of steric blocking phosphorodiamidate morpholino antisense agents directed against c-myc. Antisense Nucleic Acid Drug Dev 10:163–176
48. Nasevicius A, Ekker SC (2000) Effective targeted gene 'knockdown' in zebrafish. Nat Genet 26:216–220
49. Greenberg DE, Marshall-Batty KR, Brinster LR, Zarember KA, Shaw PA, Mellbye BL, Iversen PL, Holland SM, Geller BL (2010) Antisense phosphorodiamidate morpholino oligomers targeted to an essential gene inhibit Burkholderia cepacia complex. J Infect Dis 201:1822–1830
50. Mellbye BL, Weller DD, Hassinger JN, Reeves MD, Lovejoy CE, Iversen PL, Geller BL (2010) Cationic phosphorodiamidate morpholino oligomers efficiently prevent growth of *Escherichia coli* in vitro and in vivo. J Antimicrob Chemother 65:98–106
51. Warren TK, Warfield KL, Wells J, Swenson DL, Donner KS, Van Tongeren SA, Garza NL, Dong L, Mourich DV, Crumley S et al (2010) Advanced antisense therapies for post exposure protection against lethal filovirus infections. Nat Med 16:991–994
52. Sazani P, Kang SH, Maier MA, Wei C, Dillman J, Summerton J, Manoharan M, Kole R (2001) Nuclear antisense effects of neutral, anionic and cationic oligonucleotide analogs. Nucleic Acids Res 29:3965–3974

53. Chen JK, Weith HL, Grewal RS, Wang G, Cushman M (1995) Synthesis of novel phosphoramidite reagents for the attachment of antisense oligonucleotides to various regions of the benzophenanthridine ring system. Bioconjug Chem 6:473–482
54. Gee JE, Robbins I, van der Laan AC, van Boom JH, Colombier C, Leng M, Raible AM, Nelson JS, Lebleu B (1998) Assessment of high-affinity hybridization, RNase H cleavage, and covalent linkage in translation arrest by antisense oligonucleotides. Antisense Nucleic Acid Drug Dev 8:103–111
55. Gryaznov SM (1999) Oligonucleotide N3′–>P5′ phosphoramidates as potential therapeutic agents. Biochim Biophys Acta 1489:131–140
56. Adams JM, Cory S (2007) The Bcl-2 apoptotic switch in cancer development and therapy. Oncogene 26:1324–1337
57. Boise LH, Gonzalez-Garcia M, Postema CE, Ding L, Lindsten T, Turka LA, Mao X, Nunez G, Thompson CB (1993) bcl-x, a bcl-2-related gene that functions as a dominant regulator of apoptotic cell death. Cell 74:597–608
58. Minn AJ, Boise LH, Thompson CB (1996) Bcl-x(S) antagonizes the protective effects of Bcl-x(L). J Biol Chem 271:6306–6312
59. Lindenboim L, Borner C, Stein R (2001) Bcl-x(S) can form homodimers and heterodimers and its apoptotic activity requires localization of Bcl-x(S) to the mitochondria and its BH3 and loop domains. Cell Death Differ 8:933–942
60. Willis SN, Fletcher JI, Kaufmann T, van Delft MF, Chen L, Czabotar PE, Ierino H, Lee EF, Fairlie WD, Bouillet P et al (2007) Apoptosis initiated when BH3 ligands engage multiple Bcl-2 homologs, not Bax or Bak. Science 315:856–859
61. Amundson SA, Myers TG, Scudiero D, Kitada S, Reed JC, Fornace AJ Jr (2000) An informatics approach identifying markers of chemosensitivity in human cancer cell lines. Cancer Res 60:6101–6110
62. Tu Y, Renner S, Xu F, Fleishman A, Taylor J, Weisz J, Vescio R, Rettig M, Berenson J, Krajewski S et al (1998) BCL-X expression in multiple myeloma: possible indicator of chemoresistance. Cancer Res 58:256–262
63. Reeve JG, Xiong J, Morgan J, Bleehen NM (1996) Expression of apoptosis-regulatory genes in lung tumour cell lines: relationship to p53 expression and relevance to acquired drug resistance. Br J Cancer 73:1193–1200
64. Olopade OI, Adeyanju MO, Safa AR, Hagos F, Mick R, Thompson CB, Recant WM (1997) Overexpression of BCL-x protein in primary breast cancer is associated with high tumor grade and nodal metastases. Cancer J Sci Am 3:230–237
65. Mercatante DR, Bortner CD, Cidlowski JA, Kole R (2001) Modification of alternative splicing of Bcl-x pre-mRNA in prostate and breast cancer cells. Analysis of apoptosis and cell death. J Biol Chem 276:16411–16417
66. Watanabe J, Kushihata F, Honda K, Mominoki K, Matsuda S, Kobayashi N (2002) Bcl-xL overexpression in human hepatocellular carcinoma. Int J Oncol 21:515–519
67. Beroukhim R, Mermel CH, Porter D, Wei G, Raychaudhuri S, Donovan J, Barretina J, Boehm JS, Dobson J, Urashima M et al (2010) The landscape of somatic copy-number alteration across human cancers. Nature 463:899–905
68. Gilbert LA, Hemann MT (2010) DNA damage-mediated induction of a chemoresistant niche. Cell 143:355–366
69. Mercatante DR, Mohler JL, Kole R (2002) Cellular response to an antisense-mediated shift of Bcl-x pre-mRNA splicing and antineoplastic agents. J Biol Chem 277:49374–49382
70. Bauman JA, Li SD, Yang A, Huang L, Kole R (2010) Anti-tumor activity of splice-switching oligonucleotides. Nucleic Acids Res 38:8348–8356
71. Olie RA, Hafner C, Kuttel R, Sigrist B, Willers J, Dummer R, Hall J, Stahel RA, Zangemeister-Wittke U (2002) Bcl-2 and bcl-xL antisense oligonucleotides induce apoptosis in melanoma cells of different clinical stages. J Invest Dermatol 118:505–512
72. Guensberg P, Wacheck V, Lucas T, Monia B, Pehamberger H, Eichler HG, Jansen B (2002) Bcl-xL antisense oligonucleotides chemosensitize human glioblastoma cells. Chemotherapy 48:189–195

73. Wacheck V, Selzer E, Gunsberg P, Lucas T, Meyer H, Thallinger C, Monia BP, Jansen B (2003) Bcl-x(L) antisense oligonucleotides radiosensitive colon cancer cells. Br J Cancer 89:1352–1357
74. Taylor JK, Zhang QQ, Wyatt JR, Dean NM (1999) Induction of endogenous Bcl-xS through the control of Bcl-x pre-mRNA splicing by antisense oligonucleotides. Nat Biotechnol 17:1097–1100
75. Yarden Y, Sliwkowski MX (2001) Untangling the ErbB signalling network. Nat Rev Mol Cell Biol 2:127–137
76. Hsieh AC, Moasser MM (2007) Targeting HER proteins in cancer therapy and the role of the non-target HER3. Br J Cancer 97:453–457
77. Wan J, Sazani P and Kole R (2009) Modification of HER2 pre-mRNA alternative splicing and its effects on breast cancer cells. Int J Cancer 124:772–777
78. Vickers SM, Huang ZQ, MacMillan-Crow L, Greendorfer JS, Thompson JA (2002) Ligand activation of alternatively spliced fibroblast growth factor receptor-1 modulates pancreatic adenocarcinoma cell malignancy. J Gastrointest Surg 6:546–553
79. Luqmani YA, Mortimer C, Yiangou C, Johnston CL, Bansal GS, Sinnett D, Law M, Coombes RC (1995) Expression of 2 variant forms of fibroblast growth factor receptor 1 in human breast. Int J Cancer 64:274–279
80. Yamaguchi F, Saya H, Bruner JM, Morrison RS (1994) Differential expression of two fibroblast growth factor-receptor genes is associated with malignant progression in human astrocytomas. Proc Natl Acad Sci U S A 91:484–488
81. Jin W, Huang ES, Bi W, Cote GJ (1999) Redundant intronic repressors function to inhibit fibroblast growth factor receptor-1 alpha-exon recognition in glioblastoma cells. J Biol Chem 274:28035–28041
82. Bruno IG, Jin W, Cote GJ (2004) Correction of aberrant FGFR1 alternative RNA splicing through targeting of intronic regulatory elements. Hum Mol Genet 13:2409–2420
83. Kastan MB, Lim DS (2000) The many substrates and functions of ATM. Nat Rev Mol Cell Biol 1:179–186
84. Gatti RA (1991) Localizing the genes for ataxia-telangiectasia: a human model for inherited cancer susceptibility. Adv Cancer Res 56:77–104
85. Ahmed M, Rahman N (2006) ATM and breast cancer susceptibility. Oncogene 25:5906–5911
86. Gilad S, Chessa L, Khosravi R, Russell P, Galanty Y, Piane M, Gatti RA, Jorgensen TJ, Shiloh Y, Bar-Shira A (1998) Genotype-phenotype relationships in ataxia-telangiectasia and variants. Am J Hum Genet 62:551–561
87. Teraoka SN, Telatar M, Becker-Catania S, Liang T, Onengut S, Tolun A, Chessa L, Sanal O, Bernatowska E, Gatti RA et al (1999) Splicing defects in the ataxia-telangiectasia gene, ATM: underlying mutations and consequences. Am J Hum Genet 64:1617–1631
88. Du L, Pollard JM, Gatti RA (2007) Correction of prototypic ATM splicing mutations and aberrant ATM function with antisense morpholino oligonucleotides. Proc Natl Acad Sci U S A 104:6007–6012
89. Williams T, Kole R (2006) Analysis of prostate-specific membrane antigen splice variants in LNCap cells. Oligonucleotides 16:186–195
90. Rajasekaran SA, Anilkumar G, Oshima E, Bowie JU, Liu H, Heston W, Bander NH, Rajasekaran AK (2003) A novel cytoplasmic tail MXXXL motif mediates the internalization of prostate-specific membrane antigen. Mol Biol Cell 14:4835–4845
91. Lupold SE, Hicke BJ, Lin Y, Coffey DS (2002) Identification and characterization of nuclease-stabilized RNA molecules that bind human prostate cancer cells via the prostate-specific membrane antigen. Cancer Res 62:4029–4033
92. Nakai K, Sakamoto H (1994) Construction of a novel database containing aberrant splicing mutations of mammalian genes. Gene 141:171–177
93. Sanford JR, Ellis J, Caceres JF (2005) Multiple roles of arginine/serine-rich splicing factors in RNA processing. Biochem Soc Trans 33:443–446
94. Mazoyer S, Puget N, Perrin-Vidoz L, Lynch HT, Serova-Sinilnikova OM, Lenoir GM (1998) A BRCA1 nonsense mutation causes exon skipping. Am J Hum Genet 62:713–715

95. Liu HX, Cartegni L, Zhang MQ, Krainer AR (2001) A mechanism for exon skipping caused by nonsense or missense mutations in BRCA1 and other genes. Nat Genet 27:55–58
96. Cartegni L, Krainer AR (2003) Correction of disease-associated exon skipping by synthetic exon-specific activators. Nat Struct Biol 10:120–125
97. Wilusz JE, Devanney SC, Caputi M (2005) Chimeric peptide nucleic acid compounds modulate splicing of the bcl-x gene in vitro and in vivo. Nucleic Acids Res 33:6547–6554
98. Villemaire J, Dion I, Elela SA, Chabot B (2003) Reprogramming alternative pre-messenger RNA splicing through the use of protein-binding antisense oligonucleotides. J Biol Chem 278:50031–50039
99. Patry C, Bouchard L, Labrecque P, Gendron D, Lemieux B, Toutant J, Lapointe E, Wellinger R, Chabot B (2003) Small interfering RNA-mediated reduction in heterogeneous nuclear ribonucleoparticule A1/A2 proteins induces apoptosis in human cancer cells but not in normal mortal cell lines. Cancer Res 63:7679–7688
100. Swanton C, Nicke B, Downward J (2004) RNA interference, DNA methylation, and gene silencing: a bright future for cancer therapy? Lancet Oncol 5:653–654
101. Downward J (2004) RNA interference. Bmj 328:1245–1248
102. Lingel A, Izaurralde E (2004) RNAi: finding the elusive endonuclease. RNA 10:1675–1679
103. Bagasra O, Prilliman KR (2004) RNA interference: the molecular immune system. J Mol Histol 35:545–553
104. Scherer LJ, Rossi JJ (2003) Approaches for the sequence-specific knockdown of mRNA. Nat Biotechnol 21:1457–1465
105. Matzke MA, Birchler JA (2005) RNAi-mediated pathways in the nucleus. Nat Rev Genet 6:24–35
106. Rand TA, Ginalski K, Grishin NV, Wang X (2004) Biochemical identification of Argonaute 2 as the sole protein required for RNA-induced silencing complex activity. Proc Natl Acad Sci U S A 101:14385–14389
107. Duxbury MS, Ito H, Zinner MJ, Ashley SW, Whang EE (2004) siRNA directed against c-Src enhances pancreatic adenocarcinoma cell gemcitabine chemosensitivity. J Am Coll Surg 198:953–959
108. Duxbury MS, Matros E, Ito H, Zinner MJ, Ashley SW, Whang EE (2004) Systemic siRNA-mediated gene silencing: a new approach to targeted therapy of cancer. Ann Surg 240:667–674 (discussion 666–675)
109. Liang Z, Yoon Y, Votaw J, Goodman MM, Williams L, Shim H (2005) Silencing of CXCR4 blocks breast cancer metastasis. Cancer Res 65:967–971
110. McCarthy BA, Mansour A, Lin YC, Kotenko S, Raveche E (2004) RNA interference of IL-10 in leukemic B-1 cells. Cancer Immun 4:6
111. Iorns E, Lord CJ, Turner N, Ashworth A (2007) Utilizing RNA interference to enhance cancer drug discovery. Nat Rev Drug Discov 6:556–568
112. Castanotto D, Rossi JJ (2009) The promises and pitfalls of RNA-interference-based therapeutics. Nature 457:426–433
113. Davis M (2009) The first targeted delivery of sirna in humans via a self-assembling, cyclodextrin polymer-based nanoparticle: from concept to clinic. Mol Pharm 6:659–668
114. Davis ME, Zuckerman JE, Choi CH, Seligson D, Tolcher A, Alabi CA, Yen Y, Heidel JD, Ribas A (2010) Evidence of RNAi in humans from systemically administered siRNA via targeted nanoparticles. Nature 464:1067–1070
115. Zimmermann TS, Lee AC, Akinc A, Bramlage B, Bumcrot D, Fedoruk MN, Harborth J, Heyes JA, Jeffs LB, John M et al (2006) RNAi-mediated gene silencing in non-human primates. Nature 441:111–114
116. Taylor MF, Weller DD, Kobzik L (1998) Effect of TNF-alpha antisense oligomers on cytokine production by primary murine alveolar macrophages. Antisense Nucleic Acid Drug Dev 8:199–205
117. Wang L, Gryaznov S, Nerenberg M (1999) Inhibition of IL-6 in mice by anti-NF-kappaB oligodeoxyribonucleotide N3′– > oligodeoxyribonnucleotide N3′ – > P5′ phosphoramidates. Inflammation 23:583–590

118. Faria M, Spiller DG, Dubertret C, Nelson JS, White MR, Scherman D, Helene C, Giovannangeli C (2001) Phosphoramidate oligonucleotides as potent antisense molecules in cells and in vivo. Nat Biotechnol 19:40–44
119. Skorski T, Perrotti D, Nieborowska-Skorska M, Gryaznov S, Calabretta B (1997) Antileukemia effect of c-myc N3′– > P5′ phosphoramidate antisense oligonucleotides in vivo. Proc Natl Acad Sci U S A 94:3966–3971
120. Tafech A, Bassett T, Sparanese D, Lee CH (2006) Destroying RNA as a therapeutic approach. Curr Med Chem 13:863–881
121. Kim R, Emi M, Matsuura K, Tanabe K (2007) Antisense and nonantisense effects of antisense Bcl-2 on multiple roles of Bcl-2 as a chemosensitizer in cancer therapy. Cancer Gene Ther 14:1–11
122. Reed J (1995) Prevention of apoptosis as a mechanism of drug resistance. Hematol Oncol Clin North Am 9:451–473
123. Coultas L, Strasser A (2003) The role of the Bcl-2 protein family in cancer. Semin Cancer Biol 13:115–123
124. Bedikian A, Millward M, Pehamberger H, Al E (2006) Bcl-2 antisense (oblimersen sodium) plus dacarbazine in patients with advanced melanoma: the oblimersen melanoma study group. J Clin Oncol 24:4738–4745
125. O'Brien S, Moore J, Boyd T, Al E (2007) Randomized phase III trial of fludarabine plus cyclophosphamide with or without oblimersen sodium (Bcl-2 antisense) in patients with relapsed or refractory chronic lymphocytic leukemia. J Clin Oncol 25:1114–1120
126. Bogdahn U, Hau P, Stockhammer G, Venkataramana NK, Mahapatra AK, Suri A, Balasubramaniam A, Nair S, Oliushine V, Parfenov V et al (2009) Targeted therapy for high-grade glioma with the TGF-beta2 inhibitor trabedersen: results of a randomized and controlled phase IIb study. Neuro Oncol 13:132–142
127. Hau P, Jachimczak P, Bogdahn U (2009) Treatment of malignant gliomas with TGF-beta2 antisense oligonucleotides. Expert Rev Anticancer Ther 9:1663–1674
128. Zellweger T, Miyake H, Cooper S, Al E (2001) Antitumor activity of antisense clusterin oligonucleotides is improved in vitro and in vivo by incorporation of 2'-O-(2-methoxy)ethyl chemistry. J Pharmacol Exp Ther 298:934–940
129. Chi KN, Hotte SJ, Yu EY, Tu D, Eigl BJ, Tannock I, Saad F, North S, Powers J, Gleave ME et al (2010) Randomized phase II study of docetaxel and prednisone with or without OGX-011 in patients with metastatic castration-resistant prostate cancer. J Clin Oncol 28:4247–4254
130. Chen J, Wu W, Tahir S, Al E (2000) Down-regulation of survivin by antisense oligonucleotides increases apoptosis, inhibits cytokinesis and anchorage-independent growth. Neoplasia 2:235–241
131. Ambrosini G, Adida C, Altieri D (1997) A novel anti-apoptosis gene, survivin, expressed in cancer and lymphoma. Nat Med 3:917–921
132. Kawasaki H, Altieri D, Lu C, Al E (1998) Inhibition of apoptosis by survivin predicts shorter survival rates in colorectal cancer. Cancer Res 58:5071–5074

Clinical Perspective on Chemo-Resistance and the Role of RNA Processing

Nancy L. Krett, Shuo Ma and Steven T. Rosen

Abstract

Pre-messenger RNA splicing is significantly changed in cancer cells leading to the expression of cancer-specific transcripts. These transcripts have the potential to be used as cancer biomarkers and also as targets for new therapeutic approaches. In addition, the cancer-specific transcripts have the potential to alter the drug response of the cancer cells creating a chemo-resistant state. This later property of alternative splicing presents a challenge to clinicians in the design of effective therapeutic regimens. When a patient's cancer relapses it is frequently refractory to standard chemotherapies resulting in a poor clinical outcome. Therefore, understanding the mechanisms of how alternative splicing can lead to chemo-resistance is critical to the effective delivery of treatment. Here, we will discuss the impact of alternative splicing variants on drug metabolism and activation; on drug interactions with cell signaling pathways; and on cell death pathways in cancer therapeutics. In addition to the initial characterization of splicing variants, the mechanisms leading to alterations in splicing are being studied in the setting of chemo-resistance and will be discussed here. The promise of therapeutic intervention to obviate the impact of these splicing variants will significantly enhance treatment options for cancer patients.

Keywords

Multi-drug resistance · Drug metabolism · Steroid receptors

N. L. Krett (✉) · S. T. Rosen
Robert H. Lurie Comprehensive Cancer Center, Northwestern University, Chicago, IL, USA
e-mail: n-krett@northwestern.edu

S. Ma
Division of Hematology and Oncology, Northwestern University, Chicago, IL, USA

J. Y. Wu (ed.), *RNA and Cancer*, Cancer Treatment and Research,
DOI: 10.1007/978-3-642-31659-3_10, © Springer-Verlag Berlin Heidelberg 2013

Contents

1 Introduction

Cancer is a disease of clonal evolution which selects for cells with enhanced proliferation and survival [1]. In the face of selective pressure of chemotherapeutics, the genetic heterogeneity of the cancer clone allows for the selection and expansion of chemo-resistant cells. This may ultimately result in relapsed disease that is refractory to standard therapeutics. This is a central problem in cancer therapy [1]. Studies in bacteria indicate that selective pressure does not cause mutations, but rather selects for mutations that are advantageous to clonal survival [2]. One mechanism the cells utilize to generate diversity is alternative splicing to produce transcripts that may have a changed function or a reduced functional capacity.

Alternative splicing is a post-transcriptional mechanism for regulating the processing of pre-mRNAs such that different combinations of splice sites can be joined to form mature mRNAs. This process contributes to the functional complexity of the human proteome that is not represented by the number of genes in the genome [3]. In a tissue-specific and developmentally regulated fashion, alternative splicing regulates gene activities involved in every aspect of cell function and survival [4]. Alternative splicing can lead to functionally antagonistic products generated from the same genetic locus with both splicing isoforms being expressed in the cell. A shift in the isoform balance can lead to changes in cellular function [5].

Alternative splicing variants have been described in a number of cancers [5, 6]. Using a bioinformatics approach, Kirschbaum-Slager et al. observed a significant shift in the expression of splicing factors in tumors indicating that these factors may be involved in oncogenic pathways [7]. There is growing evidence to suggest that some cancer-specific protein expression patterns are caused by cancer-specific alternative splicing [8] indicating that splicing variants can be used as tumor markers and that alternative splicing can accompany the process of tumorigenesis [7]. Here, we will discuss the impact of alternative splicing variants on drug metabolism and activation; on drug interactions with cell signaling pathways; and on cell death pathways in cancer therapeutics. In addition to the initial characterization of splicing variants, the mechanisms leading to alterations in splicing are being studied in the setting of chemo-resistance and will be discussed here. In summary, the control of splicing is an important component of gene regulation and alternative splicing may contribute to chemoresistance to cancer therapies.

2 Alternative Splicing and Drug Delivery

Successful drug therapy relies on the ability of the drug to enter the cell either by passive or by active mechanism and also to be retained by the cell. In passive drug uptake, molecules such as steroids can diffuse across the cell membrane without energy expenditure. Active uptake requires energy and can involve cell surface molecules such as the ATP-binding cassette transporters or ABC [9]. This process can be affected by alternative splicing. Ligand-receptor binding results in the successful delivery of drug to the cell with subsequent activation of signal transduction pathways to translate the signal of drug into cellular activity. Endocrine-based therapies are used for the treatment of a number of cancers including breast cancer, prostate cancer, and hematologic malignancies. Alternative splicing of steroid receptors has been reported in these cancers and may contribute to the resistance of the steroid-based therapies. In addition to the successful uptake of drug, the retention of drug in the cell is required for successful therapy. Mechanisms to actively remove drug from the cells result in resistance to a number of drugs and have been termed multiple drug resistance or MDR and involve the ABC transporters. The development of MDR hampers the delivery of cancer therapeutics and therefore understanding the mechanisms of MDR is important for the successful delivery of therapies. Alternative splicing has been reported to play a role in some forms of MDR [10].

2.1 Alternatively Spliced Steroid Receptors

Steroid receptors belong to a large super family of hormonally activated transcription factors. The classical activation for the steroid receptor involves binding of the steroid hormone to the hormone-binding domain allowing for translocation of the receptor monomer to the nucleus. The DNA-binding domain of the receptor binds as a dimer to its response elements allowing for the transcriptional control of gene expression. Hormonally regulated cancers have long been treated with endocrine-based therapies; however, resistance to those therapies ultimately occurs. Alterations in the steroid receptors have been described for a number of hormone-resistant cancers including alterations caused by changes in splicing. Here, we will discuss some of the reported alternatively spliced hormone receptor variants and whether they contribute to the hormone resistance observed.

Tamoxifen, a selective estrogen receptor modulator (SERM), is among the first-line endocrine therapies for estrogen receptor/progesterone receptor positive breast cancers. Analysis of tamoxifen-resistant breast cancers revealed several variants of the estrogen receptor-α (ER-α) including alternatively spliced forms [11].

Alternative splicing of ER-α with deletions for exon 2, 3, 4, 5, and 7 have been described, with the most abundant variant being the exon 7 deletion. The exon 7 deletion ($\Delta 7$) was further analyzed and found to act as a dominant negative and inhibit the actions of the wild-type receptor in transient transfection assays [12]. The $\Delta 7$ variant of ER-α has also been detected in human endometrial adenocarcinoma [13]. When the $\Delta 7$ ER-α variant adenocarcinoma is grown in a nude mouse, the tumor is not responsive to either estrogen or progesterone; however, the tumor is responsive to tamoxifen which causes an increase in the doubling time of the tumor volume. This indicates tamoxifen acts as an agonist for the $\Delta 7$ receptor in an in vivo model.

Similarly, mutations in the glucocorticoid receptor (GR) have been described in glucocorticoid-resistant hematologic malignancies. We have described an alternative splice variant of GR, GR-P, in glucocorticoid-resistant myeloma cell lines [14]. GR-P is the result of a failure to splice at the exon 7 junction and retention of intron G and is the predominant GR variant observed [15, 16]. GR-P could encode a truncated receptor with a deletion in the hormone-binding domain, a critical functional domain; however, it is not clear that GR-P is translated into protein. In transient transfection assays, GR-P is not a functional receptor, nor does it act as a dominant negative receptor to reduce the function of the wild-type GR. Further studies will be required to elucidate the potential role for GR-P in glucocorticoid resistance.

Loss of the retinoic acid receptor β (RARβ) in lung cancer cells is associated with resistance to retinoic acid-induced cell killing. An alternatively spliced form of RARβ (RAR$\beta1'$) is generated by skipping exon 2 and is expressed in lung cancer cell lines that are sensitive to retinoic acid therapy [17]. Furthermore, in paired tissue samples of normal lung and tumor tissue collected from the same patient, RAR$\beta1'$ is expressed in the normal tissue, but not in the tumor tissue. Exogenous overexpression of RAR$\beta1'$ in retinoic acid-resistant lung cancer cell lines restores retinoic acid-induced cell death. These studies indicate that identification of pharmacologic approaches to restore RAR$\beta1'$ expression could provide a basis for retinoid-based lung cancer therapy or chemoprevention [17]. Alternative splicing in association with drug resistance has also been described for other members of the steroid receptor super family including the androgen receptor [18] and the peroxisome proliferator-activated receptor [19].

2.2 Multidrug Resistance

Delivery of chemotherapeutics can also be hampered by increased activity of drug efflux. This activity allows cancer cells to sustain resistance to a number of drugs and has been termed multidrug resistance. Multidrug resistance can occur when transporters are overexpressed allowing for the efficient efflux of drug resulting in drug resistance. One such transporter is the multidrug resistance protein 1 (MRP1) which is a member of the ATP-binding cassette transporter subfamily. In a study examining tissue from ovarian cancer patients, alternatively spliced variants of

MRP1 were expressed with exon skipping detected between exons 10 and 19 [10]. Exogenous expression of three of these MRP1 variants in HEK293T cells results in expression of the variant protein in the plasma membrane conferring resistance to doxorubicin due to increased influx. The MRP1 protein undergoes alternative splicing at a higher frequency in ovarian tumors than in pair matched normal tissue from the same patient.

3 Alternative Splicing and Drug Metabolism and Activation

Several drug therapies for cancer treatment are administered as a pro-drug and require activation by the cellular metabolism to be active. For example, deoxycytidine kinase (dCK) is the rate-limiting enzyme in the activation of nucleoside analogs such as cytarabine (ara-C), gemcitabine and clofarabine [20]. Ara-C is phosphorylated by dCK to ara-C-5′monophosphate and then further converted to the triphosphate form of ara-CTP. In this form it incorporates into DNA causing chain termination, blocking DNA synthesis, and ultimately causing leukemic cell death [21]. This is the basis of the successful use of ara-C for the treatment of several leukemias including acute myeloid leukemia (AML).

A number of variants of dCK have been reported [20] including variants due to alternative splicing [22–24]. In leukemic blasts from AML patients resistant to ara-C, variants of dCK were isolated with deletions in exon 5, exons 3–4, 3–6, or 2–5 [25]. To test the functional capacity of these variants, they were introduced into dCK negative cells and their dCK activity was compared to the introduction of wild-type dCK. In each case, the alternatively spliced variants had no dCK activity and no sensitivity to ara-C. However, when the variant dCK was co-expressed with the wild-type dCK, it did not appear to reduce either dCK activity or sensitivity to ara-C. The authors conclude that resistance to ara-C may lie in a defect in the splicing machinery [22].

Another nucleoside analog which requires activation by dCK is gemcitabine (2′-2′-difluorodeoxycytidine (dFdC)). Gemcitabine is an analog that is effective against a number of solid tumors including ovarian cancer. The human ovarian cancer cell line AG6000 was found to be resistant to gemcitabine due to deficient dCK activity [24]. A dCK transcript was detected which carries an exon 3 deletion bringing into frame a premature stop codon. No gross genomic alterations were detected indicating the involvement of post-transcriptional formation of the truncated dCK transcript. Transient transfection assays indicate that the Δexon 3 transcript of dCK is not translated into protein, perhaps leading to the observed resistance to gemcitabine. When wild-type dCK transcripts were transfected into the AG6000 cells, expression of the full length dCK failed to completely reverse the resistance to gemcitabine. Parallel studies introduced the Δexon3 dCK transcript into ovarian cancer cell expressing a wild-type dCK. When tested for sensitivity to gemcitabine, there was no discernable decrease in sensitivity.

4 Alterations in the Mechanisms of Drug Action

Cancer therapeutics have been designed to target cells with abnormal growth, either through inhibition of DNA synthesis and subsequent cell division; inhibition of abnormal cell growth signals; or stimulation of programmed cell death by a number of approaches. Alternative splicing of key molecules in the drug action pathways contributes to drug resistance of chemotherapeutics.

Gastric cancers are treated with a variety of DNA damaging agents including drugs such as anthracyclines and pyrimidine analogs. Differential display to profile gene expression of the drug-resistant lines identified mitotic arrest-deficient protein 2 (Mad2) as being altered and termed Mad2-Beta [26]. Wild-type Mad2 is a key component of the mitotic checkpoint also known as spindle assembly checkpoint and functions to detect DNA damage and subsequently stop or delay chromosome segregation until repair can be effected or until the cells undergo apoptosis. Mutation of this protein in cancer cells can allow cell division to occur in the face of DNA damage, resulting in resistance to DNA damaging drugs. Mad2-Beta is generated by a deletion of the third exon which would translate into a truncated protein. Exogenous expression of the Mad2-Beta transcript in adriamycin-sensitive gastric cancer cell lines induced a decrease in adriamycin sensitivity and also reduced mitotic arrest and mitosis indicating that generation of this variant contributes to the observed drug resistance [27].

Alternative splicing variants can also contribute to resistance to targeted therapies. Chronic myelogenous leukemia (CML) expresses a specific fusion protein from the Bcr-Abl gene which causes enhanced activation of the Abl kinase activity. Imatinib, a small molecule tyrosine kinase inhibitor, has been successfully used in the treatment of CML, producing a high rate of complete remission. Unfortunately, resistance does occur usually in the form of point mutation causing substitution of critical amino acid residues in the Abl kinase domain. Among these point mutations is a C to G transversion at position 1,106 which activates a cryptic splice donor sequence [28]. Analysis of CML cells from two imatinib-resistant patients indicates the presence of the transversion at position 1,106 as well as truncated transcripts due to the alternative splicing. Detection of the splice variant may pose a diagnostic challenge when PCR product sequencing is used for detection of the resistance mutations of Bcr-Abl as it may be interpreted as mixed sequence due to reduced-quality readings and therefore withdrawn from the diagnostic procedure.

Resistance to cancer therapies can also take the form of decreased cell killing due to changes in proteins associated with programmed cell death. Acute lymphocytic leukemia (ALL) is a disease of childhood or young adults. It is frequently treated with a variety of chemotherapeutics which rely on programmed cell death for success. The extrinsic pathway of programmed cell death involves the engagement of the Fas receptor (CD95) which ultimately results in activation of the caspase cascade and cell death. Leukemic blasts isolated from infants expressed variants of CD95 that are generated by changes in splicing [29]. A variety of variants have been characterized including deletion of exon 6, an exon which encodes the transmembrane domain of Fas. Expression of the exon 6 deletion variant results in a truncated soluble Fas protein which inhibits the membrane bound Fas receptor thus decreasing Fas ligand-induced apoptosis. Alternative splicing is also responsible for the generation of the caspase-3 short form which antagonizes the activity of full length caspase 3 resulting in chemo-resistance in breast tumors [30]. Expression of alternatively spliced inhibitors of apoptosis protein (IAPs) result in more IAPs with higher activity to inhibit apoptosis in HL60 cells leading to multiple drug resistance [31, 32]. Similarly, in hepatocellular carcinoma tissues, which are drug resistant, alternatively spliced IAPs result in enhanced inhibition of apoptosis [33].

5 Mechanisms of Alternative Splicing Associated with Resistance to Cancer Therapies

Understanding the mechanisms that result in alternative splicing may identify new drug targets for the treatment of drug-resistant cancers. This is complicated by the intricacies of the splicing reaction and the number of proteins and nucleic acids that participate in the formation and regulation of the spliceosome. Direct comparison of drug-sensitive cancer cell lines with drug-resistant cell lines of the same lineage has led to the identification of some splicing factors that appear to be differentially regulated and perhaps participate in the generation of the drug-resistant state.

As discussed earlier, the alternative splicing of the MRP1 is associated with ovarian tumors resistant to doxorubicin [10]. Two splicing factors, polypyrimidine track-binding protein (PTB) and SRp20, are overexpressed in ovarian tumors in comparison to matched normal ovarian tissues and overexpression of both of these splicing factors was associated with the increased number of MRP1 splicing forms [10]. It remains to be determined whether these two splicing factors directly participate in the splicing of MRP1 [34]. However, the overexpression of PTB may function in tumor progression. To that end, PTB expression in the A2780 ovarian tumor cell line was knocked down by siRNA resulting in impaired tumor cell proliferation, anchorage-dependent growth, and in vitro invasiveness [34]. Therefore, those tumors which overexpress PTB may benefit from reducing PTB as a novel therapeutic target in the treatment of ovarian cancer.

Pre-mRNA processing factor-4 (PRP-4) is overexpressed in several paclitaxel-resistant cancer cell lines including the multi drug-resistant ovarian cancer cell lines SKOV-3_{TR} and $OVCAR8_{TR}$. PRP-4 is a serine/threonine protein kinase that plays a role in splicing of pre-mRNAs. Repression of PRP-4 with shRNA constructs leads to a reversal of paclitaxel resistance in SKOV-3_{TR} cells and conversely overexpression of PRP-4 in drug-sensitive ovarian cancer cell lines leads to a modest drug resistance to paclitaxel, doxorubicin, and vincristine. These data taken together indicate an important role for PRP-4 in the development of resistance to chemotherapeutic drugs [35].

Splicing factor 45kDa (SPF45) is associated with cyclophosphamide-resistant mouse mammary tumors. A more extensive examination of tissue microarrays from several epithelial tumors indicated overexpression of SPF45 in comparison to adjacent normal tissues [36]. Overexpression of SFP45 in Hela tissue culture cells results in drug resistance to doxorubicin and vincristine, two chemotherapeutic drugs frequently used in cancer therapies [36]. In addition to generating alternatively spliced transcripts, splicing factors can also regulate transcriptional activation of the androgen receptor resulting in resistance to androgen-based therapies [18]. PTB-associated splicing factor (PSF) and p54nrb can both play key roles in regulating the transcriptional activity of the androgen receptor in prostate cancer models.

These studies open the possibility that splicing factors may form the basis of therapeutic targeting in the treatment of cancer [37]. Wilms' tumor gene (*WT*1) has been implicated in the maintenance of malignant phenotype in leukemias and a number of solid tumors [38]. Several isoforms for the WT1 transcript are produced including an alternatively spliced form skipping exon 5. In cisplatin resistant ovarian carcinoma and testicular germ cell tumor cell lines there is an increase in WT1 transcripts. Using nuclease-resistant antisense oligonucleotides which target exon 5 of WT1 reduces that transcript specifically and also induces cell death. These studies indicate that changing the ratio of exon 5+ and exon 5− WT1 transcripts affects cell viability and may be a useful approach for treating tumors that over-express WT1 [38].

Several investigators have explored modulating phosphorylation of the SR splicing factors in preclinical investigation of novel targets for cancer therapeutics. SR proteins are a family of essential factors required for constitutive splicing of pre-mRNA and play an important role in modulating alternative splicing [39]. The SR protein function is modulated by phosphorylation. While phosphorylation of the SR protein promotes spliceosome assembly dephosphorylation of the SR protein allows the transesterification reaction to occur. SR proteins are phosphorylated by Ser/Thr kinases [40]. DNA topoisomerase I (Topo I) transiently nicks DNA strands to allow relaxation of DNA supercoil which is required for transcription, DNA replication and DNA repair. In addition to these functions, Topo I also has kinase activity phosphorylating SR proteins. A Topo I-deficient murine lymphoma cell line exhibits hypophosphorylated SR proteins and an impairment of the exonic splicing enhancer (ESE)-dependent splicing. Restoration of Topo I activity in these cells restores ESE-dependent splicing leading to the hypothesis that selective targeting of the kinase activity of Topo I may provide a means to interfere with the expression of specific genes involved in cell proliferation and/or apoptosis [41]. Serine-arginine protein kinase 1 (SRPK1) also phosphorylates SR proteins. SRPK1 is expressed in ductal epithelial cells of the human pancreas and has increased expression in pancreatic tumors [42]. Decreasing the expression of SRPK1 in pancreatic tumor cell lines decreases the phosphorylation of SR proteins and enhances the sensitivity to chemotherapeutics drugs such as gemcitabine indicating that SRPK1 may be a drug target in the treatment of cancers [42]. The Cdc2-like kinase (Clk) family has also been shown to participate in phosphorylation of the SR protein family. Inhibition of Clk activity in cell lines with a beno-thiazole compound suppressed SR protein phosphorylation and decreased Clk-dependent alternative splicing [39]. This novel inhibitor of Clk may be useful as a therapeutic to manipulate abnormal splicing associated with cancer.

6 Summary and Conclusions

In summary, alternative splicing can influence various aspects of cancer therapy. Understanding the mechanisms of alternative splicing would enable us to identify novel therapeutic targets and design new treatment modalities to enhance tumor killing and to overcome drug resistance. Here, we have provided examples where drug resistance can be traced to alterations in drug uptake, metabolism, and mechanisms of action. It is likely that increased interest in the relationship of alternative splicing will uncover additional examples of drug resistance related to cancer therapeutics.

References

1. Merlo LM, Pepper JW, Reid BJ, Maley CC (2006) Cancer as an evolutionary and ecological process. Nat Rev Cancer 6:924–935
2. Luria SE, Delbruck M (1943) Mutations of bacteria from virus sensitivity to virus resistance. Genetics 28:491–511
3. Graveley BR (2001) Alternative splicing: increasing diversity in the proteomic world. Trends Genet 17:100–107
4. Wu JY, Tang H, Havlioglu N (2003) Alternative pre-mRNA splicing and regulation of programmed cell death. Prog Mol Subcell Biol 31:153–185
5. Venables JP (2006) Unbalanced alternative splicing and its significance in cancer. BioEssays 28:378–386
6. Venables JP (2004) Aberrant and alternative splicing in cancer. Cancer Res 64:7647–7654
7. Kirschbaum-Slager N, Lopes GM, Galante PA, Riggins GJ, de Souza SJ (2004) Splicing factors are differentially expressed in tumors. Genet Mol Res 3:512–520
8. Okumura M, Kondo S, Ogata M et al (2005) Candidates for tumor-specific alternative splicing. Biochem Biophys Res Commun 334:23–29
9. Jones PM, George AM (2004) The ABC transporter structure and mechanism: perspectives on recent research. Cell Mol Life Sci 61:682–699
10. He X, Ee PL, Coon JS, Beck WT (2004) Alternative splicing of the multidrug resistance protein 1/ATP binding cassette transporter subfamily gene in ovarian cancer creates functional splice variants and is associated with increased expression of the splicing factors PTB and SRp20. Clin Cancer Res 10:4652–4660
11. Zhang QX, Hilsenbeck SG, Fuqua SA, Borg A (1996) Multiple splicing variants of the estrogen receptor are present in individual human breast tumors. J Steroid Biochem Mol Biol 59:251–260
12. Fuqua SA, Fitzgerald SD, Allred DC et al (1992) Inhibition of estrogen receptor action by a naturally occurring variant in human breast tumors. Cancer Res 52:483–486
13. Horvath G, Leser G, Helou K, Henriksson M (2002) Function of the exon 7 deletion variant estrogen receptor alpha protein in an estradiol-resistant, tamoxifen-sensitive human endometrial adenocarcinoma grown in nude mice. Gynecol Oncol 84:271–279

14. Moalli PA, Pillay S, Weiner D, Leikin R, Rosen ST (1992) A mechanism of resistance to glucocorticoids in multiple myeloma: transient expression of a truncated glucocorticoid receptor mRNA. Blood 79:213–222
15. Krett NL, Pillay S, Moalli PA, Greipp PR, Rosen ST (1995) A variant glucocorticoid receptor messenger RNA is expressed in multiple myeloma patients. Cancer Res 55:2727–2729
16. Sanchez-Vega B, Krett N, Rosen S, Gandhi V (2006) Glucocorticoid receptor transcriptional isoforms and resistance in multiple myeloma cells. Mol Cancer Ther 5:3062–3070
17. Petty WJ, Li N, Biddle A et al (2005) A novel retinoic acid receptor beta isoform and retinoid resistance in lung carcinogenesis. J Natl Cancer Inst 97:1645–1651
18. Dong X, Sweet J, Challis JR, Brown T, Lye SJ (2007) Transcriptional activity of androgen receptor is modulated by two RNA splicing factors, PSF and p54nrb. Mol Cell Biol 27:4863–4875
19. Kim HJ, Hwang JY, Kim HJ et al (2007) Expression of a peroxisome proliferator-activated receptor gamma 1 splice variant that was identified in human lung cancers suppresses cell death induced by cisplatin and oxidative stress. Clin Cancer Res 13:2577–2583
20. Lamba JK, Crews K, Pounds S et al (2007) Pharmacogenetics of deoxycytidine kinase: identification and characterization of novel genetic variants. J Pharmacol Exp Ther 323:935–945
21. Kufe DW, Major PP, Egan EM, Beardsley GP (1980) Correlation of cytotoxicity with incorporation of ara-C into DNA. J Biol Chem 255:8997–9000
22. Veuger MJ, Heemskerk MH, Honders MW, Willemze R, Barge RM (2002) Functional role of alternatively spliced deoxycytidine kinase in sensitivity to cytarabine of acute myeloid leukemic cells. Blood 99:1373–1380
23. Veuger MJ, Honders MW, Spoelder HE, Willemze R, Barge RM (2003) Inactivation of deoxycytidine kinase and overexpression of P-glycoprotein in AraC and daunorubicin double resistant leukemic cell lines. Leuk Res 27:445–453
24. Al-Madhoun AS, van der Wilt CL, Loves WJ et al (2004) Detection of an alternatively spliced form of deoxycytidine kinase mRNA in the 2′-2′-difluorodeoxycytidine (gemcitabine)-resistant human ovarian cancer cell line AG6000. Biochem Pharmacol 68:601–609
25. Veuger MJ, Honders MW, Landegent JE, Willemze R, Barge RM (2000) High incidence of alternatively spliced forms of deoxycytidine kinase in patients with resistant acute myeloid leukemia. Blood 96:1517–1524
26. Yin F, Hu WH, Qiao TD, Fan DM (2004) Multidrug resistant effect of alternative splicing form of MAD2 gene-MAD2beta on human gastric cancer cell. Zhonghua Zhong Liu Za Zhi 26:201–204
27. Yin F, Du Y, Hu W et al (2006) Mad2beta, an alternative variant of Mad2 reducing mitotic arrest and apoptosis induced by adriamycin in gastric cancer cells. Life Sci 78:1277–1286
28. Gruber FX, Hjorth-Hansen H, Mikkola I, Stenke L, Johansen T (2006) A novel Bcr-Abl splice isoform is associated with the L248V mutation in CML patients with acquired resistance to imatinib. Leukemia 20:2057–2060
29. Wood CM, Goodman PA, Vassilev AO, Uckun FM (2003) CD95 (APO-1/FAS) deficiency in infant acute lymphoblastic leukemia: detection of novel soluble Fas splice variants. Eur J Haematol 70:156–171
30. Vegran F, Boidot R, Oudin C, Riedinger JM, Bonnetain F, Lizard-Nacol S (2006) Overexpression of caspase-3s splice variant in locally advanced breast carcinoma is associated with poor response to neoadjuvant chemotherapy. Clin Cancer Res 12:5794–5800
31. Notarbartolo M, Cervello M, Dusonchet L, Cusimano A, D'Alessandro N (2002) Resistance to diverse apoptotic triggers in multidrug resistant HL60 cells and its possible relationship to the expression of P-glycoprotein, Fas and of the novel anti-apoptosis factors IAP (inhibitory of apoptosis proteins). Cancer Lett 180:91–101
32. Notarbartolo M, Cervello M, Poma P, Dusonchet L, Meli M, D'Alessandro N (2004) Expression of the IAPs in multidrug resistant tumor cells. Oncol Rep 11:133–136

33. Notarbartolo M, Cervello M, Giannitrapani L et al (2004) Expression of IAPs and alternative splice variants in hepatocellular carcinoma tissues and cells. Ann N Y Acad Sci 1028:289–293
34. He X, Pool M, Darcy KM et al (2007) Knockdown of polypyrimidine tract-binding protein suppresses ovarian tumor cell growth and invasiveness in vitro. Oncogene 26:4961–4968
35. Duan Z, Weinstein EJ, Ji D et al (2008) Lentiviral short hairpin RNA screen of genes associated with multidrug resistance identifies PRP-4 as a new regulator of chemoresistance in human ovarian cancer. Mol Cancer Ther 7:2377–2385
36. Sampath J, Long PR, Shepard RL et al (2003) Human SPF45, a splicing factor, has limited expression in normal tissues, is overexpressed in many tumors, and can confer a multidrug-resistant phenotype to cells. Am J Pathol 163:1781–1790
37. Pajares MJ, Ezponda T, Catena R, Calvo A, Pio R, Montuenga LM (2007) Alternative splicing: an emerging topic in molecular and clinical oncology. Lancet Oncol 8:349–357
38. Renshaw J, Orr RM, Walton MI et al (2004) Disruption of WT1 gene expression and exon 5 splicing following cytotoxic drug treatment: antisense down-regulation of exon 5 alters target gene expression and inhibits cell survival. Mol Cancer Ther 3:1467–1484
39. Muraki M, Ohkawara B, Hosoya T et al (2004) Manipulation of alternative splicing by a newly developed inhibitor of Clks. J Biol Chem 279:24246–24254
40. Manley JL, Tacke R (1996) SR proteins and splicing control. Genes Dev 10:1569–1579
41. Soret J, Gabut M, Dupon C et al (2003) Altered serine/arginine-rich protein phosphorylation and exonic enhancer-dependent splicing in Mammalian cells lacking topoisomerase I. Cancer Res 63:8203–8211
42. Hayes GM, Carrigan PE, Beck AM, Miller LJ (2006) Targeting the RNA splicing machinery as a novel treatment strategy for pancreatic carcinoma. Cancer Res 66:3819–3827

MIX
Papier aus verantwortungsvollen Quellen
Paper from responsible sources
FSC® C105338

If you have any concerns about our products,
you can contact us on
ProductSafety@springernature.com

In case Publisher is established outside the EU,
the EU authorized representative is:
Springer Nature Customer Service Center GmbH
Europaplatz 3, 69115 Heidelberg, Germany

Printed by Libri Plureos GmbH
in Hamburg, Germany